Cholinesterases
Fundamental and Applied Aspects

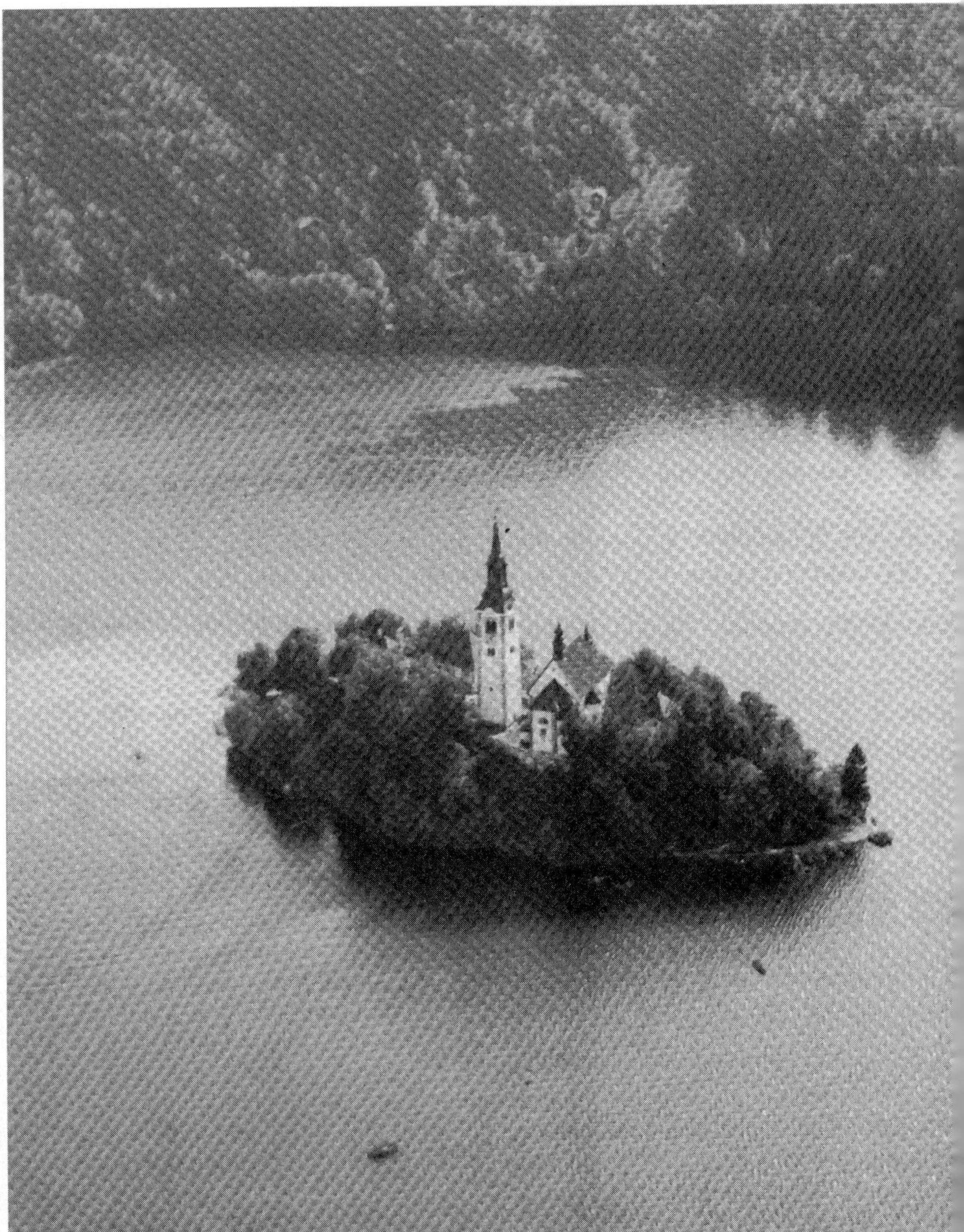

Cholinesterases

Fundamental and Applied Aspects

Proceedings of the Second International Meeting
on Cholinesterases
Bled, Yugoslavia (September 17th to 21st, 1983)

Editors
Miro Brzin · Eric. A. Barnard · Dušan Sket

Walter de Gruyter
Berlin · New York 1984

Editors
Miro Brzin, Professor, Ph. D.
Institute of Pathophysiology
School of Medicine
Edvard Kardelj University
61105 Ljubljana
Yugoslavia

Eric A. Barnard, Professor, FRS
Department of Biochemistry
Imperial College of Science and Technology
London SW7 2AZ
United Kingdom

Dušan Sket, Assistant Professor, Ph. D.
Institute of Pathophysiology
School of Medicine
Edvard Kardelj University
61105 Ljubljana
Yugoslavia

Keywords: Cholinesterase
Acetylcholinesterase
Anticholinesterases
Neurotoxic Esterase

Published in cooperation with Mladinska Knjiga, Ljubljana

CIP-Kurztitelaufnahme der Deutschen Bibliothek

Cholinesterases: fundamental and applied aspects;
proceedings of the 2. Internat. Meeting on Cholinesterases Bled,
Yugoslavia (September 17th to 21st, 1983)/
ed. Miro Brzin ... – Berlin; New York: de Gruyter, 1984.
ISBN 3-11-009873-3
NE: Brzin, Miro [Hrsg.]; International Meeting on
Cholinesterases <02, 1983, Bled>

Library of Congress Cataloging in Publication Data

International Meeting on Cholinesterases
(2nd : 1983 : Bled, Slovenia)
Cholinesterases, fundamental and applied aspects.
Includes indexes.
1. Cholinesterases--Congresses. I. Brzin, Miro.
II. Barnard, Eric A., 1927–. III. Sket, Dušan. IV. Title.
[DNLM: 1. Cholinesterases--congresses.
W3 IN756M 2nd 1983C / QU 136 I597 1983C]
QP609.C 4I58 1983 599'.019'253 84-12062
ISBN 3-11-009873-3

Preface

140 scientists from many countries (chemists, biochemists, cell biologists, physiologists, clinical scientists, neuroscientists, toxicologists) gathered in Bled, Yugoslavia, to discuss a single enzyme and its inhibitors. This surely, can only occur on such a scale with acetylcholinesterase: we doubt that any other enzyme has so large an international following. It held our attention unfailingly through several days of a crowded programme, from early morning until late at the night, and never ceased to amaze, excite or charm us with its wide ramifications, unexpected roles, or postulates thereof, strange forms and complex inhibition.

This book represents the distilled wisdom of that gathering. It attempts to show the range and power of current studies of AChE. The contributors provide an unparalleled account of our knowledge of this enzyme and of its organophosphate inhibitors. We believe that it represents most of the major current approaches in these fields and shows the new directions which they are taking. It should make it more widely understood why this enzyme system has such a band of devotees.

This was the Second International Meeting on Cholinesterases , the first, held also in Yugoslavia in 1975, covered acetylcholine receptors, both nicotinic and muscarinic, as well as AChE. It would be impossible today to do justice to all of those fields in depth at a single meeting. AChE studies have come of age, and have demanded and obtained their own arena.

The Meeting was sponsored by the Union of the Yugoslav Biochemical Societies, the Slovene Academy of Sciences and Arts and the Slovenian Physiological Society. The Union of the Republic and Province Self-Managing Communities of Interest for Research Activity in the SFRJ is thanked for financial support. The Organizers wish to express their particular gratitude to the Wellcome Trust, the Shell International Petroleum Co. Ltd., the U.S. Air Force Office of Scientific Research and the U.S. Army Medical Research and Development Command for the help with travel funds for invited participants.

Ljubljana - London, January 1984

M. Brzin

E.A. Barnard

D. Sket

List of abbreviations

ACh	acetylcholine
AChE	acetylcholinesterase
cAMP	cyclic 3´- 5´adenosine monophosphate
AThCh	acetylthiocholine
ATP	adenosine triphosphate
BuCh	butyrylcholine
BuChE	butyrylcholinesterase
BuThCh	butyrylthiocholine
BW284C51	1:5-bis(4-allyldimethylammoniumphenyl)-pentane-3-on
CAT	choline acetyltransferase
nsChE	non-specific cholinesterase
ΨChE	non-specific cholinesterase
ChEs	cholinesterases in general
ChR	cholinoreceptor
DFP	diisopropyl phosphorofluoridate
EDTA	ethylenediaminetetraacetate
ER	endoplasmic reticulum
LD_{50}	median lethal dosis
MeCh	acetyl-β-methylcholine
iso-OMPA	tetramonoisopropylpyrophosphortetramide
PAM	pralidoxime
2-PAM	pralidoxime
mRNA	messenger RNA
SCG	superior cervical ganglion

Contents

V Anticholinesterases: Toxicology and Structure-Function Relationships of Inhibitors and Antidotes

I. CHEMISTRY AND CATALYTIC ACTIVITY OF CHOLINESTERASES

INTRODUCTION TO SESSION I

Elsa Reiner

Institute for Medical Research and Occupational Health,
M. Pijade 158, 41000 Zagreb, Yugoslavia

The session on "Chemistry and catalytic activity of cholinesterases" comprised five lectures. Four of them were included into the Proceedings.

Only one paper dealt with the chemical composition of cholinesterases and it concerned the sequencing of amino acids in human serum cholinesterase. The other papers concerned the catalytic activity of the enzyme. Binding of ligands to the peripheral sites and active site and their effect upon conformational changes and catalytic activity were discussed in several papers; one paper spoke about photosuicide inhibition and one paper about accelerators of enzyme acylation and dehydration of the active site.

The subject of catalytic activity was also discussed in several papers from the other sessions and on many poster presentations. Two topics belonging to this session - stereospecificity of cholinesterases and ageing of the phosphorylated enzymes - were presented only on posters.

AMINO ACID COMPOSITION AND SEQUENCE OF HUMAN SERUM CHOLINESTERASE: A PROGRESS REPORT

Oksana Lockridge

Pharmacology Department, University of Michigan Medical School, Ann Arbor, MI 48109. USA

Introduction

The amino acid sequences of ChE and AChE are unknown. The only sequences reported for these proteins are short fragments of the active-site from horse serum ChE (1), eel AChE (2), and human serum ChE (3). We are presently sequencing the entire ChE protein isolated from human serum. Sequence results reported here are incomplete and preliminary. In future publications certain sequences may appear slightly altered. Parentheses indicate those sequences that need to be confirmed.

Results

Table I. Purification of human serum ChE.

	Total Units	Specific Activity	Fold Purification
10 liters plasma	5,000	0.02 u/mg	-
pH 4.0 DEAE	2,400	10	500 x
Procainamide affinity column	2,400	200	10,000 x

ChE was purified from outdated human plasma with a yield of 12 mg ChE from 10 liters of plasma (4,5,6). The purified ChE appeared to be 100% clean on SDS gels, on non-SDS gels, and also on thin-layer isoelectric-focusing gels from LKB, pH range 3.5 to 9.5. However, on 2D gels, where the 1st dimension was isoelectric-focusing in 8 M urea, from pH 3.5 to 10, and the 2nd dimension was gradient (11 to 14%) polyacrylamide electrophoresis in 0.1 % SDS, about 100 tiny contaminant spots were seen with silver staining when a large amount of ChE was applied. The % contamination was very small, probably on the order of 1%.

On the 2D gel ChE appeared as a set of 9 to 12 adjacent bands, thus revealing the microheterogeneity conferred by its 25% carbohydrate content.

The amino acid composition of this highly purified ChE preparation is in Table II. The results of Muensch et al (7) for human ChE, Main et al for horse ChE (8) and Teng et al for horse ChE (9) are compared in Table III with our results. There is fair agreement between these analyses though our human ChE seems to differ from Muensch et al in Met, Tyr, Pro, Gly and Ala.

To date we have sequenced 421 residues contained in 48 tryptic peptides. This accounts for 70% of the estimated 580 residues per subunit. The 160 unsequenced residues may be contained in 10 peptides for which we have only partial sequences.

Table II. Amino acid composition of human serum ChE.

	umoles	Residues per subunit (M_r 85,000 25% carbohydrate
Ala	0.393	34.8
Arg	0.288	25.5
Asp	0.741	65.7
Cys/2	0.0924	8.2
Glu	0.637	56.5
Gly	0.532	47.2
His	0.0738	6.5
Ile	0.317	28.1
Leu	0.594	52.7
Lys	0.350	31.0
Met	0.123	10.9
Phe	0.439	38.9
Pro	0.414	36.7
Ser	0.457	40.5
Thr	0.399	35.3
Trp	0.138	12.2
Tyr	0.205	18.2
Val	0.354	31.4
Total	6.547	580

Table III. Comparison of amino acid analyses.

	Lockridge[a]	Muensch (7)[a]	Main (8)[b]	Teng (9)[b]
		mol/100 mol		
Asp	11.32	9.59	10.68	11.17
Thr	6.09	5.11	6.72	5.67
Ser	6.98	6.67	7.08	6.20
Glu	9.73	9.60	10.68	11.35
Pro	6.32	4.47	5.34	6.38
Gly	8.13	10.05	7.51	7.45
Ala	6.00	7.64	5.93	5.67
Cys/2	1.41	1.37	1.63	1.06
Val	5.41	4.84	5.83	5.50
Met	1.88	1.09	1.77	1.77
Ile	4.84	3.93	3.69	3.72
Leu	9.07	7.40	8.55	9.22
Tyr	3.13	5.11	3.37	3.55
Phe	6.70	4.75	5.53	6.38
Lys	5.35	7.76	6.40	6.03
His	1.13	1.82	1.53	0.89
Arg	4.40	5.36	5.09	5.32
Trp	2.11	3.38	2.67	2.66

a. human serum ChE
b. horse serum ChE

The <u>N-terminal sequence</u> of the ChE protein is:

Glu Asp Asp Ile Ile[5] Ile Ala Thr Lys AsN[10] Gly

(Gly Val ? Gly[15] Met AsN Leu Thr Val[20] Phe Gly)
CHO

Residue 14 is probably Arg or Lys. Cycle 17 is thought to be AsN linked to carbohydrate. Cycle 17 gave a blank in manual Edman degradation. A blank cycle is typical of carbohydrate attached to AsN. The presence of Thr at cycle 19 supports this assignment.

The early cycles of Edman degradation yielded only one amino acid per cycle. This means that the protein was clean and furthermore suggests that the 4 subunits of ChE are identical. If significant contamination or non-identical subunits had been present, then more than one amino acid would have been released at each cycle. Teng et al (9) also found Glu at the N-terminal of horse ChE.

The <u>C-terminal sequence</u> of ChE is likely to be:

Glu Ser Cys Val Gly Leu

where Leu is the C-terminal. The possibility that this is the C-terminal peptide is based on the fact that this is the only tryptic peptide whose sequence did not end in Arg or Lys. Assignment of this peptide to the C-terminal has not yet been confirmed by identification of released amino acids following digestion of the intact ChE protein with carboxypeptidase.

The presence of Cys in this peptide is of particular interest. This cysteine may have the function of linking two subunits in an interchain disulfide bond. In an earlier paper (6) we presented evidence that the interchain disulfide linkage was located near the terminal of the subunit.. We did not know whether it was near the N or the C-terminal. We had observed that trypsin selectively clipped out the interchain-disulfide linkage from native, undenatured ChE, and that this cleavage did not change subunit molecular weight. ChE activity was also unaffected. Since the N-terminal sequence does not contain Cys in the 1st 22 residues, while the C-terminal region does contain Cys as well as a trypsin-cleavage site, we hypothesize that the Cys in the C-terminal is the interchain-disulfide Cys. This is a working hypothesis that needs to be confirmed.

This hypothesis is useful for explaining a purification artifact. Purification methods from different laboratories often yield ChE preparations partially depleted of interchain-disulfide bonds. This shows up on SDS gels. The complete protein migrates as a dimer of M_r 180,000 in the absence of reducing agents. ChE depleted of interchain-disulfides has a high percentage of monomers of M_r 90,000 despite omission of mercaptoethanol from the sample and the SDS gel. Our interpretation is that during purification proteases clipped off the 6 residue C-terminal peptide containing the interchain-disulfide linkage.

The <u>active-site tryptic peptide</u> has the sequence:

Ser Val Thr Leu Phe^{5} Gly Glu Ser Ala Gly^{10}
(P under Ser)

Ala Ala(Ser Val Ser^{15}Leu Phe His Leu Leu^{20}

Ser Pro Gly Ser His^{25}Leu Thr Ser Arg^{29})

The tryptic peptide is 29 residues long. It contains an extraordinarily high amount of Ser and Thr. The 7 Ser and 2 Thr comprise over 30% of its residues. The DFP label alkylates Ser located at cycle 8.

A comparison of our active-site sequence with others is in Table IV.

Table IV. Active-site sequences.

<u>Human ChE</u>	
Lockridge '83	SVTLFGES*AG^{10}AA(SVSLFHLL^{20}SPGSHLTSR^{29})
Yamato '83	GES*AG AS AVSL
<u>Horse ChE</u>	
Jansz '59	FGES*AG (AA S)
<u>Eel AChE</u>	
Schaffer '73	GGES*SE GA AG

(* printed above the active-site S)

Our results differ from those of Yamato et al (3) in that residues 12 and 13, Ala and Ser, are reversed in order. While the horse and human ChE sequences appear to be identical, the eel AChE differs in 6 out of 10 residues.

Supported by DAMD17-82-C-2271.

References

1. Jansz,H.S., Brons,D., Warringa,M.G.P.J. Biochem. Biophys. Acta 34, 573-575 (1959)
2. Schaffer,N.K., Michel,H.O., Bridges,A.F. Biochemistry 12, 2946-2950 (1973)
3. Yamato,K., Huang,I., Muensch,H., Yoshida,A., Goedde,H.W., Agarwal,D.P. Biochem. Genet. 21, 135-145 (1983)
4. Lockridge,O., La Du, B.N. J. Biol. Chem. 253, 361-366 (1978)
5. Lockridge,O., Eckerson,H.W., La Du,B.N. J. Biol. Chem. 254, 8324-8330 (1979)
6. Lockridge, O., La Du,B.N. J. Biol. Chem. 257, 12012-12018 (1982)
7. Muensch,H., Goedde,H.W., Yoshida,A. Eur.J.Biochem. 70, 217-223 (1976)
8. Main,A.R., Soucie,W.G., Buxton,I.L., Arinc,E. Biochem.J. 143, 733-744 (1974)
9. Teng,T.L., Harpst,J.A., Lee,J.C., Zinn,A., Carlson, D.M. Arch. Biochem. Biophys. 176, 71-81 (1976)

PHOTOSUICIDE INHIBITION OF ACETYLCHOLINESTERASE

Brigitte Kieffer, Maurice P. Goeldner, Christian G. Hirth
Centre de Neurochimie du C.N.R.S., 5 Rue Blaise Pascal
67084 Strasbourg Cedex, France

Introduction

By analogy with suicide inhibitors (1, 2, 3), photosuicide inhibitors are defined as photoactivatable ligands which are photodecomposed through the physicochemical properties of the enzyme while bound to its active site. This regioselective photoactivation should lead to a highly reactive species which can irreversibly react with the residues of the active site (4). Two different kinds of photosuicide inhibition of AChE are described. The first one uses the selective photodecomposition of the ligand in a more hydrophobic environment within the active site (phase transfer photoinactivation). The second implies the presence of a tryptophan residue in the vicinity of the binding site which, after excitation, transfers its energy to the bound photosensitive ligand (energy transfer photoinactivation).

Results

A) Phase transfer photoinactivation. Methyl (acetoxymethyl) nitrosamine (MAN) and methyl (butyroxymethyl) nitrosamine (MBN) are respectively substrate ($K_M = 10^{-2}$ M) and competitive inhibitor ($K_i = 2.10^{-3}$ M) of Electric Eel AChE. Irradiation of an incubation mixture of this enzyme with either nitrosamines lead to an irreversible loss of activity with a pseudo first order kinetic, which can be slowed down by competitive inhibitors (Fig. 1).

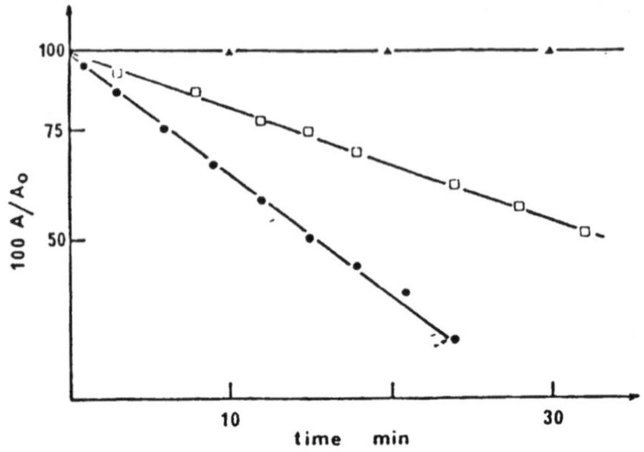

Figure 1: Inactivation of AChE by MAN (pH 7.2) in the presence of light (λ = 350 nm ; I = $12,6.10^{-6}$ einstein s^{-1} cm^{-2}). Concentration of MAN were (▲) 0 ; (●) $2,5.10^{-4}$ M ; (□) $2,5.10^{-4}$ M plus 10^{-3} M tetramethyl ammonium iodide. A_0 is the initial activity, A is the residual activity at the indicated time.

When partially purified AChE was incubated with ^{14}C MAN in the presence of light (λ = 350 nm) the number of active sites inhibited was directly proportional to the amount of radioactivity incorporated. Incorporation of 1 mole of ^{14}C methyl per mole of active site is sufficient to fully inactivate the enzyme.

Several evidence agree with the following mechanism (Scheme 1):

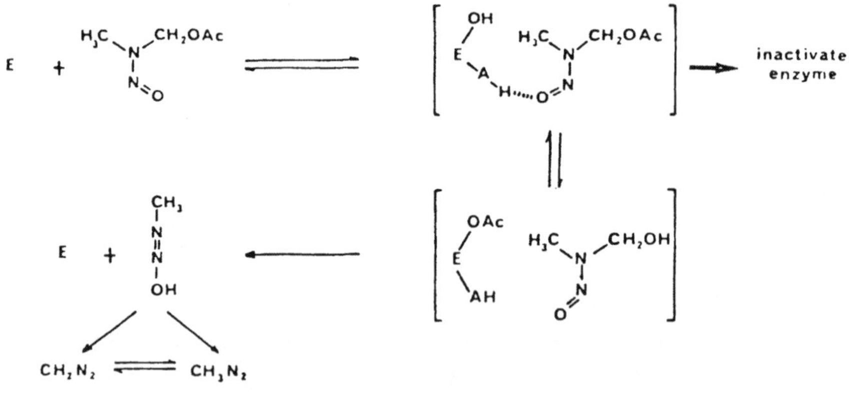

- in the absence of light, formation of diazomethane during enzyme catalyzed MAN hydrolysis was detected. However, this chemical as well as its precursor (diazoic acid) are not involved in the irreversible inactivation of AChE since the wavelength dependence of inactivation shows a maximum at 335 nm where diazomethane does not absorb (Fig. 2).

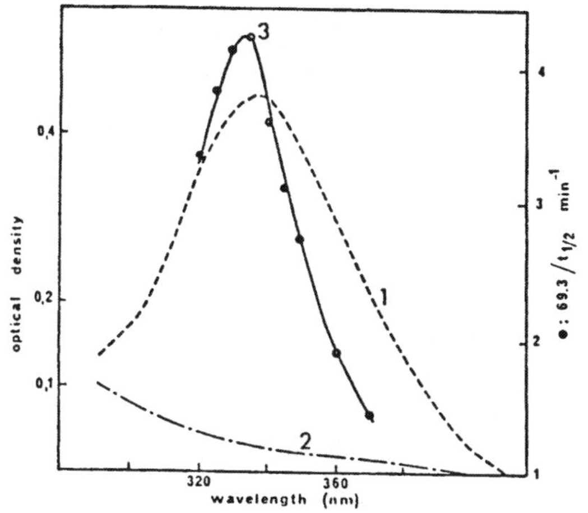

Figure 2: (1) UV spectrum of MAN in heptane (6.10^{-3} M) in the presence of 0,9 M CF_3OO_2H ; (2) same after the irradiation (λ = 350 nm ; I = $12,6.10^{-6}$ einstein $s^{-1}cm^{-2}$) ; (3) inactivation of AChE by MAN ($2,5.10^{-4}$ M) as a function of irradiation wavelength.

- detailed kinetic studies of the rate of inactivation as a function of light intensity favour a mechanism in which irreversible binding occurs in the enzyme-substrate complex prior to hydrolysis.
- finally MBN, which is a competitive inhibitor and not a substrate, inactivates very efficiently AChE in the same conditions as MAN.

Such a scheme implies that MAN which is photochemically stable in water at neutral pH becomes highly photosensitive while bound to the active site. It is known that a weak acidic medium (pH 1-3) increases the photosensitivity of nitrosamines (5) leading to the formation of nitrosyl and aminium radicals:

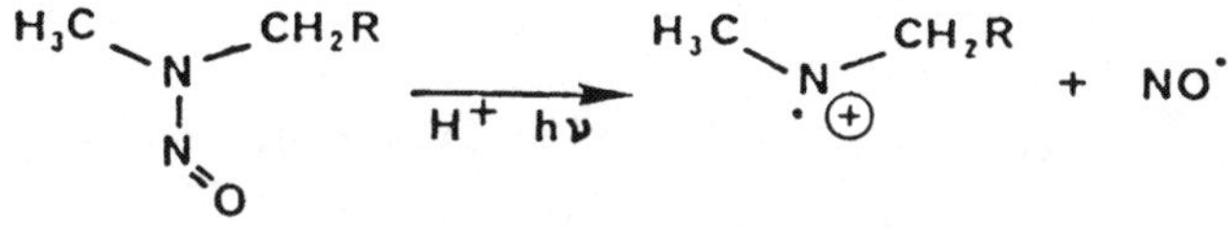

This photosensitivity is dramatically increased in low dielectric constant media ($\varepsilon \sim 2$-5) in the presence of acids. In fact the absorption spectrum of MAN in heptan-trifluoracetic acid fits the action spectrum of the enzyme inactivation by MAN as a function of irradiation wavelength (Fig. 2) suggesting that the nitrosamine was specifically photoactivated after association with an acidic hydrogen in the active site (6).

B) Energy transfer photoinactivation. Electric Eel AChE is known to have at least one tryptophan residue in the vicinity of the acetylcholine binding site (7). Thus, selective activation of bound ligand by an energy transfer reaction between the excited donor (Trp) and the acceptor (photosensitive reagent) becomes possible (Scheme 2).

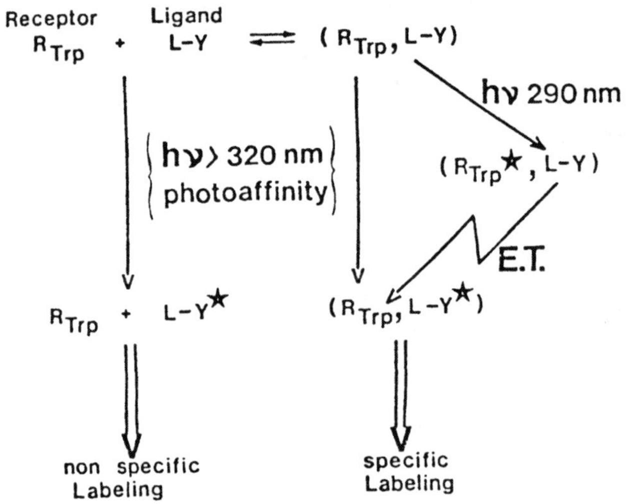

Several conditions are required for successful labeling of AChE under energy transfer conditions: i) the photosensitive ligand should possess all the properties of a good photoaffinity reagent ii) it must be stable at tryptophan excitation wavelength but highly photosensitive at tryptophan emission wavelength iii) it should be an efficient tryptophan fluorescence quencher.

We found that some aryldiazonium salts meet all these criteria (Table I).

Table I

ARYL DIAZONIUM SALTS — Structure / Properties	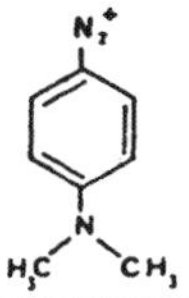	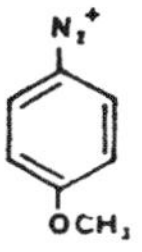	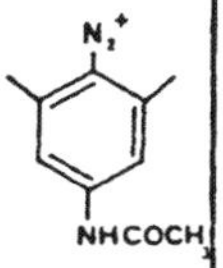
Stability at pH 7.2 $T_{1/2}$ (hours)	3 5	> 2 4	> 72
λ max (nm) ε	379 37500	313 23500	338 22500
photolysis in water phenol yield quantum yield	 92 0.59	 80 0.46	 90 0.33
affinity for Acetylcholine-Esterase ; K_i (M)	competitive $2\ 10^{-5}$	competitive $4\ 10^{-5}$	non competitive $8\ 10^{-6}$
% irreversible inactivation by 5 K_i $Ar-N_2^+$ in the dark under irradiation time of irradiation mn	 0 78 2.5	 < 10 63 3.5	 < 10 0 4
protection against inactivation by $\overset{+}{N}[Et]_4$	+	+	

In the dark they are reversible inhibitors of AChE and by irradiation they give rise to an aryl cation which is a highly reactive species able to react with amino acids residues as well as the amide bond (Scheme 3).

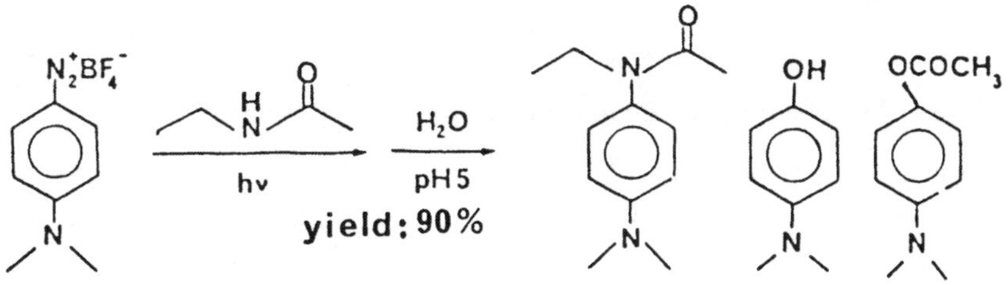

1 9

In the following, we shall focus our attention on the inactivation of AChE by p-N,N-dimethylamino benzene diazonium fluoroborate (DDF). There is a good overlap between the UV absorption spectrum of DDF and the AChE fluorescence emission spectrum from which a critical distance R_0 = 28 Å, according to Förster, was estimated. Thus DDF can be a good acceptor in energy transfer processes via Coulombic interaction.

In fact Fig. 3 shows a comparison of the rate of irreversible inactivation of AChE by DDF in normal photoaffinity conditions and in energy transfer conditions using the same number of incident photons.

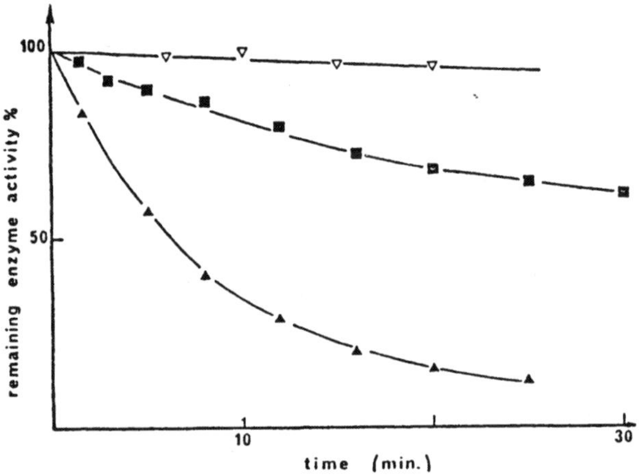

Figure 3: AChE inactivation in the presence of 2.10^{-5} M DDF at pH 7.2 by irradiation at λ = 295 nm ($I = 6.10^{5}$ einstein s^{-1} cm^{-2}) ; by irradiation at λ = 410 nm ($I = 10^{5}$ einstein s^{-1} cm^{-2}). Stability of AChE irradiated at 295 nm in the absence of DDF.

Clearly the energy transfer method (λ_{exc} = 290 nm) gives a large increase in the rate of inactivation as compared to the normal photoaffinity labeling condition (λ_{exc} = 410 nm). In both conditions, tetraethylammonium iodide (4.10^{-3} M) protects against inactivation (results not shown).

The stoichiometries of the inactivation of purified AChE with methyl [^{3}H] DDF are shown in Table II.

Table II

		mole of $|^3H|$ DDF incorporated by mole of inactivated enzyme binding site	
		Photoaffinity	Energy transfer
($|^3H|$ DDF)	2.10^{-5} M	1.2	1
	10^{-4} M	3.9	2.4

Enzyme concentration 2.2 10^{-6} M ; each value is an average of three determinations for enzyme inactivation ranging from 25 % to 80 %.

For two different concentrations of DDF, a better stoichiometry of inactivation was observed in energy transfer conditions. At 10^{-4} M of DDF non specific labeling is increased due to a larger amount of uncomplexed ligand. To a lesser extent this is also true for energy transfer conditions since DDF slightly absorbs at 295 nm (ε = 1000) and can be directly photodecomposed (8).
Finally highly purified AChE was inactivated by methyl $[^3H]$ DDF and submitted to successive proteolysis with trypsin, Staphylococcus aureus protease and pepsin. A short peptide representing more than 20 % of the overall incorporated radioactivity found in the medium was purified. Its sequence was determined using microsequencing techniques (9, 10, 11):

NH_2-Gly-Ser-X-Phe-COOH

X being the amino acid residue modified by DDF which structure remains to be elucidated.
Interestingly this sequence does not overlap with the sequence of the polypeptide containing the activated serine residue (12). It is believed that DDF, a competitive inhibitor of AChE, because of its positive charge due to the diazonium function, binds to the quaternary ammonium site involved in the binding of acetylcholine, and that the isolated tetrapeptide belongs to this site.

Conclusion

In this communication, we describe the irreversible inactivation of Electric Eel AChE by means of photosuicide labeling. Even if the precise mechanisms of inactivation remains to be elucidated, photosuicide inhibition allowed us i) to isolate a small peptide which is part of the acetylcholine binding site ii) to favour the hypothesis that this site is hydrophobic iii) to show that photosuicide inhibitors, as well as suicide inhibitors, can be used successfully despite a low affinity.

References

1. Bloch, K.: Acc. Chem. Res. 2, 193-202 (1969).
2. Rando, R.R.: Science 185, 320-324 (1974).
3. Abeles, R.H., Maycock, A.L.: Acc. Chem. Res. 9, 313-319 (1976).
4. Goeldner, M.P., Hirth, C.G., Kieffer, B., Ourisson, G.: Trends Biochem. Sci. 7, 310-312 (1982).
5. Chow, Y.L.: Acc. Chem. Res. 6, 354-360 (1973).
6. Eid, P., Goeldner, M.P., Hirth, C.G., Jost, P.: Biochemistry 20, 2251-2256 (1981).
7. Shinitzky, M., Dudai, Y., Silman, I.: FEBS Letters 30, 125-128 (1973).
8. Goeldner, M.P., Hirth, C.G.: Proc. Natl. Acad. Sci. USA 77, 6439-6442 (1980).
9. Chang, J.Y., Knecht, R., Ball, R., Alkan, S.S., Braun, D.G.: Eur. J. Biochem. 127, 625-629 (1982).
10. Chang, J.Y., Knecht, R., Braun, D.G.: Biochem. J. 203, 803-806 (1982).
11. Chang, J.Y.: Biochem. J. 199, 537-545 and 557-564 (1981).
12. Shaffer, N.K., Michel, H.O., Bridges, A.F.: Biochemistry 12, 2946-2950 (1973).

ROLE OF DEHYDRATION OF THE ESTERATIC SITE IN ACYLATION OF CHOLINESTERASES

Miloš R. Pavlič and Matjaž Zorko
Institute of Biochemistry, Medical Faculty,
Ljubljana, Yugoslavia

Introduction

Many years ago Kitz and Wilson found (1) that some reversible cationic competitive inhibitors of AChE (acetylcholine hydrolase,EC 3.1.1.7) such as tetramethylammonium (TMA) and tetraethylammonium (TEA) did not inhibit the acylation of this enzyme by methanesulfonylfluoride (MSF) but did accelerate this reaction. The phenomenon is interesting in itself and, besides, it seems important because the same acceleration mechanism may be involved in the acylation of both AChE and of BuChE (acylcholine acyl-hydrolase,EC 3.1.1.8) by their natural substrates since the acylation of ChEs by MSF is analogous to the acylation of these enzymes by their substrates (2-4; Figs. 1-2).

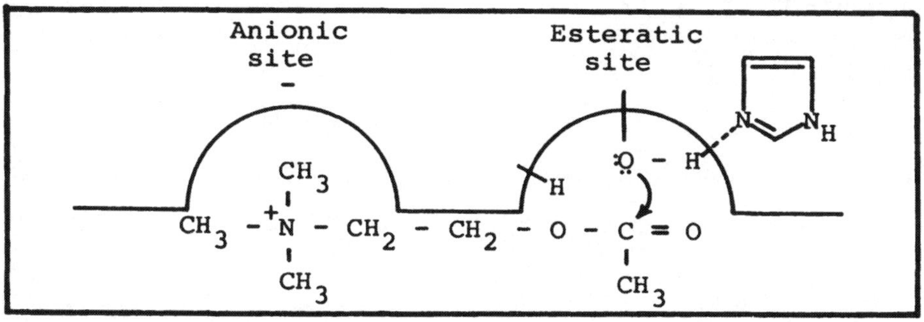

Fig. 1. Schematic representation of the hydrolytic mechanism of AChE (from 5).

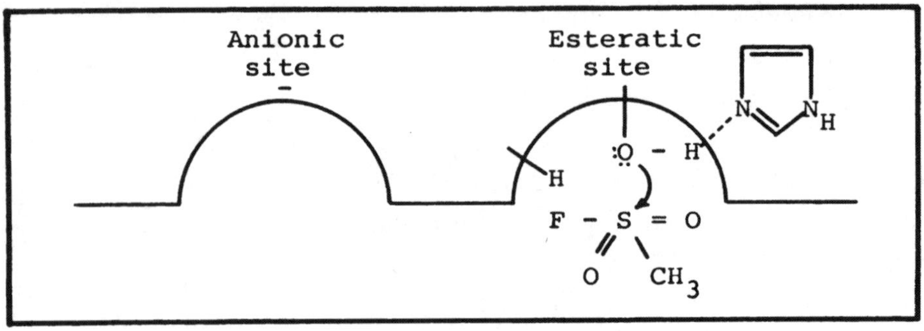

Fig. 2. Schematic representation of the mechanism of the sulfonylation of AChE by MSF (from 5).

In order to elucidate the mechanism of acceleration various investigations have been made in our laboratory in the last few years. The course of these investigations and the main results are described below.

Mechanism of acceleration of the acylation of ChEs by MSF

The acylation of ChEs by MSF may be represented by the following schemes and equations (cf. 2, 6-9)

$$E + I \underset{k_{-1}}{\overset{k_{+1}}{\rightleftharpoons}} EI \xrightarrow{k_{+2}} E' + P_1 \qquad (1)$$

$$E + I \xrightarrow{k} E' + P_1 \qquad (2)$$

$$k = \frac{k_{+1}\ k_{+2}}{k_{-1}} = \frac{k_{+2}}{K_i} \qquad (3)$$

$$\ln\frac{(E)}{(E)_o} = -\frac{k_{+2}\ t}{1 + \frac{K_i}{(I)}} = -k_{app}\ t \qquad (4)$$

$$\frac{1}{k_{app}} = \frac{1}{k_{+2}} + \frac{K_i}{k_{+2}} \frac{1}{(I)} \tag{5}$$

$$\ln\frac{(E)}{(E)_o} = - k\ (I)\ t = - k_{app}\ t \tag{6}$$

where E is the enzyme, I the irreversible inhibitor MSF, EI the complex between E and I, E´ the acylated enzyme, P_1 the product (HF), K_i the dissociation constant for the binding of I to E, and k´s the rate constants.

In the presence of an accelerator, A, the following additional schemes and equations apply (cf. 1, 10-11)

$$E + A \overset{K_A}{\rightleftharpoons} EA \tag{7}$$

$$EA + I \underset{k'_{-1}}{\overset{k'_{+1}}{\rightleftharpoons}} EAI \xrightarrow{k'_{+2}} E' + P_1 \tag{8}$$

$$EA + I \xrightarrow{k_A} E' + P_1 \tag{9}$$

$$k_A = \frac{k'_{+1}\ k'_{+2}}{k'_{-1}} = \frac{k'_{+2}}{K'_i} \tag{10}$$

$$\ln\frac{(E)}{(E)_o} = - k \frac{1 + \frac{k_A}{k} \frac{(A)}{K_A}}{1 + \frac{(A)}{K_A}} (I)\ t = - k_a\ (I)\ t \tag{11}$$

$$\frac{k_a - k_A}{k - k_a} = K_A \frac{1}{(A)} \tag{12}$$

where EA is the complex between enzyme and accelerator, EAI the ternary complex between enzyme, accelerator and

MSF, K_A the dissociation constant for the binding of A to E, and k´s the rate constants.

In order to elucidate the mechanism of acceleration, the inhibition of AChE and BuChE, respectively, by MSF in relatively high concentrations was followed (cf. 9), with added accelerators TMA, TEA and decamethonium (C-10) and the experimental results analysed by means of equations listed above. Experimental conditions in these and all other experiments were as follows. The temperature was 25° C. The universal buffer solution of Britten and Robinson (12) was used; its ionic strength was adjusted to 0.2 M by addition of NaCl. The pH of the buffer was 8.4, which is the optimal value for methanesulfonylation of AChE and BuChE at 25°C (3,8).Enzymes used were AChE from the electric organ of *Electrophorus electricus*, Worthington, 4000 units/mg and BuChE from horse serum, Worthington, 11 units/mg. The main findings of these investigations can be summarized by free energy profiles for the acylation of ChEs in the absence and presence of accelerators, as shown for the case of TEA in Figs. 3 and 4.

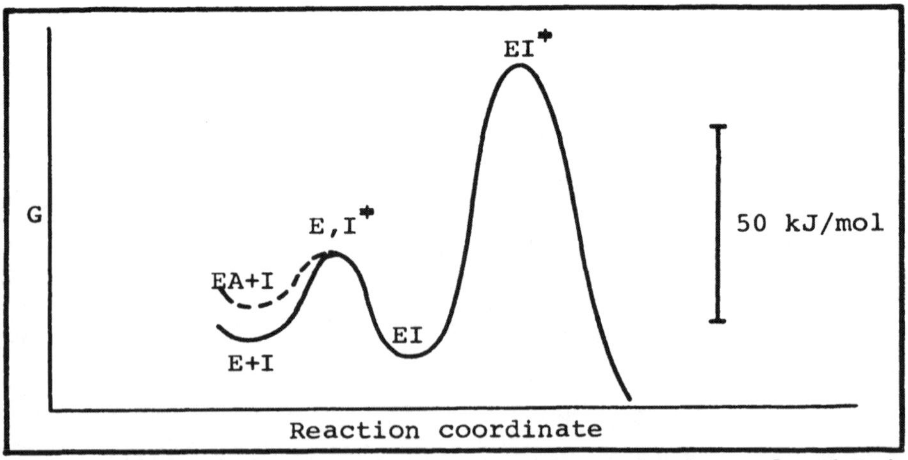

Fig. 3. Free energy profile for the acylation of AChE in the absence (full line) and presence (interrupted line) of accelerator TEA.

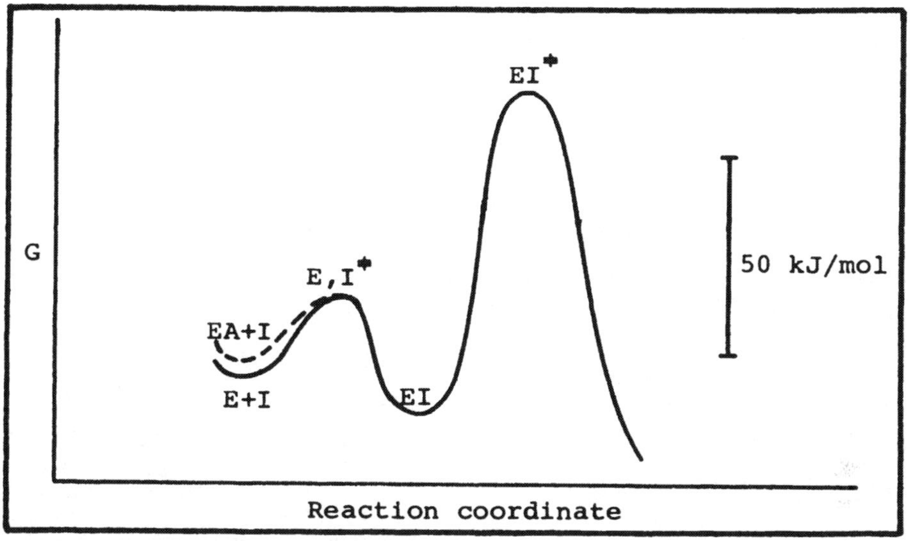

Fig. 4. Free energy profile for the acylation of BuChE in the absence (full line) and presence (interrupted line) of accelerator TEA.

It can be seen that the accelerator accelerates the acylation by improving the binding between the enzyme and the acylating agent without affecting the first-order acylation rate constant.

Acceleration site

In order to determine the site(s) from which accelerators accelerate the reaction, two sets of experiments were performed and analysed. Firstly, methanesulfonylation of AChE and BuChE, respectively, in the presence of all possible pairs of accelerators TMA, TEA and C-10 was followed and the results compared with a theoretical curve based on Eq. 13 calculated for pure competitive competition between two accelerators (cf. 10).

$$\ln\frac{(E)}{(E)_o} = -k\,\frac{1+\frac{k_A}{k}\frac{(A)}{K_A}+\frac{k_B}{k}\frac{(B)}{K_B}}{1+\frac{(A)}{K_A}+\frac{(B)}{K_B}}\,(I)\,t = -k_{ab}\,(I)\,t \quad (13)$$

In Eq. 13, k_{ab} is the second-order rate constant for the acylation of the enzyme by MSF in the presence of two (competing) accelerators A and B. Secondly, the dissociation constants, K_A´s, for the binding of accelerators to AChE and BuChE, respectively, were determined according to Eq. 12 and compared with the corresponding inhibition constants of these ligands (cf. 10).

In the case of AChE the results of these experiments are as follows (10). The accelerators compete in acceleration with each other. The values of the dissociation constants for the binding of accelerators to the enzyme are in good agreement with the values of the dissociation constants of these ligands as inhibitors of AChE. The conclusion is that accelerators accelerate from the same site on AChE and this site is the catalytic anionic site of AChE (10).

In the case of BuChE the results (in preparation) are not so clear. TMA and TEA compete with each other in acceleration; C-10 and TMA as well as C-10 and TEA, however, act together and the joint acceleration is neither the sum nor the product of individual accelerations. The value of the dissociation constant for the binding of TMA as accelerator (K_A = 0.54 mM) is similar to the value of the inhibition constant for this ligand (K_i = 0,75 mM, ref. 13); the corresponding values for TEA are different (K_A = 3.4 mM; K_i = 0.54 mM, ref. 14). In the case of C-10 two acceleration binding constants exist (K_{A1} = 26 µM,

K_{A2} = 1.3 mM); the value of one of these constants is close to the value of the inhibition constant of C-10 (K_i = 28 μM, calculated from I_{50} of ref. 15). These findings indicate that the acceleration site for TMA and TEA is the same for both ligands and that C-10 accelerates from two other sites on BuChE which, however, are distinct from the common acceleration site for TMA and TEA. It seems likely that the acceleration site of TMA and TEA is the catalytic anionic site as in the case of AChE but a proof for this is lacking.

Hydration changes in acceleration

Some features of the acceleration mechanism (cf. 16) and some other evidence (17-18) indicated that water may be somewhat involved in the process of acceleration. In order to test this assumption, the influence of the monovalent cations and anions of the Hofmeister series on the acylation by MSF of AChE and BuChE, respectively, was investigated (11, 19, in preparation).

It was found that all tested cations accelerate the acylation of both enzymes and that the acceleration is in accordance with their position in the Hofmeister series. In acceleration of AChE, the cations compete with each other and with specific accelerators TMA, TEA and C-10; in the case of BuChE the cations compete with each other but not with specific accelerators. The tested anions have no effect on the acceleration by the cations. It follows that the cations of the Hofmeister series accelerate specifically and in accordance with their position in the series.

The parallelism between the position of the cations in the Hofmeister series and their acceleration effect speaks for an involvement of water in the process of acceleration since the position of the cations reflects their ability to associate with water. We searched for and did find some other and even more indicative correlations. The most illustrative of them is shown, for the case of AChE, in Fig. 5 and others are displayed in Table 1.

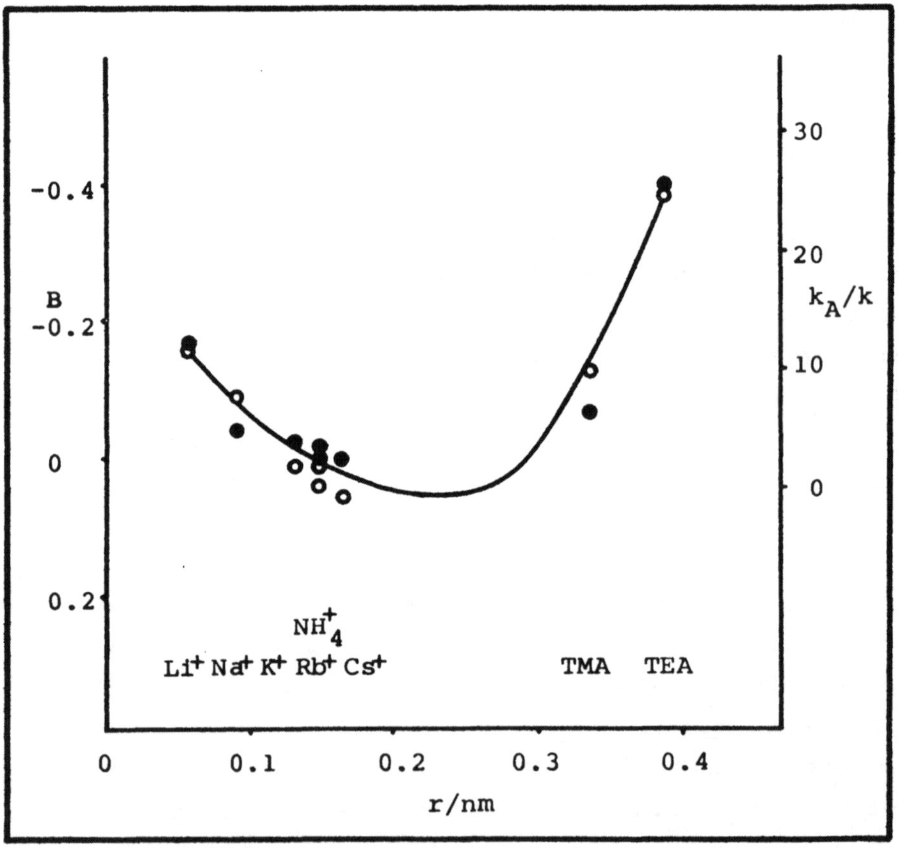

Fig. 5. The dependence of the Jones and Dole parameter, B, on ionic radius, r, (from 20) compared with the corresponding acceleration factors, k_A/k, (our data, ●). Note that the correlation between B and k_A/k is very good (r = 0.94, p 0.01).

Table 1. Acceleration of the acylation of AChE and BuChE by the cations of the Hofmeister series and some other relevant characteristics of the cations.

Cation	Acceleration (k_A/k) of AChE	of BuChE	r(cr) nm	r(s) nm	B	ΔS(ex) J/K mol
NH_4^+	1.94	1.28	0.148	0.125	-0.007	—
Cs^+	2.7	1.90	0.169	0.119	-0.045	81.2
Rb^+	3.9	2.13	0.148	0.118	-0.030	74.9
K^+	2.9	2.57	0.133	0.125	-0.007	58.2
Na^+	3.2	3.17	0.095	0.183	0.086	42.7
Li^+	10.3	6.3	0.060	0.237	0.150	-14.7

r(cr) is crystal ionic radius (from 21); r(s), solvated ionic radius (from 21); B, viscosity coefficient (from 22); ΔS(ex), extra entropy of hydration (from 22).

It can be seen that the acceleration is well correlated with crystal ionic radia ($r = 0.81$, $p < 0.05$ for AChE and $r = 0.92$, $p < 0.01$ for BuChE), solvated ionic radia ($r = 0.86$, $p < 0.05$ for AChE and $r = 0.94$, $p < 0.01$ for BuChE), viscosity coefficient B ($r = 0.80$, $p < 0.05$ for AChE and $r = 0.90$, $p < 0.01$ for BuChE) and extra entropy of hydration ($r = 0.91$, $p < 0.05$ for AChE and $r = 0.99$, $p < 0.01$ for BuChE). So, the very same phenomenon must be involved both in the acceleration and in the above mentioned characteristics of accelerators. Since these characteristics are undoubtedly related to the hydration of cations, the underlying phenomenon must be hydration. Consequently, the acceleration of the acylation of ChEs by MSF must reflect hydration changes under the influence of accelerators. It should be noted here that the best accelerators are the small (when not hydrated) Li^+ and the large TMA and TEA. On the other hand, bulkier analogs of TMA or TEA do not accelerate (tetra-n-propylammonium, ref. 1) or even inhibit (tetra-n-butylammonium, ref. 1) methanesulfonylation of AChE. This indicates that the hydration changes, electrostatic in the case of Li^+

and hydrophobic in the case of TMA and TEA (cf. 17, 23), occur around 0.4 nm from the center of the bound accelerator.

Site of hydration changes

It is evident that the hydration changes in acceleration are geometrically connected with the position of the bound accelerator at the active site of the enzyme. The site of hydration changes must be therefore somewhere in or at the active site of the enzyme. MSF molecule approaching the enzyme surface can not be excluded as the site of hydration changes. However, this possibility seems unlikely because the changes in free energy connected with acceleration are not low in some instances and, on the other hand, the hydration of MSF must be weak since its solubility is low. So, it seems very likely that the site of hydration changes is the enzyme (cf. 9). The acylation of ChEs by MSF occurs at the esteratic site of the enzyme (3, 4, 6). Consequently, hydration changes in acceleration must take place in the esteratic site of the enzyme. There are three groups in the esteratic site of ChEs (cf. 24) which come into consideration as the site(s) of hydration changes: the basic and the acidic group and the nucleophilic -OH group of serine. In order to get an indication about the group(s) involved, pH profiles of the methanesulfonylation of AChE and BuChE, respectively, were determined in the absence (3, 8) and presence (cf. 25) of accelerator TEA.

Fig. 6 shows the result of these experiments for the case of AChE. The diagram (and an analogous one for the case of BuChE) shows that the pH profile in the presence of

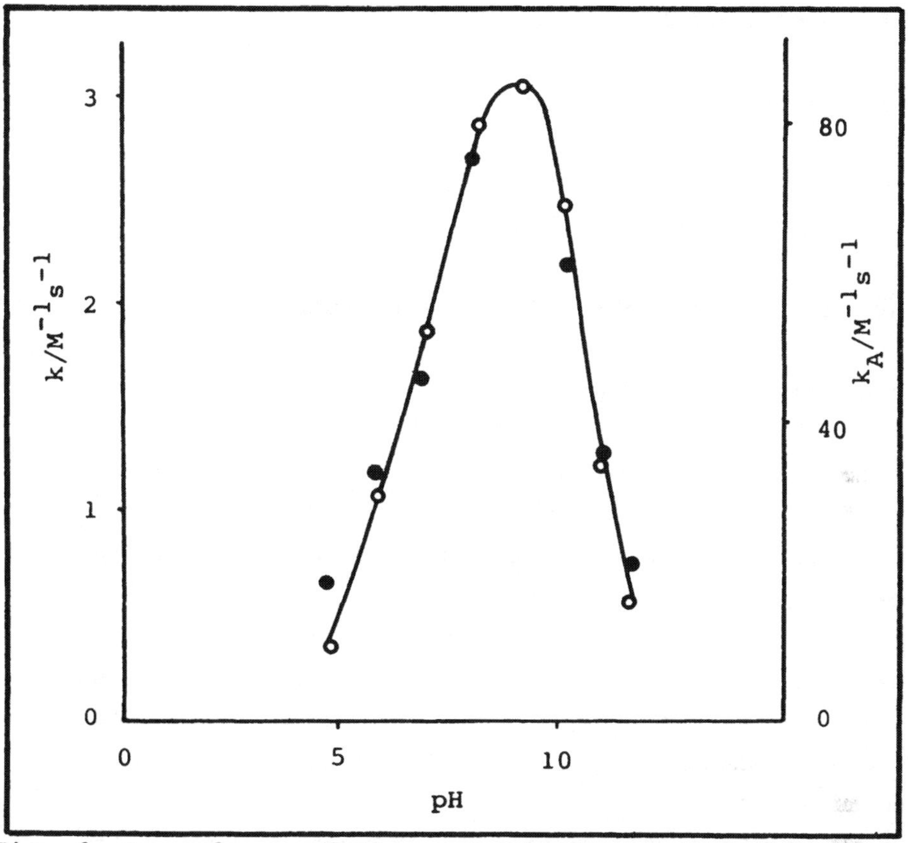

Fig. 6. Dependence of the second-order rate constant, k or k_A, for the acylation of AChE by MSF in the absence (o) and presence (●) of TEA on pH.

accelerator is identical, when normalized, with the pH profile without accelerator. This indicates that the acceleration does not affect the basic and the acidic group in the esteratic site since in this case a change in the shape of the pH profile would result from the presence of accelerator unless the two groups are affected quite equally. Consequently, it must be the -OH group of serine where hydration changes during acceleration take place. This seems even more probable because it is this group which directly binds MSF molecule (2-4, 6), and, besides, because this group is situated around 0.6 nm from the catalytic anionic site, a distance which is consistent with the distance between the center of the bound accelerator and the site of hydration changes.

Molecular events in acceleration

Our investigations seems to have well established the following:

1.) accelerator improves the binding between ChE and MSF,
2.) accelerator binds to the (catalytic) anionic site of the enzyme,
3.) accelerator brings about hydration changes, and
4.) hydration changes occur at the serine -OH group in the esteratic site of the enzyme.

Accordingly (cf. 25), accelerator binds to the catalytic anionic site of ChE and changes the hydration of the serine -OH in the esteratic site of the enzyme which results in a faster formation of the complex between ChE and MSF.

It seems plausible that hydration changes at the serine -OH group consist in a (partial) dehydration of the group what makes it more reactive towards the acylating agent (cf. 26). Having in mind that hydration is a fast dynamic process (cf. 22) and that the neighboring accelerator probably competes for vicinal water with the serine -OH, the dehydration of the serine -OH under the influence of the nearby accelerator possibly consists in a shift of the dynamic equilibrium between H_2O and -OH towards less hydrated -OH according to the schemes

$$EA + H_2O \overset{K}{\rightleftharpoons} \overset{*}{E}A \qquad (14)$$

$$EA + H_2O \overset{K'}{\rightleftharpoons} E\overset{*}{A} \qquad (15)$$

$$\overset{*}{E}A : E\overset{*}{A} = \frac{1}{K} : \frac{1}{K'} \qquad (16)$$

where $\overset{*}{E}A$ and $E\overset{*}{A}$ are the complexes between enzyme and accelerator in which hydration water is bound to E and A, respectively, and K´s are dissociation constants for the binding of water.

The shift of the dynamic equilibrium as described by schemes 14 - 16 seems likely but needs experimental support. As a matter of fact, our experiments with BuChE and pairs of accelerators seems to give some support to the proposed schemes. As stated before, in acceleration of methanesulfonylation of BuChE by the accelerator pairs C-10 - TMA and C-10 - TEA, the joint acceleration is higher than each individual acceleration. It is important to note that the joint maximal acceleration is less than the product of individual accelerations: $k_{AB}/k = 11.5 < (k_A/k) \times (k_B/k) = 6.3 \times 4.7$ for the pair C-10 - TMA; $k_{AB}/k = 12.8 < 6.3 \times 5.2$ for the pair C-10 - TEA. This is exactly what follows from schemes

$$EAB + H_2O \overset{K_1}{\rightleftharpoons} \overset{*}{E}AB \qquad (17)$$

$$EAB + H_2O \overset{K_2}{\rightleftharpoons} E\overset{*}{A}B \qquad (18)$$

$$EAB + H_2O \overset{K_3}{\rightleftharpoons} EA\overset{*}{B} \qquad (19)$$

$$\overset{*}{E}AB : E\overset{*}{A}B : EA\overset{*}{B} = \frac{1}{K_1} : \frac{1}{K_2} : \frac{1}{K_3} \qquad (20)$$

analogous to schemes 14 - 16, developed for the case of joint acceleration. Namely, in this system, k_{AB}/k is less than $(k_A/k) \times (k_B/k) = \exp((\Delta\Delta G_A^o + \Delta\Delta G_B^o)/RT)$. Here EAB represents the ternary complex between enzyme and two accelerators A and B, * hydration water bound to E, A or B, respectively, and $\Delta\Delta G^{o}$ the difference in the standard free energy changes for the binding between E and MSF in presence and absence of accelerator, which is equal to the difference between the free energies of activation of the reaction in absence and presence of accelerator (cf. Figs. 3 - 4).

A summary of our findings about the molecular events in acceleration may be presented by following scheme (Fig. 7)

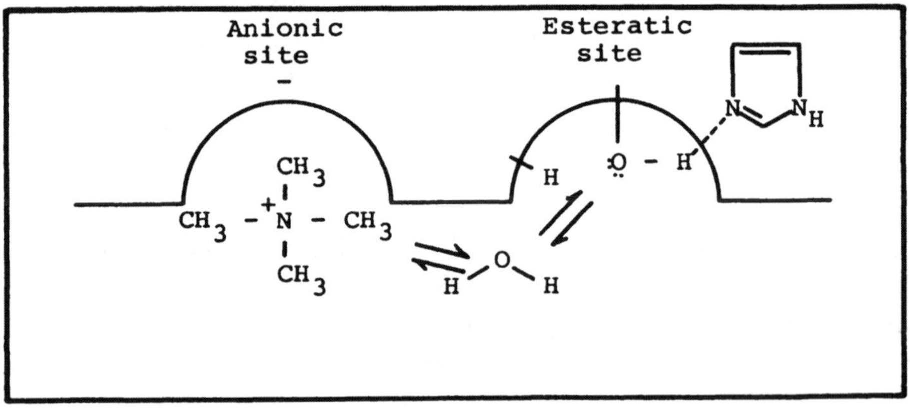

Fig. 7. Schematic representation of the molecular events in acceleration of the acylation of ChEs by MSF.

Relevance to hydrolysis of substrates

Since the cationic head of ACh corresponds in the structure, in the size and in the site of binding (cf. Figs. 1 and 7) to specific accelerators, it seems probable indeed that "ACh molecule can accelerate its own hydrolysis through its quaternary ammonium function" (5). The same is true of other substrates. And the molecular mechanism of this acceleration seems to consist in a shift of the dynamic equilibrium between water of hydration and the nucleophilic -OH group of serine in the esteratic site in favour of a less hydrated -OH, as described before.

Keeping in mind that the concentration of AChE in the synaptic cleft is in the order of 10^{-5} M and the effective maximum concentration of ACh is about half the enzyme concentration (27), the described acceleration phenomenon might be not only theoretically but also physiologically important.

References

1. Kitz, R., Wilson, I. B.: J. Biol. Chem. 238, 745-748 (1963).
2. Kitz, R., Wilson, I. B.: J. Biol. Chem. 237, 3245-3249 (1962).
3. Pavlič, M. R.: Period. biol. 73, 69-74 (1971).
4. Pavlič, M. R.: Vestnik SKD 20, 39-47 (1973).
5. Wilson, I. B.: Ann. N. Y. Acad. Sci. 144, 664-674 (1967).
6. Pavlič, M. R.: Biochim. Biophys. Acta 198, 389-391 (1970).
7. Iverson, F.: Mol. Pharmacol. 7, 129-135 (1971).
8. Pavlič, M. R.: Biochim. Biophys. Acta 284, 435-440 (1972).
9. Pavlič, M. R., Wilson, I. B.: Biochim. Biophys. Acta 523, 101-108 (1978).
10. Pavlič, M. R., Zorko, M.: Biochim. Biophys. Acta 524, 340-348 (1978).
11. Pavlič, M. R. in Enzyme Regulation and Mechanism of Action (Mildner, P., Ries, B., eds.) pp. 113-122, Pergamon Press, Oxford and New York 1980.
12. Britten, H. T. S., Robinson, R. A. in Biochemisches Taschenbuch (Rauen, H. M., ed.) pp. 649, 651, 654, Springer Verlag, Berlin 1956.
13. Grigoreva, G. M.: Biokhimiya 30, 415-422 (1964).
14. Kulikova, A. I., Kupriyanov, V. A., Rozengart, V. I.: Biokhimiya 37, 1041-1047 (1972).
15. Bergmann, F., Segal, R.: Biochem. J. 58, 692-698 (1954).

16. Pavlič, M. R.: Croat. Chem. Acta 47, 355-359 (1975).

17. Belleau, B.: Ann. N. Y. Acad. Sci. 144, 705-719 (1967).

18. Low, P. S., Somero, G. N.: Proc. Nat. Acad.Sci USA 72, 3305-3309 (1975).

19. Pavlič, M. R., Zorko, M.(in press) Proc. 2nd Int. Conf. on Water and Ions in Biological Systems, Bucharest 1982, Rumania, Plenum Press.

20. Podolsky, R. J.: J. Am. Chem. Soc. 80, 4442-4451 (1958).

21. Monk, C. B.: Electrolytic Dissociation, p. 271, Acad. Press, London and New York 1961.

22. Gordon, J. E.: The Organic Chemistry of Electrolyte Solutions, pp. 186, 197, 204, John Wiley and Sons, New York, London, Sidney and Toronto 1975.

23. Jencks, W. P.: Catalysis in Chemistry and Enzymology, McGraw-Hill Book Company, New York, St. Louis, San Francisco, London, Sidney, Toronto, Mexico and Panama, p. 388, 1969.

24. Krupka, R. M., Laidler, K. J.: J. Am. Chem. Soc. 83, 1458-1460 (1961).

25. Pavlič, M. R.: Period. biol. 82, 449-453 (1980).

26. Weaver, W. M., Hutchison, J. D.: J. Am. Chem. Soc. 86, 261-265 (1964).

27. Barnard, E. A., Rymaszewska, T., Wieckovski, J. in Cholinergic Ligand Interactions (Triggle, D. J., Moran, J. F., Barnard, E. A., eds.), Acad. Press, New York 1971.

SITES FOR REVERSIBLE BINDING OF ACYLATING INHIBITORS TO ACETYLCHOLINESTERASE EVALUATED FROM KINETIC STUDIES

Elsa Reiner

Institut za medicinska istraživanja i medicinu rada
Zagreb, Jugoslavija

It has been shown earlier that some organophosphorus compounds (AB) form complexes with acetylcholinesterase which have different properties than the Michaelis complex between the enzyme and AB which precedes phosphorylation (1, 2, 3). The differentiation between the two types of complexes discussed in this paper will be based upon the effect of substrates (S) and reversible inhibitors (R) upon reversible binding of AB and upon phosphorylation by AB.

The theoretical equations are based upon the following assumptions concerning binding of AB and substrates to the enzyme (E) (4). AB and S can bind to the enzyme in the active site (E-AB and E-S; dissociation constants K_a and K_s), in a peripheral site (AB-E and S-E; dissociation constants K_i and K_{ss}) and in both sites (AB-E-AB and S-E-S; dissociation constants K_a, K_i, K_s, K_{ss}). It is assumed that the sites are independent as far as binding is concerned, i.e. that the dissociation constants in the ternary complexes AB-E-AB and S--E-S are the same as in the binary complexes. It is also assumed that the active site cannot be acylated

Cholinesterases, © Walter de Gruyter & Co., Berlin - New York, 1984

when the peripheral site is occupied, and this in turn precludes that the binding of the substrates to the peripheral site causes substrate inhibition.

Although the postulated assumptions very probably oversimplify the properties of the binding sites on acetylcholinesterase, by the approach discussed here two different types of complexes formed with acylating agents can be satisfactorily distinguished.

For the reaction between E and AB two schemes will be considered:

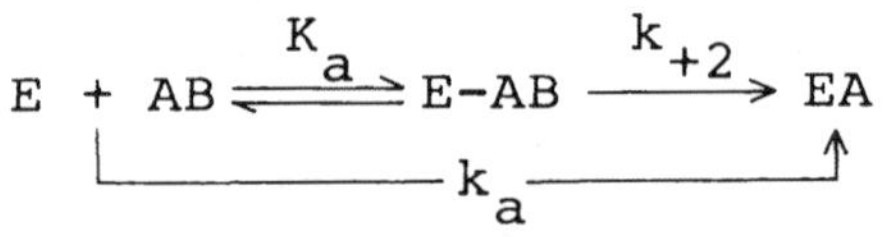

Scheme I

$$k = ab.k_{+2}/(K_a+ab) \qquad k_a = k_{+2}/K_a \qquad (1)$$

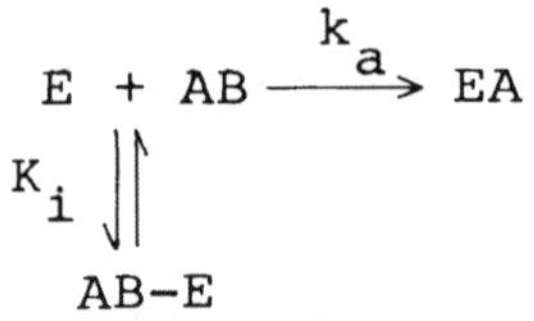

Scheme II

$$k = ab.k_a.K_i \ / \ (K_i+ab) \qquad (2)$$

In Scheme II it is assumed that the concentration of the Michaelis complex E-AB is too small to be measurable; the only measurable complex is therefore between the enzyme and AB in the peripheral site, AB-E. The corresponding dissociation constants are K_a and K_i; $\underline{k}$ and k_a are the first - and second - order rate constants of phosphorylation, EA is the phosphorylated enzyme and $\underline{ab}$ the concentration of AB.

Schemes I and II cannot be differentiated from each other by measuring the rates of phosphorylation in absence of S or R, because equations (1) and (2) are kinetically indistinguishable. Substrates and reversible inhibitors, however, will have the following different effects upon the two types of reaction.

If AB reacts according to Scheme I, the rate constant in presence of a substrate, which causes substrate inhibition, will be:

$$k = \frac{ab \cdot k_{+2} / K_a}{(1+s/K_m)(1+s/K_{ss}) + (ab/K_a)(1+s/K_{ss})} \qquad (3)$$

and if AB reacts according to Scheme II:

$$k = \frac{ab \cdot k_a}{(1+s/K_m)(1+s/K_{ss}) + (ab/K_i)(1+s/K_m)} \qquad (4)$$

At a given substrate concentration the maximum rate of phosphorylation is little affected by the substrate (slope of the line in Fig. 1) when Scheme I holds, but the dissociation constant of AB is apparently increased (intercept on the abscissa in Fig. 1). For Scheme II the dissociation constant remains almost unaltered at concentrations which considerably decrease the maximum rate (Fig. 2).

If the substrate does not cause substrate inhibition, the equations (3) and (4) will simplify to:

$$k = \frac{ab \cdot k_{+2}/K_a}{1 + s/K_m + ab/K_a} \qquad (5)$$

$$k = \frac{ab \cdot k_a}{1 + s/K_m + (ab/K_i)(1 + s/K_m)} \qquad (6)$$

At a given substrate concentration the maximum rate of phosphorylation remains unaltered by the substrate when Scheme I holds, but the dissociation constant of AB is apparently increased by a factor of $1+s/K_m$. For Scheme II the dissociation constant remains unaltered, while the maximum rate decreases by a factor of $1+s/K_m$.

The effect of reversible inhibitors (R) upon phosphorylation will depend upon the sites of binding of both R and AB. If AB reacts according to Scheme I and the reversible inhibitor binds only to the active site (with a dissociation constant $K_{a,R}$), the rate constant will be:

$$k = \frac{k_{+2}}{1 + (K_a/ab)(1+r/K_{a,R})} \qquad (7)$$

If AB reacts according to Scheme II and the reversible inhibitor binds only to the peripheral site (with a dissociation constant $K_{i,R}$), the rate constant in presence of R will be:

$$k = \frac{ab \cdot k_a}{1 + ab/K_i + r/K_{i,R}} \qquad (8)$$

If AB reacts according to Scheme I and the reversible inhibitor binds only to the peripheral site (with a dissociation constant $K_{i,R}$), the rate constant will be:

$$k = \frac{k_{+2}}{(1+K_a/ab)\ (1+r/K_{i,R})} \qquad (9)$$

If AB reacts according to Scheme II and the reversible inhibitor binds only to the active site (with a dissociation constant $K_{a,R}$), the rate constant will be:

$$k = \frac{ab \cdot k_a}{(1+ab/K_i)(1+r/K_{a,R})} \qquad (10)$$

It follows from the above equations that when AB and R bind reversibly to the same site on the enzyme (which can be either the active or the peripheral site) the maximum rate of phosphorylation will remain unaltered, but the dissociation constant will apparently increase (Fig. 3). When AB and R bind to different sites, the dissociation constant for AB remains unaltered, but the maximum rate of phosphorylation decreases (Fig. 4).

The effect of substrate upon reversible binding of AB can also be studied when there is no phosphorylation: AB is added to the reaction medium containing the enzyme and the substrate, and the initial rate of substrate hydrolysis is measured; the rate must remain constant during enzyme assay. Equation (11) should then hold when AB reacts according to Scheme I, and eqn. (12) when it reacts according to Scheme II (v_o and $\underline{v}$ are the enzyme activities in absence and presence of AB).

$$K_{app} = v.ab/(v_o-v) = K_a + K_a.s/K_m \qquad (11)$$

$$K_{app} = v.ab/(v_o-v) = K_i + K_i.s/K_{ss} \qquad (12)$$

According to both equations the apparent dissociation constants should be linear functions of the substrate concentration with intercepts on the abscissa which are either K_m or K_{ss}. The intercepts on the ordinate are either K_a or K_i, and should have the same numerical values as those obtained from the kinetics of phosphorylation. The same equations should hold for inhibition by any reversible inhibitor irrespective of whether it is an acylating or non-acylating agent.

Figure 1. (refers to eqn. 3)

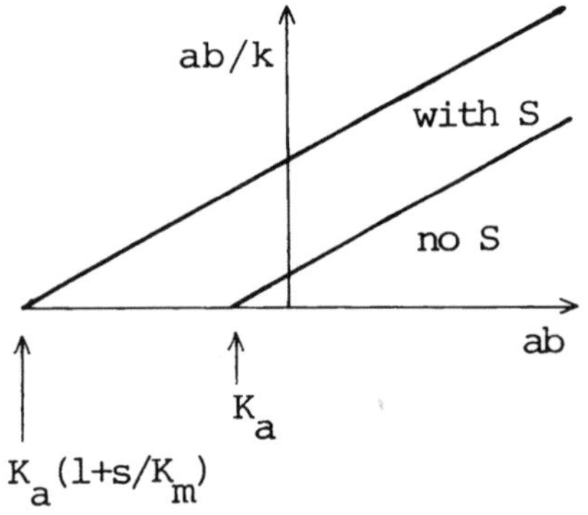

Slope in presence of S = $(1+s/K_{ss})/k_{+2}$

Figure 2. (refers to eqn. 4)

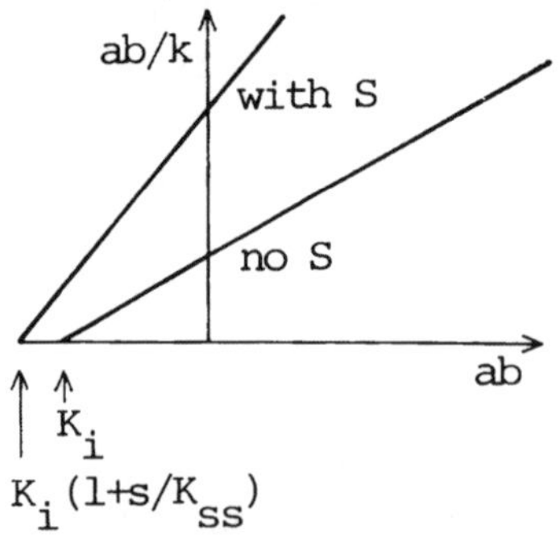

Slope in presence of S = $(1+s/K_m)/(k_a K_i)$

Figure 3. (refers to eqns. 7 and 8)

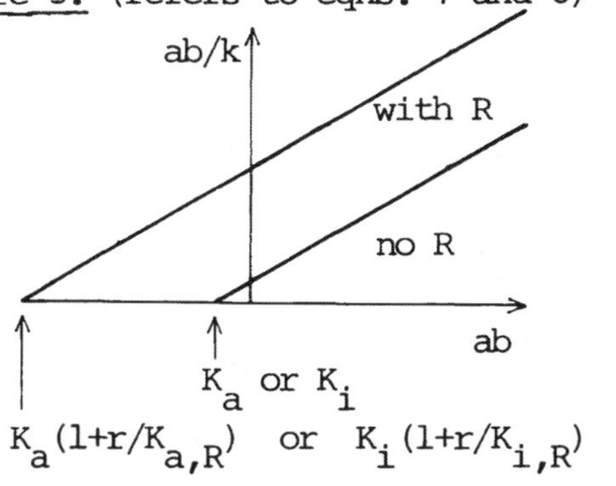

Slope in presence of $\underline{R}$ =
$1/k_{+2}$ or $1/(k_aK_i)$

Figure 4. (refers to eqns. 9 and 10)

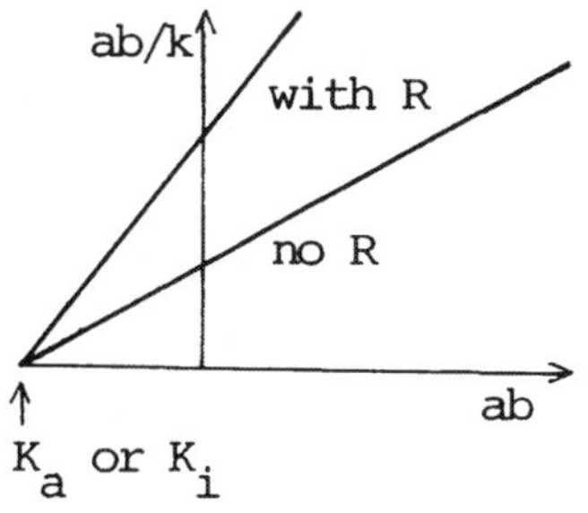

Slope in presence of $\underline{R}$ =
$(1+r/K_{i,R})/k_{+2}$ or
$(1+r/K_{a,R})/(k_aK_i)$

The outlined approach for the differentiation of two types of complexes between acetylcholinesterase and organophosphorus compounds has been applied to reactions of haloxon (di-2-chloroethyl 3-chloro-4-methylcoumarin-7-yl phosphate), coroxon (di-ethyl 3-chloro--4-methylcoumarin-7-yl phosphate), phosphostigmine (3-N-trimethylanilinium diethylphosphate methyl sulphate) as phosphorylating agents, tetramethylammonium (TMA), edrophonium (3-hydroxy-N-ethyl dimethyl anilinium chloride) and coumarin (the leaving group in haloxon and coroxon) as reversible inhibitors, and acetylcholine and acetylthiocholine as substrates. The enzyme was from bovine and human erythrocytes.

From the effect of acetylthiocholine, TMA, edrophonium and coumarin upon inhibition by phosphostigmine it was concluded that phosphostigmine reacts according to Scheme I (5). From the effect of acetylthiocholine and acetylcholine upon inhibition by haloxon, coroxon and coumarin it was concluded that haloxon and coroxon react according to Scheme II (1, 2, 3); the effect of TMA and edrophonium upon phosphorylation by haloxon complies with the same scheme (5). The results outlined above point to be conclusion that reversible inhibition by haloxon and coroxon, and substrate inhibition by acetylcholine and acetylthiocholine both occur at a peripheral site of acetylcholinesterase.

References

1. Aldridge, W. N., Reiner, E.: Biochem. J. 115, 147-162 (1969).

2. Reiner, E., Simeon, V.: Croat. Chem. Acta 47, 321-331 (1975).

3. Simeon, V., Kobrehel, Dj., Reiner, E.: Croat. Chem. Acta 50, 331-334 (1977).

4. Aldridge, W. N., Reiner, E.: Enzyme Inhibitors as Substrates. Interaction of esterases with esters of organophosphorus and carbamic acids. North Holland, Amsterdam (1972).

5. Radić, Z., Reiner, E., Simeon, V.: submitted for publication to Biochem. Pharmacol.

II. MULTIPLE MOLECULAR FORMS OF ACETYLCHOLINESTERASE: STRUCTURE, REGULATION AND MOLECULAR GENETICS

INTRODUCTION TO SESSION II

Eric A. Barnard

Department of Biochemistry, Imperial College, London SW7, UK

One of the fascinations of AChE is its highly developed polymorphism. There is a beauty about this range of structures and its culmination in the tailed dodecamer. This unusual structure invites speculation on its assembly, significance and the interactions it makes *in situ* with other components. The range of possibilities inherent in the multiple forms of AChE led to the need for two Sessions (2a and 2b) to accommodate the lectures relating to them.

The multiple forms were originally recognised electrophoretically and much work in the past used that technique; this must now be largely discarded since the heavy forms do not penetrate the usual gels and since the charge differences are not fundamental in this series. Every one of the speakers in Session 2 employed sedimentation velocity on sucrose gradients to analyse the forms: the introduction of that method to this problem by Jean Massoulié and François Rieger at the early stage of 1969 can now be seen as a prescient advance in this field. Several lectures in this Session considered the detailed protein structure of the tailed assembly. Important contributors to our knowledge of this structure were gathered together: J. Massoulié, T.L. Rosenberry, I. Silman and P. Taylor. The number of polypeptides involved in the assembly is still uncertain. The accumulation of amino acid sequence data on the catalytic subunits of both AChE and ψ ChE is now proceeding, as the collected papers here (and in Session 3) show.

cDNA cloning for more rapid sequencing is now being actively sought in several of these laboratories, and is becoming a major interest in this field. The discussions left us with the feeling that we can expect structural elucidation of AChE to come thus with explosive force in the fairly near future. Indeed, also, that an era of new and profound insights into AChE structures by means of molecular-genetics is likely to break on us with surprising rapidity. This approach is also necessary for the study of the cellular control of the AChE forms. Synthesis of these by injected mRNA in the Xenopus oocyte system (N. Razon et al.; E.A. Barnard et al.) has begun to show how assembly can occur. Stages in the processing and assembly in cultured cells (R.L. Rotundo) are also becoming much clearer.

An important functional correlation was fortunately provided by L.G. Magazanik, who showed us how measurements on ACh-gated channels in muscle cell membranes can be related to the local arrangement of AChE molecules. This physiological approach was directly relevant to discussions of the roles of the forms in some of the lectures and posters.

The multiple forms separated by sedimentation, originally thought to constitute a series, are now being seen as dividing into several different series. Different hydrophobic and hydrophilic elements are probably involved, an emphasis of a number of both the lectures and the poster presentations. This analysis is important for consideration of the cellular location of the various forms. This Session (and part of the succeeding one) brought forth a range of new information on these questions, which is beginning to make sense of the puzzle of the molecular forms and their complex cellular distributions.

MULTIPLE MOLECULAR FORMS OF ACETYLCHOLINESTERASE AND THEIR RELATIONSHIP TO MUSCLE FUNCTION

Eric A. Barnard, Penelope J. Barnard, Jonathan Jarvis, Jolanta Jedrzejczyk, Josephine Lai, John A. Pizzey and William R. Randall

Department of Biochemistry, Imperial College, London SW7, UK

Israel Silman

Weizmann Institute, Rehovot, Israel

Introduction

The molecular forms of AChE in vertebrate striated muscles comprise (in decreasing size order) the asymmetric collagen-tailed "heavy" (H) forms (H_{2C} and minor H_{1C}) and the globular forms M, L_2 and L_1. H_{2C} corresponds to A_{12} in the nomenclature of J. Massoulié and colleagues, this having $s_{20,w}$ of 20 S in birds and 16 S in mammals; L_2 corresponds to G_2, etc. We do not yet know for certain that there are 12 catalytic subunits in the heaviest form in vertebrate muscle - the nomenclature having been based on the structure deduced for fish electric organ AChE (1) - so we prefer the phenomenological classification of H, L, etc., forms and we indicate the two main classes by the suffix C for the collagen-tailed class (2). All the evidence to date on AChE in vertebrate muscles shows that forms fitting the above-mentioned 5 designations can occur in all muscles, although the $s_{20,w}$ value of one form can vary between species, and so, presumably, can the size of the polypeptides. This scheme may be partly a simplification; a hydrophobic dimer similar in size to L_2 (or G_2) has been detected in <u>Torpedo</u> (3) and other hydrophobic variants may occur in vertebrate muscle. Likewise there may be both tailed and non-tailed forms of the tetramer (4), although the former are generally difficult to detect in muscle. That the H_{2C} and H_{1C} forms are collagenous in the birds as well as the mammals and fish has been demonstrated by the collagenase sensitivity of their hydrodynamic behaviour (2,5). The latter statement applies also to the $H_{2C}\psi$ChE in the muscle (2).

In vertebrate skeletal muscles the 16 - 20 S form, H_{2C}, is now familiar as the form of AChE associated with the endplates. This attribution is based principally upon the selective occurrence of H_{2C} AChE in neural segments of muscle seen in many studies, its partial removal therefrom by collagenase, and the loss of H_{2C} following denervation and its reappearance upon re-innervation (reviewed in (4)). However, we wish to emphasise the observation that when different mammalian (including human) muscles are analysed for these forms of AChE, a variety of sedimentation profiles are obtained which generally contain a mixture of various L, M and H types. An example is given in Fig. 1A. The variations seen in the ratios of these forms between different muscles and animal species are wide and complex. Certainly, the H (tailed) forms do not predominate in published analyses of the AChE of these muscles. In a recent review (4) Bon and Massoulié note that the tailed forms "generally constitute only a small fraction of the enzyme". For example, in mature animals the fraction of H_{2C} reported present (taking the total extracted AChE in a muscle as 100%) varies from 3-7% in rat gastrocnemius or rectus muscles (6,7) to 15-20% in rat extensor digitorum longus (EDL) muscles (8,9), up to a maximum of about 30% reported for human intercostal muscle (10) or mouse diaphragm or EDL (11). Endplate-specific H forms in rat diaphragm were found to be 12% (12). Can we make any sense of this complexity and the low proportion of the "endplate form" of AChE?

We can firstly note that AChE profiles for the same species and muscle can differ considerably between different authors, and commonly between the same muscle in different species. Secondly, in our own analyses of AChE chicken twitch muscles (2,13,14), H_{2C} is not minor but is 80%-90% of the total. However, our methods differed in certain respects from those used in all of the studies on mammalian muscles known to us. This, and the variability mentioned, raise the question whether the low amounts of H_{2C} in the mammalian muscles are real or an artefact of the methods used. Finally, we observed that in a quite different fibre type in chicken muscles, the slow tonic fibres, the H_{2C} contribution to the high total AChE content of those fibres could become vanishingly small (15). We address here, therefore, the questions:

(i) What is the true occurrence of tailed and globular forms of AChE in a range of mammalian muscles?

(ii) Can we interpret the differences in AChE forms between muscles in terms of their varying fibre type compositions, or in some other systematic manner?

(iii) Which forms truly occur in the endplate, in muscles with different profiles of forms?

(iv) What regulatory and functional influences upon the amount and location of the various AChE forms can be identified as acting on the muscle when in the animal?

Results

<u>Precautions for the extraction of native forms of AChE.</u> Investigation showed that the following are of value: (a) prior perfusion (2) of the animal with 10mM EDTA/ isotonic saline to remove blood AChE and ψChE and proteases; (b) homogenisation in 1% Triton X-100/1M NaCl/10mM EGTA (pH 7)

for full extraction (13); (c) an array of protease inhibitors (essential) during the extraction; (d) rapid processing, such that the sample is placed on a sucrose density gradient within one hour after death. For (c), we now use: aprotinin (0.2mg/ml), bacitracin (1mg/ml), benzamidine (2mM), EGTA (5mM), N-ethylmaleimide (5mM), leupeptin (0.04 mg/ml), ovomucoid (chicken, 0.02mg/ml) pepstatin (0.02mg/ml), lima bean trypsin inhibitor (0.1mg/ml). In some cases (where mast cell proteases are active) Vipera ammodytes snake venom protease inhibitor (0.1mg/ml) is added. To obtain this, the crude venom (from Sigma, or other snake venom suppliers) is gel-filtered (16) in a volatile buffer; the last-eluted protein peak contains the inhibitors, which are freeze-dried and stored at 4°C. Freezing or storage of the muscle or its extract, must be avoided.

When these precautions are employed, the proportion of H_{2C} in mammalian muscular AChE can become quite large. Dropping some of them produces a definite trend to reduction in H_{2C} and appearance of L forms (Fig.1). The proportion of L_1 (~4 S) is low in the native state in most muscles, L_2 (~6 S) being the main L form; when any proteolysis occurs L_1 grows at the expense of L_2 and H forms. The greater changes which are produced when anti-protease protection is lessened have been demonstrated earlier on avian muscle (2, 17).
All analyses were made on such extracts by sucrose density gradient centrifugation (13); profiles are shown with the heavier forms on the right, and with the catalase internal marker (11.4 S) shown by an arrow.

Relationship to muscle fibre type. Almost all mammalian skeletal muscles contain the general fibre types I (slow-twitch-oxidative), IIA (fast-twitch-oxidative-glycolytic) and IIB (fast-twitch-glycolytic) (18,19), usually mixed. We

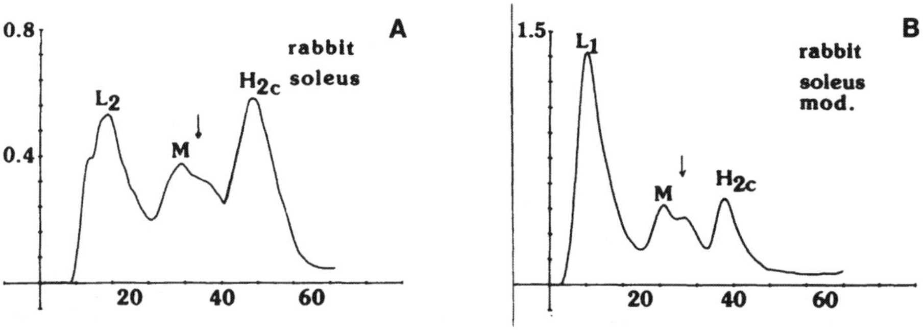

Fig. 1 Forms of AChE in rabbit soleus muscle. A: Fully protected. B: Modified due to less protection - only bacitracin, benzamidine and N-ethylmaleimide were used, and the period before applying to gradient tube was 4 hr. In this and all subsequent gradient profiles, abscissa shows fractions (on SW40 Ti rotor at 39,000 rpm) and ordinate shows activity (absorbance change or cpm).

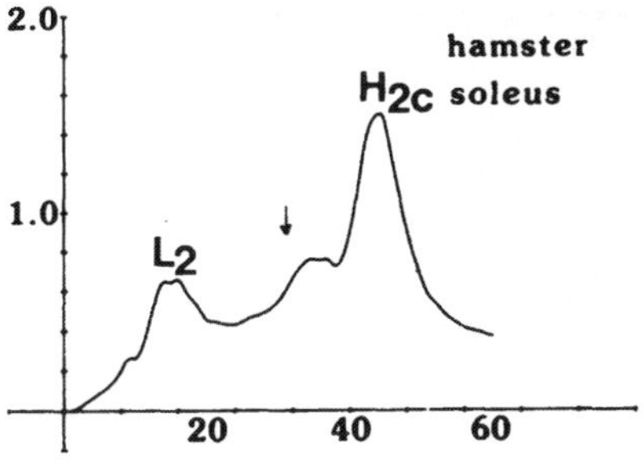

Fig. 2 Forms in hamster soleus muscle (80% type I fibres).

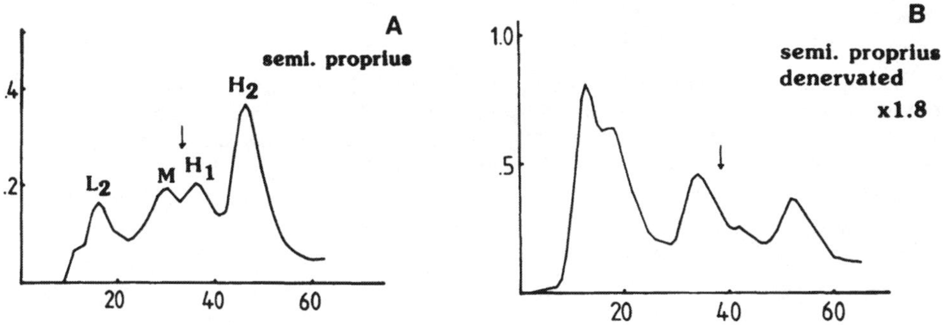

Fig. 3 Forms in rabbit semimembranosus proprius (99% type I) muscle. A: Normal. B: After 4 weeks total denervation (1.8 times the activity used in A was applied in B).

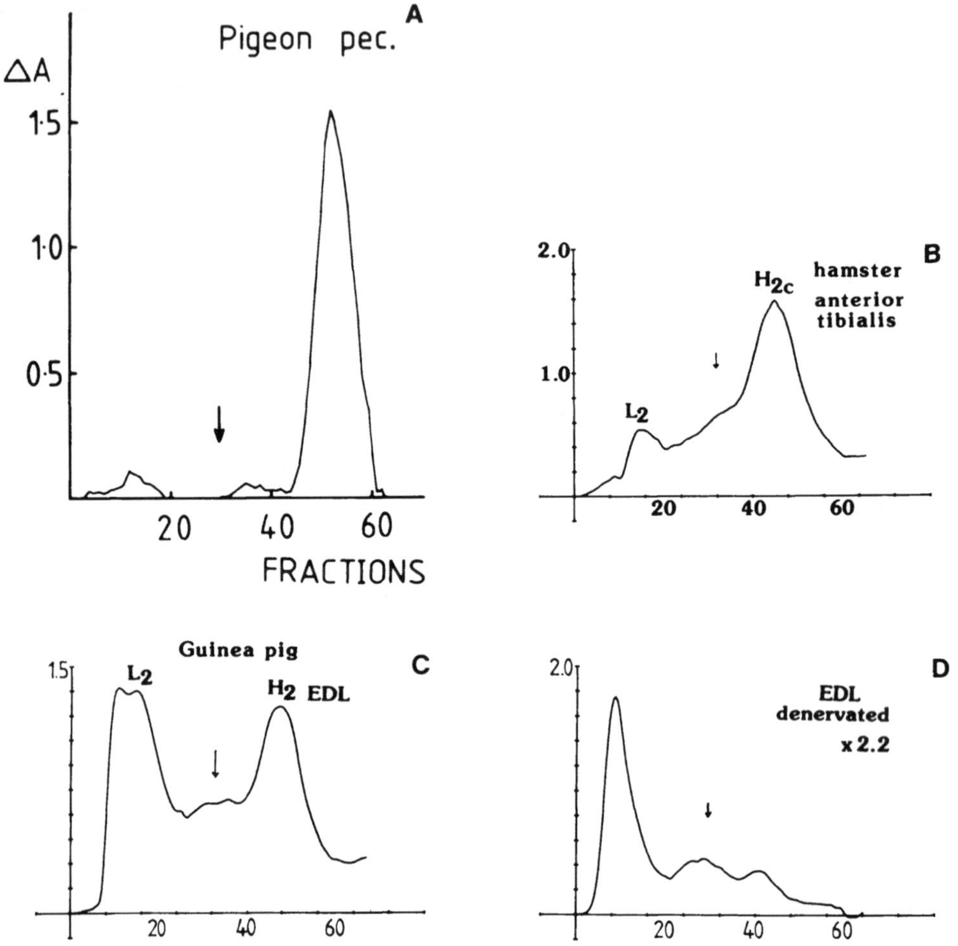

Fig. 4 A: Pigeon pectoral (100% type II) muscle. B: Hamster anterior tibialis (type II). C: Guinea pig EDL (94% type II). D: Guinea pig EDL, 4 weeks denervated (2.2 times the activity used in C was applied).

have selected certain muscles which are nearly pure for one fibre type. In the slow-twitch muscles very rich in type 1 fibres, the H forms (i.e. H_{2C} + H_{1C}) contribute most of the AChE in all species examined. Examples are shown in Figs. 1A, 2, 3A. Nevertheless, L can be quite significant in some of these muscles (Fig. 1A).

For muscles having virtually only type II fibres, we have firstly studied birds, where such pure muscles are more common. In the mature chicken pectoral muscle 99% of the fibres are type IIB, and 90% of its AChE was found in the H_{2C} form (13). The pigeon pectoral is different in sub-type, being oxidative (because it is used for sustained flight), i.e. is $>$ 90% type IIA, but likewise has 95% of its AChE in the H_{2C} form (Fig. 4A). A great predominance of the H_{2C} form is also found in several other type IIB and type IIA avian muscles (14). In general, there is little difference between type IIA and type IIB avian fibres in their AChE pattern, although in some type IIA muscles rather more of the M and L forms are present. In some mammalian muscles very rich in type II fibres (group (i)), the same pattern of high H_{2C} content is found (Fig. 4B). However, in some other type II-rich muscles (group (ii)), L and H forms contribute about equally (Fig. 4C).

There are thus two main groups of mammalian fast-twitch muscles, with respect to the AChE forms they maintain. (We cannot exclude the possibility that some proteases for which as yet an inhibitor has not been applied might still affect the detailed distribution in particular cases). In the mammals, as in the birds, the sub-types IIA and IIB are not the origin of the differing patterns of AChE forms in different fast-twitch muscles (Table I). Muscles with more mixed fibre types, e.g. the rat diaphragm (45% I, 27% IIA, 28% IIB), give a gradient profile between that of the types I and II profiles, but it is difficult to predict the pattern

Table I. Forms (% of total AChE) in vastus lateralis muscles

Muscle (guinea pig)	Fibre types	% H	% L
vastus l. (red sector)	78% IIA, 18% IIB	57	26
vastus l. (white sector)	29% IIA, 71% IIB	58	29

in advance because we do not know which group of type II fibres is present. Group (ii), with higher L AChE, may be a sub-type of type II having a high protein turnover rate, producing a pool of the precursor L form. Sub- types within the populations of fibre types IIA and IIB have been detected by more subtle differences, e.g. on the basis of myosin isoform variants (20,21) and such differentiations need to be compared to the AChE profile sub-types.

Another muscle type which is essentially pure in the birds is the slow-tonic type, composed of a specific fibre type, III (14). These fibres are multiply-innervated and contract very slowly and sustain a tetanus. During growth of the bird the tonic muscles lose all or most of their H_{2C} content, their AChE finally being in the L and M forms, mainly L_2 (15). Hence, the situation in the tonic fibres is the converse of that in the twitch fibres, with L AChE predominating in the tonic muscles.

<u>AChE forms located in the endplates</u>. Direct evidence on the forms localised at the endplates was obtained by micro-dissection of individual endplates and analysis of their extracts (fully protected from proteolysis) on gradients (22). This showed unequivocally that the fast-twitch (type II) muscle endplate in the mature chicken contains the H_{2C} form of AChE and a very small amount of H_{1C} (Fig.5A). The low but definite L AChE content of the whole muscle is almost entirely extra-synaptic. In mammalian type II <u>and</u> type I fibre endplates, essentially the same result has been

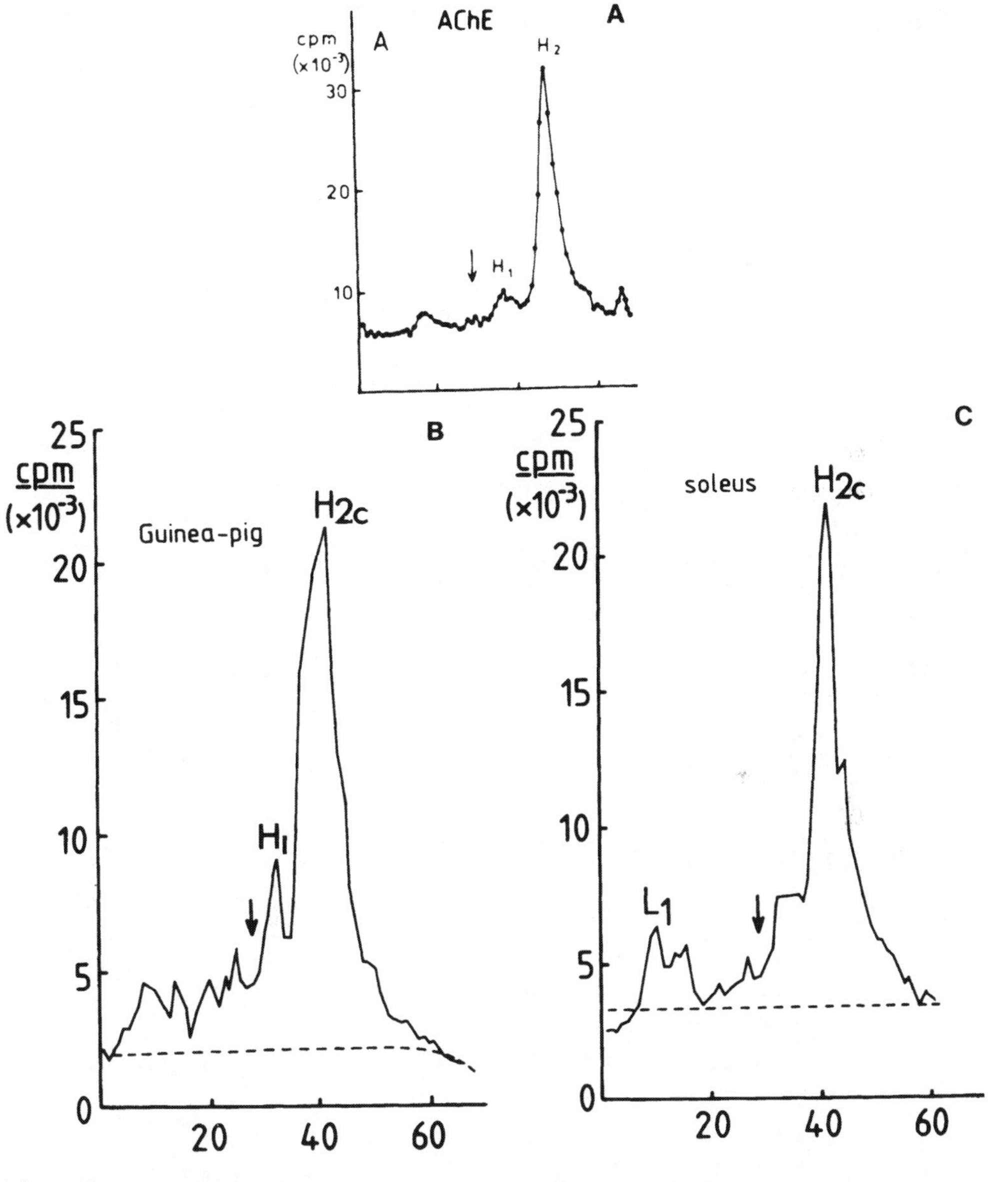

Fig. 5 Endplates were micro-dissected, fully extracted, analysed and fractions assayed with [^{3}H]ACh plus 10^{-4}M iso-OMPA (22). A: Endplates of the chicken PLD (type II) fibres. (From (22); control cpm not subtracted).
B: Endplates of guinea pig EDL (type II). Broken line in this and other plots shows a parallel control (i.e. sample with AChE and ΨChE totally inhibited in the assays).
C: Endplates of rat soleus (type I).

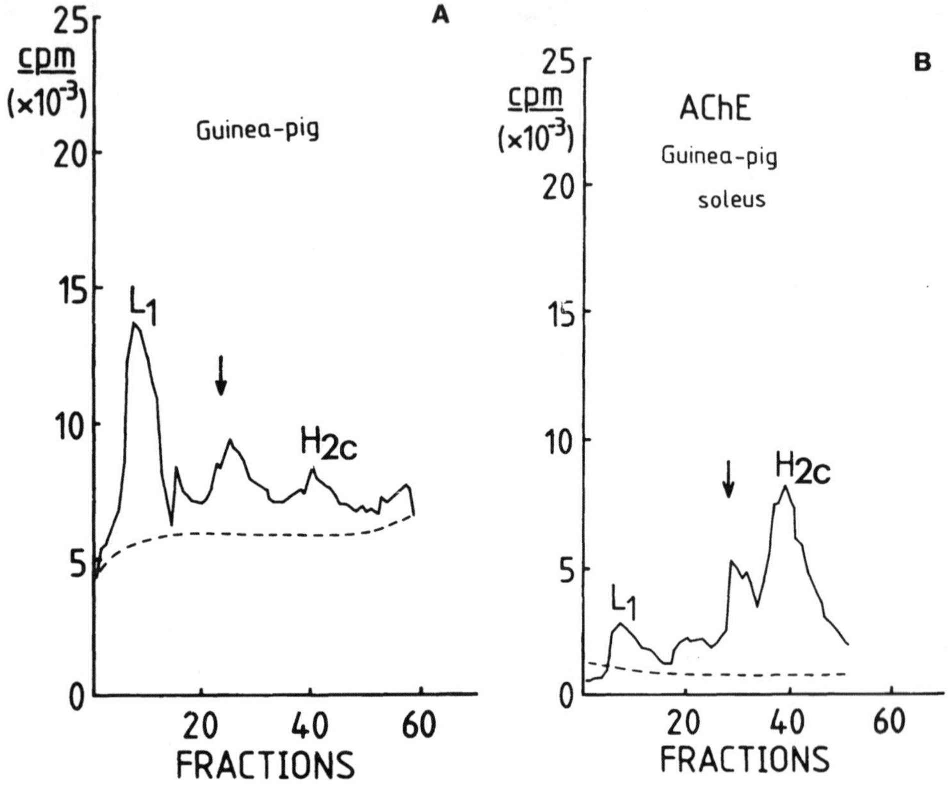

Fig. 6 Zones free of endplates were micro-dissected, as far as possible from the endplates but not in the tendon area. As in Fig. 5, but with at least 10 times more fibre length used. A: Guinea pig EDL. B: Guinea pig soleus.

obtained (Fig. 5B,C). The endplate contains a high concentration of H_{2C}, and some H_{1C}, AChE, in all twitch muscles examined. In the slow-twitch fibres, however, a definite L component is also found (Fig. 5C). Outside (and far from) the endplates, micro-dissection shows that in group (i) muscles of type II (see above) the AChE concentration is extremely low, this being in the L form with no H forms at all; likewise in group (ii) muscles of type II, the L form predominates, but the M form is distinctly present (Fig.6A).

In contrast, in the mammalian slow-twitch fibres, H_{2C} AChE definitely occurs throughout the length of the fibre (Fig. 6B). Extra-junctional H AChE has been established to occur previously only in rare cases (apart from immature muscle); most notably in human intercostal muscle, where a gross separation of the endplate-containing zones is feasible, the H_{2C} concentration is high extra-synaptically (10). Rat diaphragm also shows a small effect of that type (12). Those muscles are mixed, but human muscle fibres of all types may contain substantial extra-synaptic H AChE.

Since the slow-tonic avian (type III) fibres lose nearly all of their H forms of AChE (see above), it is of interest to enquire into the situation at their endplates, which definitely retain the usual strong histochemical staining for AChE. In fact, these endplates have a high content of L_2 AChE (Fig.7). A moderate amount of M is there also, and a small amount of H remains. The ratios of the forms found outside the endplates are the same as inside them. The tonic fibre is the only case known where the major form in the endplate is not H AChE.

Effects of denervation on AChE. In chronic denervation, the total AChE content is known to decrease in all of the muscles in several mammalian species but, exceptionally, to

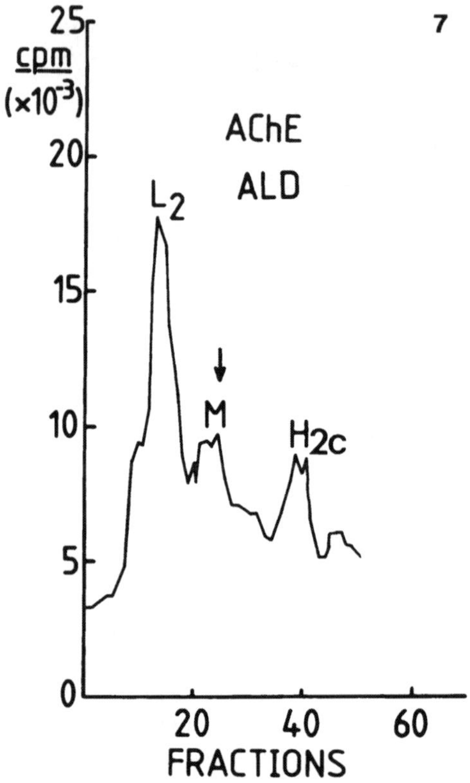

Fig. 7 Forms in the endplates of ALD (tonic) muscle of mature chicken. (Background not subtracted.)

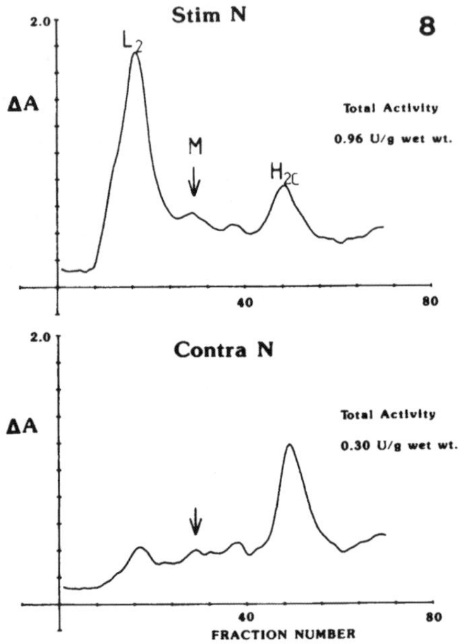

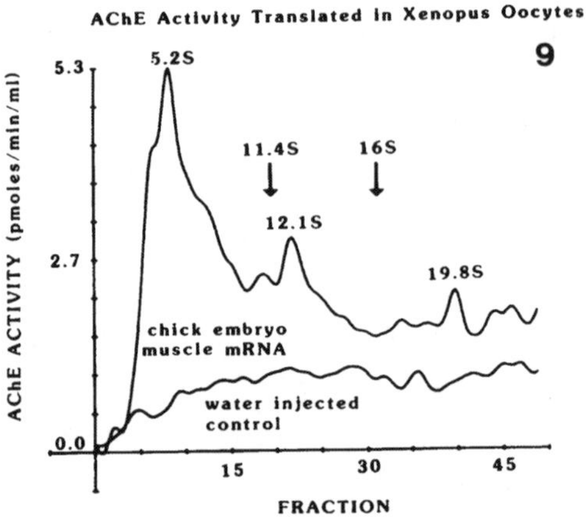

Fig. 8 The forms in the PLD muscle of an 8-week chicken, after chronic stimulation at 10Hz for 3 weeks. The contralateral PLD, not stimulated, is analysed in the lower panel (using 1.7 times the amount of muscle used above). (Controls not subtracted.)

Fig. 9 Sedimentation of the forms of AChE produced 24 hr after micro-injection into Xenopus oöcytes of poly(A)$^+$mRNA extracted from 19-day embryonic chick pectoral muscle. For the lower trace, a parallel set were injected with water. [^{3}H]ACh + 10^{-4}M iso-OMPA was used in the assays. (Backgrounds not subtracted.)

increase in chicken (23) and rabbit (24) muscles. We have found that it also increases in the guinea pig, e.g. by 2.6-fold in a fast-twitch muscle or 2.5-fold in the soleus (after 4 weeks). When analysed with due precautions, it was verified that H_{2C} AChE almost disappears from the denervated muscle, in the fast-twitch fibres of all species, including those where an increase in AChE occurs overall (Fig.4D). In the slow-twitch fibres in all of the species used here, H_{2C} AChE also declines as a fraction of the total, but a significant amount persists. As would be expected, the absolute amount of AChE present in the H forms does not decline so much in the species where an overall increase in this enzyme occurs in response to denervation. A test case here is the semimembranosus proprius (the "conoidal" or core sector) in the rabbit, which has 100% type I fibres, since Bacou et al. (25) found that after 4 weeks denervation thereof a large increase apparently occurred in the proportion of H_{2C} in the total AChE and in the absolute amount of H_{2C} in the muscle. We have found that in reality no increase occurs, if steps are taken to preserve the high original content of H_{2C} when the innervated muscle is analysed and if both the sciatic and the obturator innervations of the muscle are severed (Fig. 3). Partial denervation, by sciatic scission only (25), can lead to the decline in H_{2C} being retarded. Hence, still no exception is known to the finding that the maintenance of H AChE at the twitch endplate depends upon continuing neural input.

The finding that H_{2C} AChE persists, at a lower but significant level, throughout chronic denervation in the slow-twitch fibres may be related to the occurrence of that form outside the endplates in the innervated fibres of type I. It was confirmed by micro-dissection that in the rabbit semimembranosus proprius the same pattern of extra- synaptic forms of AChE is present as in the other type I muscles. Neural control can be expected to be lower at extra-synaptic locations.

Control of AChE by muscle electrical activity. Neural control of muscle is divisible into the direct effect of neurally-secreted factors and the indirect effect via the nerve-evoked muscle action potentials (26). We have tested for an effect of the latter component in the regulation of AChE forms, by employing prolonged repetitive stimulation, in situ in the living chicken, of a muscle through its nerve. Silver electrodes were implanted in contact with the PLD nerve, and impulses at 10 Hz were delivered to them from a totally-implanted, encapsulated printed-circuit stimulator. This neural stimulation was continuous for 4 weeks. The animals moved and fed freely. The stimulation produced a characteristic increase in the total AChE of the muscle (from 0.3U/g to 0.96U/g) and a marked increase in the content of L_2 AChE (Fig.8). The absolute amount of H_{2C} was also augmented. Under these conditions, changes are known to occur in the myosin isoforms with an increase in muscle total protein synthesis (27). The results found here, as exemplified in Fig.8, suggest that the synthesis of catalytic subunits of AChE is stimulated by increased electrical activity of the muscle fibre.

This result extends to the in vivo level the observations previously reported on cells in culture, that synaptic blockers such as d-tubocurarine retard the synthesis of muscle cell AChE and especially of H_{2C} (28) and that tetrodotoxin blockade of the action potentials in cultured myotubes acts in a similar direction on the H_{2C} AChE (29).

Production of mRNA for muscle AChE. To investigate the effects of neural factors on muscle AChE synthesis, measurement under various conditions of the mRNAs coding for this protein has begun. The *Xenopus* oocyte translation system is used, since conventional cell-free translations of mRNA do not permit the processing and assembly of membrane-bound or secreted proteins. Poly(A)$^+$mRNA was isolated from 19-day embryonic chick muscle, micro-injected into oocytes and shown to give rise to new AChE activity therein. This was analysed on sucrose density gradients (Fig. 9). A considerable proportion of L_2 AChE is produced, along with a small but reproducible amount of H_{2C} AChE. The production of this is not due to a stimulation of the expression of oocyte AChE genes, since the amphibian H_{2C} AChE has $s_{20,w}$ of 17.5 S, distinct from the 19.8 S form produced here, the latter being identical in size to the chicken H_{2C} AChE. The level of host cell AChE (which is first selectively inhibited by a mercurial inhibitor) is seen to be negligible, in the profile from the water-injected controls run in parallel (Fig.9, lower trace). Hence, we can conclude that mRNAs coding for the various polypeptides of the collagen-tailed AChE structure can be extracted, translated and their products processed and assembled in the oocyte. This system can, therefore, probe the factors which control the production of the various forms of AChE in different muscle types.

Discussion

We have seen that when the native forms of AChE are preserved (so far as present knowledge permits), some of the anomalies noted from earlier studies disappear. The situation had been complicated by the fact that in some muscles proteolytic effects on the AChE forms occur during their analysis much more readily than in others. The H_{2C} and H_{1C} forms together *are* the major species in most twitch muscles, both avian and mammalian.

In all twitch fibres studied, both in birds and in mammals, AChE at the endplate is entirely (in type II fibres) or mainly (type I fibres) in the H forms. This fraction is under neural control and decreases after denervation, without known exception. Substantial amounts of L and M forms occur extra-synaptically, but only in certain muscles. In addition, type I fibres contain significant amounts of H_{2C} AChE all along their length. It is known that these slow-twitch fibres also differ from the fast-twitch in that they contain a low but definite concentration of ACh receptor along their sarcolemma, have a lower resting potential and receive _in vivo_ a constant stream of nerve impulses (26,30). For comparison, chronic nerve stimulation in the same frequency range, applied to the fast-twitch muscle, appears to evoke the production of AChE polypeptides (Fig.8) and of other proteins and RNA (27,31). Hence, in a similar manner the extra-synaptic AChE may be merely a consequence of a natural higher general protein synthesis in certain muscles, but this remains to be explored. In the dystrophic chicken there is a genetically determined major de-regulation of muscle AChE levels, and both the H_{2C} and L_2 forms accumulate extra-synaptically, with excess H_{2C}, especially, becoming located around the endplates (22). On the view just suggested, wherever extra-synaptic AChE is found in muscles it is incidental to muscle activity and not of functional importance; nevertheless a true but unknown function for it has not been excluded. One such possibility is that slow muscles may require to be constantly ready to accept another nerve terminal, and the fibre type plasticity which is known (26,31,32) to exist may require a pool of ACh receptor and AChE throughout slow fibres. In any case, fibre type composition is seen to be a major factor in governing both the proportions and the locations of the AChE forms in a muscle.

It is also seen that dimeric (and some tetrameric) AChE is capable of replacing H_{2C} AChE in functional endplates, as in the ALD muscle. A fraction of the L_2 and M forms, in various sources, has been shown to be detergent-soluble and external, suggesting a location in the cell membrane (3,4,32-35). In the mature ALD muscle only one-third of the total AChE is water-soluble, despite the near-absence of H forms (2). At the ALD endplate the globular forms, therefore, may be on the post-synaptic membrane. It is not yet excluded that instead, they remain in the synaptic basal lamina as the residue of a degradation of the H_{2C} form, which is present there in the embryo.

Function of the forms at the endplate. AChE action is well known to play a vital role in the removal of ACh from the synaptic cleft of fast-twitch fibre endplates to terminate transmission there, aiding diffusion loss (36). This is shown by the lethal effect of anti-cholinesterases, and is measurable by the prolongation of the endplate current by such a drug - best examined by the effect of an irreversible organophosphate after the excess is washed away (37). In the article by L.G. Magazanik in this Volume, work from his laboratory is reviewed showing the extent and the physiological significance of that effect in fast-twitch fibre endplates, and the different behaviour, indicating less efficient removal of ACh, at the endplates of the slow-tonic muscles of the chick or frog (without AChE inhibition). There is a smaller effect in the same direction at the endplates of the slow-twitch, compared to the fast-twitch, mammalian muscles (38). Can we relate these adaptions to differing physiological needs to differences in the AChE?

No difference, qualitative or quantitative, has been detected between the various forms of muscle or electric organ AChE, tailed or globular, hydrophobic or hydrophilic, with respect to the catalytic properties (including the substrate inhibition behaviour) when examined in detergent-salt extracts (6,9,34,35). However, their respective effective activities could nevertheless be modified by different in situ locations. Four parameters are particularly important for analysis of the function of AChE at the endplate: (i) the forms present there, and their ratio; (ii) the location of AChE on the basal lamina or on, or in, one or more synaptic membranes; (iii) the local density (molecules per μm^2 of post-synaptic membrane area) of each form at those locations; (iv) whether that density is maintained constant, relative to the entire folded post-synaptic membrane, or is graded or discontinuous.

For factor (i), micro-dissection of single endplates with negligible amounts of surrounding regions of the fibre has provided accurate data, as illustrated here, for the various types of vertebrate endplate. For factor (ii), current information, as reviewed by others in this Volume (and see also (33)) strongly supports the view that H_{2C} AChE is anchored to the synaptic basal lamina. As noted above, in the cases where L_2 AChE is present at the endplate, it may be on the postsynaptic membrane where, it has been suggested (35), it may distribute itself uniformly. The questions involved under headings (iii) and (iv) have been addressed in previous studies, employing quantitative electron microscope autoradiography at endplates. Specific AChE was shown thus to be at the density of 3000 catalytic centres per μm^2 in several types of mouse fast-twitch muscle and to lie uniformly over the whole synaptic cleft, in both folded and unfolded post-synaptic zones (39,40). This latter feature is consistent with some attachment to the synaptic basal lamina.

In contrast, a parallel method has shown that the ACh

receptors are not distributed uniformly through the cleft. They are located almost exclusively on the crests of the synaptic folds, being virtually absent in the lower part of the folds; the local density on the crest is 22,000 α-bungarotoxin-binding sites per μm^2 (39, 41-43). It is now fully established that there are 2 α-subunits and hence 2 α-bungarotoxin-binding sites per muscle ACh receptor molecule (44). Therefore, there are about 11,000 receptor molecules per μm^2 (a density which agrees with recent freeze- fracture particle counts). For fast-twitch fibre endplates, all the AChE is H_{2C} and this is assumed to have 12 catalytic centres per molecule, so there are ~250 AChE molecules per μm^2, or only one for every 88 ACh binding sites on the receptors, as we have pointed out previously (45). Hence a possible reason for the specialisation of the H_{2C} form of AChE is that this high ratio reduces the interception by cleft AChE of the released ACh to a manageable proportion. We suggest that this ratio of receptor sites to AChE may have developed to be optimal, so as to provide sufficient total AChE at the synapse for a high margin of safety and rapid post-activation hydrolysis, without too high a local AChE density to impede receptor activation by the ACh. However, whether an advantage is actually gained from increase in this ratio is difficult to determine until all the parameters of the time-course of receptor activation (36) are fully established. Neumann and Bernhardt (46) have deduced a model for this in which sequential processing of ACh by the receptor and then AChE occurs, with a micro-separation of these, in agreement with the above suggestion of the "ratio advantage", but Rosenberry (47) has fitted similar endplate current data to a quite different, single-phase model, and the question remains open. If the true kinetics permit the ratio advantage to operate, then the physiological effects at the slow endplates can be readily explained. The dimers, distributed uniformly on the membrane, would not possess the ratio advantage of the dodecamers in the cleft, so the tonic endplates would deal with ACh less efficiently. The type I fibre endplate has a mixture of H_{2C} and L_2, and so is intermediate in its effectivness. The alternative explanation is based on factor (iii) above: if the absolute density of AChE is much lower at the slow endplates than at those on fast fibres, then their low efficiencies could be equally well explained. In this interpretation, the functional reason for anchoring the H_{2C} structure at the fast endplates is to maintain a higher overall concentration of AChE in the cleft while minimising the number of attachment sites which must be provided for it. At the post-synaptic crests, in the fast-twitch endplate the membrane is already packed with the receptors and associated proteins, and it could be that secretion and extra-cellular attachment of very large AChE units is the most economic way of exposing the enzyme to the cleft. If receptor density is much lower at slow-tonic endplates, then an anchoring of the AChE in the membrane, also at a lower density, could account for the hydrophobic smaller forms there.

Present knowledge is insufficient to decide between these two models. Determination of the actual density of each form of AChE at the endplate, and of the receptors and their distribution there, is in progress at various slow-fibre endplates, to provide all of the parameters listed above. These are needed before a definitive account of AChE synaptic function can be constructed.

Acknowledgements. This work was supported by the Muscular Dystrophy Group of Great Britain and by the S.E.R.C. (U.K.).

References

1. Bon, S., Rieger, F., Massoulié, J.: Eur. J. Biochem. 35, 372-379 (1973).

2. Lyles, J.M., Silman, I., Di Giamberardino, L., Couraud J.Y., Barnard, E.A.: J. Neurochem. 38, 1007-1021 (1982).

3. Lee, S.L., Camp, S.J., Taylor, P.: J. Biol. Chem. 257, 12302-12309 (1982).

4. Massoulié, J., Bon, S.: Ann. Rev. Neursci. 5, 57-106 (1982).

5. Bon, S., Vigny, M., Massoulié, J.: Proc. Natl. Acad. Sci. USA 76, 2546-2550 (1979).

6. Vigny, M., Koenig, J., Rieger, F.: J. Neurochem. 27, 1347-1353 (1976).

7. Fernandez, H.L., Duell, M.J., Festoff, B.W.: J. Neurobiol. 10, 441-445.

8. Senni, M., Biagoni, S., Marini, P., Scarsella, G.: Neurochem. Res. 6, 1291-1298 (1981).

9. Groswald, D.E., Dettbarn, W.D.: Neurochem. Res. 8, 983-995 (1983).

10. Carson, S., Bon, S., Vigny, M., Massoulié, J., Fardeau, M.: FEBS Lett. 97, 348-352 (1979).

11. Skau, K.A., Brimijoin, S.: J. Neurochem. 35, 1151-1154.

12. Younkin, S.G., Rosenstein, C., Collins, P.L., Rosenberry, T.L.: J. Biol. Chem. 257, 13630-13637 (1982).

13. Lyles, J.A., Silman, I., Barnard, E.A.: J. Neurochem. 33, 727-738 (1979).

14. Barnard, E.A., Lyles, J.M., Pizzey, J.A.: J. Physiol. 331, 333-334 (1982).

15. Lyles, J.M., Barnard, E.A.: FEBS Lett, 109, 9-12 (1980).

16. Turk, V., Ritonja, A., Gubenšek, F.: Toxicon 17 (Suppl.1), 195 (1979).

17. Silman, I., Lyles, J.M., Barnard, E.A.: FEBS Lett. 94, 160-170 (1978).

18. Brooke, M.H., Kaiser, K.K.: Archs. Neurol. 23, 369-379 (1970).

19. Peter, J.B., Barnard, R.J., Edgerton, V.R., Gillespie, C.A., Stempel, K.E.: Biochemistry 11, 2627-2633 (1972).

20. Lutz, H., Weber, H., Jenny, E: Nature 281, 142-144 (1979).

21. Pierbon-Bormioli, S., Satore, S., Dalla Libera, L., Vitadello, M., Schiaffino, S.: J. Histochem. Cytochem. 29, 1179-1188 (1981).

22. Jedrzejczyk, J., Silman, I., Lyles, J.M., Barnard, E.A.: Biosci. Rep. 1, 45-51 (1981).

23. Wilson, B.W., Kaplan, M.A., Merhoff, W.C., Mori, S.S.: J. Exp. Zool. 174, 39-54 (1970).

24. Tennyson, V.M., Kremzner, L.T., Brzin, M.: J. Neuropath. Exp. Neurol. 36, 245-275 (1977).

25. Bacou, F., Vigneron, P., Massoulié, J.: Nature 296, 661-664 (1982).

26. Vrbová, G., Gordon, T., Jones, R.: Nerve-Muscle Interactions, Chapman and Hall, London 1979.

27. Heilig, A., Pette, D: FEBS Lett. 151, 211-214 (1983).

28. Rubin, L. L., Schuetze, S.M., Weill, C.L., Fischbach, G.D.: Nature 283, 264-267 (1980).

29. Rieger, F., Koenig, J., Vigny, M.: Develop. Biol. 76, 358-365 (1980).

30. McArdle, J.J., Albuquerque, E.X.: J. Gen. Physiol. 61, 1-23 (1973).

31. Salmons, S., Henriksson, J.: Muscle Nerve 4, 94-105 (1981).

32. Pette, D. (ed): Plasticity of Muscle, Walter de Gruyter, Berlin, New York 1980.

33. Inestrosa, N.C., Silberstein, L., Hall, Z.W.: Cell 29, 71-79 (1982).

34. Bon, S. Vigny, M. Massoulié, J.: Proc. Natl. Acad. Sci. USA 77, 4464-4468 (1979).

35. Viratelle, O.M., Bernhard, S.A.: Biochemistry 19, 4999-5007 (1980).

36. Kordaš, M.: J. Physiol. 270, 133-150 (1977).

37. Kuba, K., Albuquerque, E.X., Daly, J., Barnard, E.A.: J. Pharm. Exp. Therap. 189, 499-512 (1974).

38. Magazanik, L.G., Fedorov, V.V., Snetkov, V.A.: Prog. Brain Res. 44, 225-240 (1979).

39. Porter, C.W., Barnard, E.A.: J. Membrane Biol 20, 31-49 (1975).

40. Salpeter, M.M., Rogers, A.W., Kasprzak, H., McHenry, F.A.: J. Cell Biol. 78, 274-285 (1978).

41. Albuquerque, E.X., Barnard, E.A., Porter, C.W., Warnick, J.: Proc. Natl. Acad. Sci. USA 71, 2818-2822 (1974).

42. Fertuck, J.C., Salpeter, M.M.: J. Cell Biol. 69, 144-158 (1976).

43. Matthews-Bellinger, J., Salpeter, M.M.: J. Physiol. 279, 197-213 (1978).

44. Barnard, E.A., Dolly, J.O.: Trends Neurosci. 5, 325-327 (1982).

45. Barnard, E.A., Lamprecht, J., Lo, M., Nockles, E., Sumikawa, K., Cavanagh, J., Dolly, J.O., in: Synaptic Constituents in Health and Disease (eds. M. Brzin, D. Sket, H. Bachelard), pp. 224-240, Pergamon Press, Oxford 1980.

46. Neumann, E., Bernhardt, J.: J. Physiol. (Paris) 77, 1061-1072 (1981).

47. Rosenberry, T.L.: Biophys. J. 26, 263-289 (1979).

THE POLYMORPHISM OF CHOLINESTERASES:
Classification of molecular forms; Interactions and solubilization characteristics; Metabolic relationships and regulations.

Jean Massoulié*, Suzanne Bon*, Monique Lazar**, Jacques Grassi***, David Marsh*, Khaled Meflah****, Jean Pierre Toutant*, François Vallette*, and Marc Vigny*.

*Laboratoire de Neurobiologie, Ecole Normale Supérieure, 46 rue d'Ulm 75005 Paris, France.
**Laboratoire de Biochimie Cellulaire, Collège de France, 11 place Marcelin Berthelot, 75005 Paris, France.
***Laboratoire d'Etudes Radioimmunologiques, Centre d'Etudes Nucléaires de Saclay, 91191 Gif sur Yvette, Cedex, France.
****Laboratoire de Biochimie Médicale, Faculté de Médecine, 1, rue Gaston Veil, 44000 Nantes, France.

INTRODUCTION

In Vertebrate tissues, cholinesterases display an extensive polymorphism (for a review, see Massoulié and Bon, 1982) : they occur in a number of molecular forms which possess distinct structural characteristics and interactions, but share essentially identical catalytic properties.

The molecular forms of acetylcholinesterase have been best characterized in the case of the enzyme from electric organs of Electrophorus (Bon et al., 1976, Rosenberry and Richardson 1977, Anglister and Silman, 1978). There are three globular forms and three asymmetric forms : the globular forms are the monomers dimers and tetramers of the catalytic subunits (respectively G1, G2 and G4), and the asymmetric forms consist of one two or three tetramers attached to the strands of a triple helical collagen-like tail (respectively A4, A8 and A12). It is remarkable that both acetylcholinesterase (E.C. 3.1.1.7.) and pseudocholinesterase (E.C. 3.1.1.8.) of all Vertebrate species present similar sets of molecular forms. The maintenance of this very complex polymorphism for both acetylcholinesterase and pseudocholinesterase throughout the evolution of Vertebrates suggests that it fulfils an important physiological role.

Cholinesterases, © Walter de Gruyter & Co., Berlin - New York, 1984

It is very likely that its function is to allow the precise positioning of these enzymes at various sites : for example, collagen-tailed forms may be anchored in extracellular structures such as the basal lamina in neuromuscular synaptic clefts, and globular forms which may be inserted in cellular plasma membranes.

Every tissue expresses a more or less complete set of molecular forms, in proportions which depend upon the developmental stage and physiological conditions. It is therefore important to understand as completely as possible the structural basis of this polymorphism, the manner in which it is generated, the mechanisms of biogenesis and assembly of the different forms, and the physiological factors which condition their expression. In the present chapter, we discuss several problems raised by this polymorphism in different experimental systems.

CLASSIFICATION OF CHOLINESTERASE FORMS : COLLAGEN-TAILED AND GLOBULAR FORMS ; HOMOLOGIES OF QUATERNARY STRUCTURES AND MOLECULAR DIVERSITY

We propose to classify cholinesterase molecular forms according to their general quaternary structure, and to their ionic or hydrophobic interactions, by using the following criteria :

1) The class of asymmetric forms is unambiguously characterized by a large Stokes radius ($>$12 nm), and by a specific sensitivity to collagenase digestion (Bon et al., 1979). Asymmetric forms exhibit ionic interactions, and may be quantitatively solubilized only in high salt buffers. They have not been shown to interact with non-denaturing detergents such as Triton X100. Considering their interaction properties, asymmetric forms appear to be a rather homogeneous class of molecules. Differences observed in the solubilization of these forms which may or may not require chelating agents, as reported by Ramirez and coll. in this volume, are thought to reflect their association with small molecules, rather than intrinsic differences in the enzymes themselves.

2) The class of globular forms is defined by the absence of a collagen-like tail. These forms may either interact with non-denaturing

detergents and are thus called amphipathic or amphiphilic (cf. articles by Rosenberry and by Brodbeck, this volume), or they may be detergent-insensitive. Amphipathic globular forms may be aggregated or soluble in the absence of detergent. The sedimentation coefficient of the soluble form is decreased, and their Stokes radius increased in the presence of detergent. In both cases, interactions with non-denaturing detergents may also be demonstrated by charge shift electrophoresis, i.e. modifications of migration rates in the presence of negatively charged or positively charged detergents. Amphipathic molecules may be converted by limited proteolytic digestion (pronase, proteinase K, papain) into detergent-insensitive forms (Bon & Massoulié, 1980, Grassi et al., 1981, articles by Brodbeck and by Rosenberry in this volume).

Within each class, molecules which differ in their polymerization state may be distinguished by their hydrodynamic parameters. They are frequently designated by their sedimentation coefficients. However, we find it useful to extend the terminology based on studies of Electrophorus acetylcholinesterase to the enzymes from other tissues, in order to express homologies between molecules which appear to represent similar quaternary associations. There are in fact marked variations between homologous forms of acetylcholinesterase and pseudocholinesterase in a given organism, and between corresponding enzyme forms in different species : for example, A12 forms sediment at 16-17 S in mammals, 17.4 S in Torpedo, 18.5 S in Electrophorus and 20 S in chicken. It is remarkable that all forms of chicken acetylcholinesterase have larger sedimentation coefficients than the homologous mammalian forms. The polypeptides corresponding to the catalytic subunits are approximately 30 % heavier (Rotundo, this volume). We found, however, that after cleavage by trypsin, which changes neither their catalytic properties nor their ionic or hydrophobic interactions, the chicken forms are converted into molecules which resemble the mammalian forms in their hydrodynamic parameters (Allemand et al., 1981). Acetylcholinesterase from quail is similar, although slightly heavier than chicken acetylcholinesterase (unpublished results).

Additional variations in the sedimentation coefficient depend upon experimental conditions, notably upon the presence of detergent in the case of amphipathic molecules : for example the G1 form from bovine brain sediments at 3.1 S in the presence of Triton X100 and either aggregates or sediments at 4.5 S in the absence of detergent. Thus the S values of the different forms fall in the following ranges : G1 (3-5 S), G2 (5-7 S), G4 (9-12 S), A4 (8-9 S), A8 (13-15 S), A12 (16-20 S).

Quite clearly, the proposed terminology only represents a superficial classification of quaternary structures. Allowance must be made for considerable variations between different types of molecules, which may include the following aspects :

1) Whereas the index represents the number of catalytic subunits in the An and Gn forms of Electrophorus, this is not necessarily the case in other species. Taylor and coll. have shown that in the collagen-tailed forms of Torpedo, catalytic subunits may be partially replaced by another type of globular, non catalytic subunit (Lee et al., 1982 a, Lee and Taylor, 1982).

2) Non-catalytic elements may be associated with the catalytic polymers. For example, catalytic tetramers (G4) obtained by proteolysis of the A forms of Electrophorus may or may not contain fragments of the tail peptides, covalently attached by disulfide bonds (Rosenberry et al., 1980).

3) In the case of Torpedo, a fraction of amphipathic dimers (G2) is found to be soluble in non covalent association with non catalytic proteins. These associations disappear in the presence of Triton X100, and the catalytic dimers form detergent complexes which present the same hydrodynamic characteristics as detergent soluble dimers.

4) The catalytic subunits themselves may differ in various ways, in addition to the large differences which exist between species, e.g. chicken or quail vs mammalian acetylcholinesterases.

- Different primary polypeptide sequences may exist, as suggested for example by the findings of Taylor and coll., in the case of Torpedo A and G forms (Lee et al., 1982 b, Taylor, this volume).

- Proteolytic cleavage may also occur either physiologically or experimentally : for example amphipathic forms may be converted into detergent-insensitive molecules (Bon & Massoulié, 1980, Grassi et al., 1981, Rosenberry, this volume).

- Finally, post-translational modifications such as glycosylation introduce additional variations among the catalytic subunits (Meflah, Bernard and Massoulié, in preparation).

Considering that all these possible variations in the cholinesterase molecules are not yet fully understood, the classification into asymmetric, amphipathic globular, and detergent-insensitive globular forms, as operationally defined above, and the nomenclature which expresses homologies between forms of similar quaternary structures, appear useful although incomplete.

HETEROGENEITY OF GLOBULAR FORMS; AMPHIPATHIC CHARACTER AND SOLUBILITY

A) Torpedo

Torpedo tissues offer an excellent illustration of the possible diversity of cholinesterase forms.

Acetylcholinesterase and pseudocholinesterase . A first aspect is the presence of two types of cholinesterases. Electric organs, muscles and nervous tissues contain essentially true acetylcholinesterase, which hydrolyzes acetylcholine much more rapidly than butyrylcholine, and is inhibited by 1 μM BW284C51. Heart extracts contain a pseudocholinesterase which hydrolyzes butyrylcholine and is insensitive to BW284C51.

Torpedo plasma contains the two activities in approximately equal proportions . Acetylcholinesterase corresponds to a G4 form, which does not interact with Triton X100. In this respect this naturally occurring molecule resembles the lytic forms obtained by proteolysis from native collagen-tailed or hydrophobic molecules. In contrast, plasma pseudocholinesterase is a clearly amphipathic enzyme: its sedimentation rate is shifted from 7.4 S to 6 S in the presence of Triton X100. Its electrophoretic mobility in the presence of the neutral detergent Triton X100 is increased upon addition of the anionic detergent deoxycholate, and decreased upon addition of the cationic detergent cetyltrimethylammonium. Similar observations demonstrate the amphipathic character of globular forms of pseudocholinesterase in heart extracts and of acetylcholinesterase in other tissues.

Solubility properties According to their solubility properties, the amphipathic molecular forms of acetylcholinesterase may be divided into a buffer-soluble fraction (solubilized at low ionic strength in the absence of detergent) and a detergent-soluble fraction (solubilized at low ionic strength in the presence of the non-denaturing detergent Triton X100). The two fractions occur in varying proportions in different tissues: for example; the buffer-soluble fraction represents 50% of acetylcholinesterase from skeletal muscle but only 15 % of the enzyme from spinal cord. When analyzed in the absence of detergent, the detergent-soluble molecules from various tissues form polydisperse aggregates of variable size. The buffer-soluble molecules show only reversible shifts in sedimentation, depending upon the presence or absence of detergent. However, addition of an excess of organophosphate-inactivated detergent extract from electric organs induces the aggregation of these molecules (Bon & Massoulié, 1980, Toutant & Bon, in preparation). Thus, the formation of aggregates by amphipathic cholinesterase molecules depends at least in part on the presence of hydrophobic proteins.

Differences in electrophoretic migration Although the G2 molecular forms of the various tissue extracts are very similar in their hydrodynamic properties and present apparently equivalent amphipathic properties, electrophoresis in non denaturing conditions reveals large differences in their mobility. This is, for example, the case for the G2 forms from electric organs, muscle and spinal cord. Electrophoresis even reveals an heterogeneity within the muscle G2 form, which is resolved into two distinct bands. These electrophoretic differences are maintained after pronase digestion, which converts the amphipathic molecules into detergent-insensitive forms. They are therefore not related to the hydrophobic interaction of these molecules, but probably reflect differences in the charges of the polypeptides themselves or in their glycosylation.

Differences in catalytic polypeptides We have also studied the acetylcholinesterase forms from electric organs by electrophoresis in the presence of sodium dodecylsulfate, with and without reduction. It is possible to differentiate several types of catalytic subunits, which may be revealed by protein staining, or by autoradiography after radioactive labeling with diisopropyl- fluorophosphate. The buffer-soluble fraction contains a minor band which, in contrast to all others, appears as a monomer even in non reducing conditions, and is heavier than disulfide-linked subunits. This subunit has an apparent molecular weight of 76 Kilodaltons in 7.5 % polyacrylamide gels, and probably corresponds to the low salt soluble enzyme described by Witzemann and Boustead (1983). The corresponding native enzyme may be dimeric, although not disulfide-bridged. In our hands this is only a minor component : the buffer-soluble fraction contains mainly disulfide-linked dimers. The reduced acetylcholinesterase subunits from the different fractions present the following order of apparent molecular weights: subunits from collagen-tailed A forms (72 K), subunits from detergent-soluble G2 dimers (69 K), subunits from buffer-soluble G2 dimers (68 K), and lytic subunits obtained after pronase digestion of G2 dimers (67 K) (Toutant and Bon, in preparation). This order is in good agreement with the findings of other authors (Lee et al., 1982 b, Witzemann and Boustead, 1983). It does not necessarily correspond to real molecular weight differences, since the relative electrophoretic mobilities change with the polyacrylamide concentration (Lee et al., 1982 b).

Differences in electrophoretic migration may be partially due to differences in glycosylation of the subunits. For example, we found that in the presence of Triton X100, although they appear hydrodynamically undistinguishable, buffer-soluble and detergent-soluble G2 dimers may be differentiated by their interactions with lectins : only buffer-soluble dimers are retained on wheat germ agglutinin immobilized columns and the reverse is observed with Lens culinaris agglutinin columns.

B) Globular forms of mammalian acetylcholinesterase

Secreted amphipathic enzyme In a former study of acetylcholinesterase forms in cultures of murine neural cells (T28 cell line) we characterized the enzyme recovered in the culture medium as detergent-insensitive G1 and G4 forms, while the corresponding cellular forms were amphipathic (Lazar and Vigny, 1980). In more recent experiments, with the same cell line, we found that the secreted G form was clearly amphipathic (shifting from 4.6 S in the absence of detergent to 3.8 S in the presence of Triton X100) and that secreted G4 possessed both amphipathic and detergent-insensitive components (Lazar et al, in press). This difference may be due to uncontrolled proteolysis in the former experiments, or to subtle changes in culture conditions, e.g. in the composition of the medium. In any case, these observations show that amphipathic soluble cholinesterase forms may be released by living cells into the medium. This is consistent with the occurrence, *in vivo* , of both types of molecules in Torpedo plasma.

Buffer-soluble and detergent-soluble fractions: aggregation properties
We studied the amphipathic properties of the globular forms of acetylcholinesterase from bovine tissues, principally the caudate nucleus (Grassi et al., 1982). Sequential extractions without, and with Triton X100 produced a buffer-soluble fraction containing amphipathic G1 and both amphipathic and detergent-insensitive G4, and a detergent-soluble fraction containing amphipathic forms, mainly G4, which aggregate in the absence of detergent. However, partially purified detergent-soluble G4 no longer aggregates but only shifts in sedimentation, from 9.7 S in the presence of Triton X100, to 11.5 S in the absence of detergent, like the corresponding buffer-soluble amphipathic G4. It should be noted that this non aggregating amphipathic

form was not pure, and possibly formed soluble associations with small hydrophobic proteins or with small amounts of detergent. Self-aggregation was probably prevented by the low concentration of the tissue extracts. The partially purified G4 fraction aggregated when mixed with an organophosphate-inactivated detergent extract indicating, as in the case of Torpedo, that aggregation depends in part upon interaction with hydrophobic proteins.

Molecular properties and immunological relationships of buffer-soluble and detergent-soluble enzymes The amphipathic G1 and G4 molecular forms recovered in the buffer-soluble and detergent-soluble fractions presented identical hydrodynamic parameters in the presence of Triton X100, and yielded indistinguishable detergent-insensitive lytic forms after pronase digestion. The only intrinsic difference between the two fractions therefore appeared to be the presence of a detergent-insensitive soluble G4 form in the buffer-soluble extract.

However, we attempted to detect immunological differences between buffer-soluble and detergent-soluble enzymes, as reported by other groups (Zanetta et al., 1981 Sorensen et al., 1982). We found that an antiserum prepared against purified rat amphipathic G4 presented the same reactivity with both fractions from rat brain : it showed the same partial inhibition of activity and the same precipitation titer. Moreover, the two fractions were equivalent in competition experiments with radiolabeled G4 (Marsh et al., in preparation). We also found that a monoclonal antibody (C5) obtained by Fambrough and coll (1982) against human erythocyte acetylcholinesterase recognized G4 and G1 forms in both buffer-soluble and detergent-soluble extracts.

Interconversion of buffer-soluble and detergent-soluble molecules In the case of bovine caudate nucleus, differential solubilization in the absence or presence of detergent cannot be simply related to subcellular compartments. In agreement with previous observations of Hollunger and Niklasson (1973) and Adamson and coll., (1975, 1977), we found that repeated extractions considerably increased the solubilization of activity in the absence of detergent : the yield of a second extraction may in fact be higher than that of the first, indicating that the process does not simply exhaust a defined cellular pool. Therefore, in this tissue, the buffer-soluble and detergent-soluble fractions are partially interconvertible, depending upon solubilization procedures.

The same experiments showed that the ratio of G1 to G4 forms obtained was considerably greater when the tissue was repeatedly extracted in the absence, and finally in the presence of detergent, than for a simple quantitative extraction in the presence of detergent. This observation demonstrates that artefacts may also modify the composition of molecular forms, and questions the physiological significance of these forms. However we found that while the proportion of molecular forms varied when solubilization was incomplete, i.e. in the absence of detergent or with relatively inefficient detergents (such as deoxycholate) it was constant when a quantitative solubilization was obtained in the presence of detergent such as cholate or Triton X100.

A definitive proof that molecular forms solubilized in the presence of Triton X100 represent distinct cellular entities is given for example by the observed correspondance, in T28 cells, of G1 with endocellular activity and G4 with ectoactivity, as indicated below (Lazar and Vigny, 1980).

Differences in glycosylation Different cellular compartments of acetylcholinesterase may correspond to differences in glycosylation, as already mentioned in the case of *Torpedo* . For example, we found that G1 and G4 forms in bovine muscle extracts do not bind lectins in the same manner : in particular G1 does not interact with wheat germ agglutinin while G4 does, suggesting that only the polymeric forms possess complex polysaccharides (Meflah et al, in preparation).

The specificity of lectin binding also revealed differences between isologous, membrane-bound forms, obtained from different tissues or cell types. This is for example the case for the G2 forms associated with the plasma membranes of bovine erythrocytes and lymphocytes. The two enzymes appear to be immunologically equivalent in their reaction with an anti-serum, raised against rat G4 acetylcholinesterase. However the lymphocyte enzyme, but not the erythocyte enzyme, interacts with lectins such as concanavalin A, Lens Culinaris agglutinin or wheat germ agglutinin. In addition the lymphocyte enzyme has a higher Km value for acetylthiocholine, and requires a higher level of Triton X100 for its solubilization. Such differences are possibly related to glycosylation (Meflah et al., in preparation).

IONIC INTERACTIONS OF THE COLLAGEN-TAILED FORMS. RELATIONSHIP BETWEEN THE COLLAGEN-LIKE TAIL AND EXTRACELLULAR MATRIX COMPONENTS

The collagen-tailed forms are capable of ionic interactions that cause them to aggregate, in physiological conditions, in the presence of polyanionic compounds such as glycosaminoglycans (Bon et al., 1978). Their quantitative solubilization therefore usually requires a high ionic strength buffer. In addition, divalent ions such as Ca^{++} are thought to play a role in the interactions of some of the A forms, which can only be solubilized in the presence of chelating agents, as shown by Ramirez and coll. (this volume, Gómez-Barriocanal et al.,1981).

In Torpedo, the salt concentration which is required to solubilize collagen-tailed acetylcholinesterase from electric organs increases with the maturation of the embryos (Bon,1982, Witzemann and Boustead, 1982). This of course indicates that the interactions which anchor these forms in situ vary with the nature of other components and possibly with the organization of the extracellular matrix. In contrast, A12 acetylcholinesterase is solubilized at a constant lower salt concentration from the electric lobes of the central nervous system, which command the electrical discharge. In this tissue, acetylcholinesterase appears to be present mostly in the motoneuron cell bodies (Tsuji, 1977).

Ionic interactions of the asymmetric forms depend on the presence of the collagen-like tail since they are abolished after collagenase treatment (Bon and Massoulié, 1978). In collaboration with R. Timpl, we have examined whether the matrix proteins laminin and fibronectin, which are known to bind collagens, interact with collagen-tailed acetylcholinesterase from Electrophorus electric organs or bovine superior cervical ganglion (Grassi et al., 1983). The results have been entirely negative. We have also examined if the collagen-like tails bear some immunological relationship to collagens of various classes (collagens I, III, IV, and V of mammalian origin), using specific antisera. We have found no evidence for any specific recognition. We therefore consider that the collagen-like tail subunits not only differ in their mass from the known types of collagens (Anglister and Silman, 1978, Rosenberry et al., 1980) but probably derive from totally independent structural genes. It would be interesting to know whether they are identical in acetylcholinesterase and pseudocholinesterase A forms and whether, in addition to possible precursors of collagen-tailed cholinesterases, they occur as independent molecules, or in association with other enzymes or structural proteins.

SUBCELLULAR LOCALIZATION OF THE MOLECULAR FORMS

We have used cell cultures to analyze the distribution of acetylcholinesterase in the external (ectoactivity) and intracellular (endoactivity) compartments, according to the accessibility of the active sites to non permeating substrates (acetylthiocholine), and inhibitors (echothiopate). The T28 murine neuron-like cell line synthesizes only globular forms, essentially G1 and G4. In these cells G1 is intracellular while G4 essentially corresponds to the ectoactivity. This is true in exponential phase cultures, which contain about equal proportions of G1 and G4, as well as in stationary phase cultures, which are morphologically differentiated, are characterized by the extension of neurites, and which possess a higher level of acetylcholinesterase activity and express a higher proportion of G4 (Lazar and Vigny, 1980 and unpublished results).

Hall, Inestrosa and coll. have studied a murine muscle cell line (C2) which expresses the A12 form. They have shown that in these cells A12 corresponds to extracellular patches of activity. It is entirely accessible to collagenase (Inestrosa et al., 1982), and probably associated with basal lamina components, which are also synthesized by these cells (Silberstein et al., 1982).This form was also found to be entirely extracellular in pheochronocytoma PC12 cells (Inestrosa et al., 1981).

Primary cultures of muscle cells from 11 days chick embryos express collagen-tailed as well as globular forms of acetylcholinesterase. In these cells the main molecular forms in the myotubes are G2, G4 and A12. We found that in these cells all forms are partially endocellular and partially ectocellular in different proportions (Vallette et al., in preparation). A12 and G4 are predominantly external while G2 is mostly internal. Similar results were obtained with quail muscle cultures by Rotundo and Emmerling (private comm.), and with rat myotubes by Brockman et al., (1982). In vivo , all acetylcholinesterase forms were also found to be partially ecto and partially endo cellular (G1 being mostly internal, G4 ands A12 mostly external), both in rat diaphram (Younkin et al. 1982) and in rat gracilis muscle (Fernandez and Inestrosa, private comm.).

RELATIONSHIPS BETWEEN MOLECULAR FORMS: MULTIPLICITY OF METABOLIC POOLS

We have applied the method of heavy isotope labeling (Devreotes et al., 1977) to an analysis of acetylcholinesterase metabolism in steady state, differentiated cultures of the murine neural T28 cell line (Lazar, Salmeron, Vigny and Massoulié, in press). This method is ideally suited for studying minor proteins which may be identified by their specific activity. In this case we were able to satisfactorily resolve heavy and light components of each of the major G1 and G4 forms by sedimentation in sucrose gradients. We followed in this manner the replacement of pre-existing light molecules by newly synthesized heavy enzyme, after a shift from light to heavy medium. The observed kinetics led us to the following conclusions :

1) an inactive precursor with a short half life is synthesized before the appearance of active G1 acetylcholinesterase.

2) G1 is renewed much faster than G4 (50 % replacement after about 4 and 40 hours, respectively).

3) most of the cellular G1 form is not converted into G4 or secreted, but degraded.

4) each form consists of several metabolically distinct pools.

5) G4 does not derive from the bulk of cellular G1, but from a rapidly turning over subcompartment of G1 or inactive precursor.

6)a comparison of the kinetics of secretion with the evolution of the cellular enzyme forms suggests that a fraction of the enzyme which appears in the medium as secreted G4 derives from a pool of cellular G1, so that there may be a partial coupling between polymerization and secretion.

7) newly synthesized heavy molecules appear in the medium after a delay of about 3 hours, suggesting that this represents the duration of transport processes within the cell to the external medium.

Our analysis has been based on kinetic models in which a small number of cellular compartments are being fed and emptied according to characteristic rate constants. This type of analysis is not logically opposed to models in which transport is considered to occur along linear assembly lines, but it cannot be readily translated in terms of time intervals. We found that our data could be adequately simulated by models which incorporate 3 pools of G1 either derived in parallel from an inactive precursor, or sequentially derived from each other, and with 2 pools of G4. More complex models, with for example a larger number of enzyme pools, and possibly distinct inactive precursors for several of them, e.g. G1 and G4, cannot of course be excluded.

Our results present several features in common with the findings of Rotundo and Fambrough (1980, a, b) who found that in cultures of chick muscle cells the intracellular enzyme is renewed much faster than the membrane-bound enzyme, and that newly formed molecules reach the cell surface after about 3 hours. We find further similarities with the recent work of Rotundo, who studied the metabolism of acetylcholinesterase by radioactive labeling (private comm., cf. this volume). In the case of primary chick muscle cultures Rotundo demonstrated the existence of inactive polypeptides which were rapidly degraded. Active enzyme destined to be localized at the external membrane and/or secreted, appeared to be stable. In chick muscle as well as in T28 cells, therefore, rapid degradation is important (at least 70 % of the synthesized enzyme in T28 cells) and appears to operate on both active and inactive components. The synthesized polypeptides thus do not follow a linear process of successive maturation and polymerization steps, but face one or several branching points leading to different fates.

The multiplicity of metabolic pools of acetylcholinesterase, at least three for the intracellular G1 form in T28 cells probably corresponds to a subcellular compartmentalization of the enzyme and/or to the fine structural differences of the enzymes, e.g. in their glycosylation. In any case, it is clear that the different forms are not homogeneous entities and cannot be considered to derive in a simple manner from one another. It is therefore not surprising that their proportions may vary widely in vivo .

PHYSIOLOGICAL EXPRESSION OF ACETYLCHOLINESTERASE MOLECULAR FORMS

The well established role of cholinesterases in the inactivation of the neurotransmitter acetylcholine must be fulfilled by extracellularly accessible enzymes, i.e. by amphipathic molecules inserted in pre or post-synaptic membranes, by collagen-tailed molecules associated with matrix components (e.g. in the basal lamina at neuromuscular junctions), or possibly by soluble secreted molecules. It would be tempting to associate each type of molecule with specific aspects of this function. One way to attempt such an interpretation is of course to examine possible correlations between the expression of particular enzyme forms, and physiological characteristics of synapses. It is however difficult at the moment to understand why collagen-tailed forms constitute a large proportion of acetylcholinesterase in the central nervous system of fishes, amphibians and reptiles, but only a very minor fraction in the brains of birds and mammals.

Early results suggested that in skeletal muscles innervation regulates the biosynthesis of the collagen-tailed forms. It was very attractive therefore to consider these characteristic molecules as biochemical markers of neuro-muscular interactions ("endplate forms"). This hypothesis was based on the following evidence :

1) While globular forms are present very early during embryonic development in rat and chicken, the appearance of collagen-tailed forms in muscles corresponds to the formation of neuro-muscular contacts.

2) The A forms are not expressed in cultures of muscle cells obtained from rat or chick embryo limbs before innervation, but their biosynthesis can be triggered by coculture with motoneurons (Koenig and Vigny, 1978; Rubin et al.,1980).

3) In adult rat, the A forms are localized preferentially at the endplate sites.

4) They disappear after denervation, in rat, where acetylcholinesterase activity globally decreases, and also in chicken, where globular forms increase several-fold.

5) In mammals, A forms exist in skeletal muscles but not in smooth muscles. The synthesis of A12, however, may be induced in the cat's nictitating membrane, where it is normally absent, by innervation with the hypoglossal nerve (Inestrosa et al., 1979).

Because, counter-examples to each of these observations have now been found, they cannot be extrapolated as general rules. In the following section, we will examine the regulation of acetylcholinesterase forms in various organisms.

Torpedo Analyses of acetylcholinesterase forms during development in Torpedo embryos (Bon, 1982; Witzemann and Boustead, 1982) showed that all forms, including the collagen-tailed forms, exist in the electric organ primordium when the cells are still in a myogenic morphological phase, i.e. before innervation. Collagen-tailed forms start to accumulate rapidly at a time when the cells have assumed a flattened electrocyte configuration, and have acquired a basal lamina, but have not yet established nerve contacts. In fact, the proliferation of nerve terminals in the electric organ, which takes places a little later, coincides with a rapid increase of amphipathic, detergent-soluble G2 acetylcholinesterase. This form then becomes predominant, together with A12, at the adult stage.

A large fraction of this G2 form, and therefore of acetylcholinesterase activity in the electric organs, appears to be inserted at the outer surface of nerve terminals (synaptosomes) (Morel and Dreyfus, 1982; Li and Bon, 1983). Electrophorus electroplaques, in contrast with Torpedo electroplaques, sustain action potentials, so that nerve terminals are far less extended. This may be related to the fact that Electrophorus electric organs contain almost exclusively collagen-tailed forms of acetylcholinesterase. Although a small proportion of amphipathic, detergent-soluble G2 form has also been shown in these organs (Bon, 1983) its presynaptic location has not been established.

<u>Chicken and quail</u> In the case of chicken, the A12 form of acetylcholinesterase appears at about the fifth day of embryonic development in the hind legs. In culture, early myoblasts produced myotubes which did not express this collagen-tailed form, in contrast with myotubes derived from later myoblasts (Toutant et al. 1983). These different cultures also expressed different sets of contractile proteins (Toutant et al., 1983). It therefore appears that successive populations of myoblasts correspond to distinct differentiation states. This is consistent with the clonal hypotheses proposed by various authors (Bonner and Hauschka, 1974; White et al., 1975). The capacity to synthesize A12 molecules did not appear after demedullation of young chick embryos, suggesting that it must be induced by neural influences <u>in vivo</u> . However we have not been able to obtain the expression of A12 acetylcholinesterase in cocultures of young myoblasts with motoneurons

in vitro (Toutant et al., 1983).

Quail embryos appear to express A12 acetylcholinesterase earlier than chick embryos : this form is present in hind leg buds at 4 days (Fauquet and Vallette, in preparation).

In order to examine the expression of acetylcholinesterase forms at earlier stages, we examined dermomyotomes in 3 day chick and quail embryos (Fauquet and Vallette, in preparation). At that stage, chick dermomyotomes did not contain any collagen-tailed acetylcholinesterase, but, after 3 days in culture, developed myotubes and produced a very significant proportion of A12 form. Quail dermomyotomes already possess A12 acetylcholinesterase at 3 days, although they do not contain any myotubes. Although there is no stable innervation in dermomyotomes of chick or quail at such early stages, transitory contacts with motoneuron fibers, or neural influence mediated by extracellular soluble or insoluble components cannot be entirely ruled out (Filagamo and Marchisio, 1971). Dermomyotomes of quail embryos from which the neural crest had been removed at 1 1/2 days (12-15 somites, before neural crest cells began to migrate) also contained A12 acetylcholinesterase, excluding the necessity of its induction by neural crest cells, but not necessarily the influence of spinal cord motoneurons.

It is interesting that the A12 forms are present in mononucleated presumptive muscle cells, because in many other cases the appearance of this enzyme appears to be correlated with the fusion of myoblasts into myotubes. For example, quail myoblasts which had been infected by a thermosensitive Rous sarcoma virus were able to fuse and produce A12 acetylcholinesterase at 41°, but not at 35° (Toutant et al., 1983). Similar observations have been reported in the case of mammalian muscle cell lines : the appearance of A12 coincides with fusion (Sugiyama, 1977), and its synthesis is suppressed if fusion is prevented in the absence of Ca^{++} (Inestrosa et al., 1983).

At early stages of chick embryogenesis, during their migration towards the sites of the various cholinergic or non cholinergic peripheral ganglia, neural crest cells present a higher level of histochemically detectable acetylcholinesterase activity than other cells (Cochard and Coltey, 1983). The migrating neural crest cells express essentially the G2 form of the enzyme.

All these observations suggest that the capacity to produce the more elaborated, collagen-tailed forms of acetylcholinesterase is characteristic of certain differentiation states, which is reached at different stages by cell populations during development and may be retained in transformed cell lines.

Mammalian muscles In rat muscles (hind legs) the proportion of the A12 form of acetylcholinesterase is higher in late embryos than in the adult (Koenig and Vigny, 1978). Around birth, the distribution of this form has been shown to extend along the entire muscle fiber (Brzin et al, 1980, Koenig and Rieger, 1981). There is a subsequent decrease in extrajunctional regions, and a concentration of this form at the endplates. Thus the nerves exert a negative, as well as a positive regulatory effect on the synthesis and localization of this form. A negative influence may also explain the regression of pseudocholinesterase in rat muscle after birth (Brzin et al., 1980). Weinberg and Hall (1979) have shown that ectopic reinnervation of a denervated rat soleus muscles led to the reappearance of collagen-tailed forms both at the new endplate and at the original endplate. This suggests that two aspects may be distinguished in the positive influence of the nerve : a) a local, permanent or long lasting influence which permits the anchoring and perhaps stabilization of A forms and may be linked to a specialization of the junctional basal lamina (Sanes and Hall, 1979) surviving the disappearance of presynaptic terminals, and b) a general influence which triggers the synthesis of A forms by the muscle fiber, and may correspond to the stimulation of contractile activity (Lømo and Slater, 1980).

In adult rat (Lømo, Massoulié and Vigny, in preparation) and mouse (Gisiger and Stephens, 1982, 1983) the patterns of acetylcholinesterase molecular forms observed clearly differ in fast and slow muscles: fast muscles contain essentially G1, G4 and A12, while slow muscles such as soleus, present a more complex pattern, with a lower proportion of G4, and a significant level of A8. It is remarkable that the muscles and their corresponding nerves present very similar patterns of acetylcholinesterase molecular forms (Gisiger and Stephens, 1982) suggesting that both are determined by common factors. The rhythm of activity, which differentiates phasic and tonic muscles, may be determinant in this regulation.

Together with T.Lømo, we have analyzed acetylcholinesterase in denervated rat soleus muscles which had been stimulated in two ways : in a "slow" mode (10 Hz), and in a "fast" mode (100 Hz bursts of 1s, with a mean frequency of 1 Hz), supposed to mimic the normal stimulation rhythms of the soleus ("slow") muscle and of a "fast" muscle such as the extensor digitorum longus (EDL). We found that both modes of stimulation induced a rapid, transitory increase in acetylcholinesterase specific activity which reached up to 200 % of a control non denervated muscle, within 2 days. The compositions in molecular forms were however different in the two cases : the pattern obtained in the "fast" stimulated soleus muscles presented a simpler pattern, resembling that of a normal EDL, whereas the pattern of the "slow" stimulated muscles was closer to that of control, non denervated soleus muscles (Lømo, Massoulié and Vigny, in preparation).

Such experiments of course do not mean that muscle characteristics can be reversibly interchanged by external factors such as stimulation. In collaboration with F. Bacou and P. Vigneron, we have studied the effects of denervation in a leg muscle of the rabbit, the semimembranosus, which is composed of an external fast glycolytic part, and an internal slow oxidative bundle. Both regions of the muscle retained their characteristic metabolic properties even after two months, in spite of extensive atrophy. Acetylcholinesterase specific activity greatly increased in both regions. However, A forms dramatically decreased in the fast region, but increased both in proportion and absolute level (25-fold after one month) in the slow region (Bacou et al, 1982).

CONCLUSION

Taken together, these observations indicate that each differentiation state corresponds to a particular capacity for the synthesis of cholinesterase catalytic subunits, their glycosylation, the cleavage of hydrophobic peptides, their polymerization into dimers and tetramers, their assembly with non catalytic components such as the collagen-like tail, as well as the transport, insertion into plasma membranes, or secretion of enzyme molecules. All these mechanisms, generating the polymorphism of cholinesterases, may operate either on the products of a single structural gene, possibly with the splicing of distinct sequences determining for example hydrophobic regions responsible for the amphipathic or detergent-insensitive characteristics of the molecules, or with sets of distinct genes which, according to immunological evidence, must be closely related.

Both genetic and post translational mechanisms are likely to contribute to the polymorphism of cholinesterases. Distinct genes, or sets of genes, most probably code for acetylcholinesterase and pseudocholinesterase which do not immunologically cross react, although they present parallel series of molecular forms. On the other hand, the large variety of molecular structures must depend at least in part on post translational modifications, e.g. glycosylation or proteolytic cleavage.

Although our present view of cholinesterase polymorphism is still incomplete in many respects, it allows us to approach the fundamental problems raised by the generation and control of this molecular diversity using the powerful methods of genetic and molecular biology.

References

Adamson, E.D., Ayers, S.E., Deussen, Z.A. and Graham, C.F. Analysis of the form adult mouse brain : Biochem. J. *147*, 205-214 (1975).

Adamson, E.D. Acetylcholinesterase in mouse brain, erythrocytes and muscles : J. Neurochem. *28*, 605-615 (1977).

Allemand, P., Bon, S., Massoulié, J. and Vigny, M. The quaternary structure of chicken acetylcholinesterase and butyrylcholinesterase : effect of collagenase and trypsin : J. Neurochem. *36*, 860-867 (1981).

Anglister, L. and Silman, I. Molecular structure of elongated forms of electric eel acetylcholinesterase. J. Mol. Biol. *125*, 293-311 (1978).

Bacou, F., Vigneron, P. and Massoulié, J. Acetylcholinesterase forms in fast and slow rabbit muscle : Nature *296*, 661-664 (1982).

Bon, S., Huet, M., Lemonnier, M., Rieger, F. and Massoulié, J. Molecular forms of *Electrophorus* acetylcholinesterase ; molecular weight and composition : Eur. J. Biochem. *68*, 523-530 (1976).

Bon, S. and Massoulié, J. Collagenase sensitivity and aggregation properties of *Electrophorus* acetylcholinesterase : Eur. J. Biochem. *89*, 89-94 (1978).

Bon, S., Cartaud, J. and Massoulié, J. The dependence of acetylcholinesterase aggregation at low ionic strength upon a polyanionic component Eur. J. Biochem. *85*, 1-14 (1978).

Bon, S., Vigny, M. and Massoulié, J. Asymmetric and globular forms of acetylcholinesterase in mammals and birds : Proc. Natl. Acad. Sci. USA *76*, 2546-2550 (1979).

Bon, S. and Massoulié, J. Collagen-tailed and hydrophobic components of acetylcholinesterase in *Torpedo marmorata* electric organ : Proc. Natl. Acad. Sci. USA *77*, 4464-4468 (1980).

Bon, S. Molecular forms of acetylcholinesterase in developing *Torpedo* embryos : Neurochem. Int. *4*, 577-585 (1982).

Bonner, P.H. and Hauschka, S.D. Clonal analysis of vertebrate myogenesis. 1. Early developmental events in the chick limb : Dev. Biol. *37*, 317-328 (1974).

Brockman, S.K., Przybylski, R.J. and Younkin, S.G. Cellular localization of the molecular forms of acetylcholinesterase in cultures embryonic rat myotubes : J. of Neurosci. *2*, 1775-1785 (1982).

Brzin, M., Sketelj, J., Grubič, Z. and Kiauta, T. Cholinesterases of neuromuscular junctions : Neurochem. Intern. *2*, 149-159 (1980).

Cochard, P. and Coltey, P. Cholinergic traits in the neural crest : acetylcholinesterase in crest cells of the chick embryo : Dev. Biol. *98*, 221-238 (1983).

Devreotes, P.N., Gardner, J.M. and Fambrough, D.M. Kinetics of biosynthesis of acetylcholine receptor and subsequent incorporation into plasma membrane of cultures chick skeletal muscle : Cell. *10*, 365-373 (1977).

Fambrough, D.M., Engel, A.G. and Rosenberry, A.G. Acetylcholinesterase of human erythrocytes and neuromuscular junctions : homologies revealed by monoclonal antibodies : Proc. Natl. Acad. Sci. USA *79*, 1078-1082 (1982).

Filogamo, G. and Marchisio, P.C. Acetylcholine system and neural development : Neurosc. Res. *4*, 29-64 (1971).

Gisiger, V. and Stephens, H.R. Acetylcholinesterase content in both motor nerve and muscle is correlated with twitch properties : Neurosci. Lett. *31*, 301-305 (1982).

Gisiger, V. and Stephens, H.R. Asymmetric and globular forms of AChE in slow and fast muscles of 129,REJ normal and dystrophic mice : J. Neurochem. in press (1983).

Gómez-Barriocanal, J., Barat, A., Escudero, E., Rodriguez-Borrajo, C. and Ramirez, G. Solubilization of collagen-tailed acetylcholinesterase from chick retina : Effect of different extraction procedures : J. Neurochem. *37*, 1239-1249 (1981).

Grassi, J., Vigny, M. and Massoulié, J. Molecular forms of acetylcholinesterase in bovine caudate nucleus and superior cervical ganglion : solubility properties and hydrophobic character : J. Neurochem. *38*, 457-469 (1982).

Grassi, J., Massoulié, J. and Timpl, R. Relationship of collagen-tailed acetylcholinesterase with basal lamina components. Absence of binding with laminin fibronectin and collagen types IV and V and lack of reactivity with different anticollagen sera : Eur. J. Biochem. *133*, 31-38 (1983).

Hollunger, E.G. and Niklasson, B.H. The release and molecular state of mammalian brain acetylcholinesterase : J. Neurochem. *20*, 821-836 (1973).

Inestrosa, N.C., Mendez, B. and Luco, J.V. Acetylcholinesterase like that of skeletal muscle in smooth muscle reinnervated by a motor nerve : Nature *280*, 504-506 (1979).

Inestrosa, N.C., Reiness, C.G., Reichardt, L.F. and Hall, Z.W. Cellular localization of the molecular forms of acetylcholinesterase in rat pheochromocytoma PC_{12} cells treated with nerve growth factor : J. Neurosci. *1*, 1260-1267 (1981).

Inestrosa, N.C., Silberstein, L. and Hall, Z.W. Association of the synaptic form of acetylcholinesterase with extracellular matrix in cultured mouse muscle cells : Cell, *29*, 71-79 (1982).

Inestrosa, N.C., Miller, J.B., Silberstein, L., Zisking-Conhaim, L. and Hall, Z.W. Development and regulation of 16 S acetylcholinesterase and acetylcholine receptors in a mouse muscle cell line. Exp. Cell Res. *147*, 393-406 (1983).

Koenig, J. and Vigny, M. Neural induction of the 16 S acetylcholinesterase in muscle cell cultures : Nature *271* : 75-77 (1978).

Koenig, J. and Rieger, F. Biochemical stability of the acetylcholinesterase molecular forms after cytochemical staining : post natal localization of the 16 S acetylcholinesterase in rat muscle : Dev. Neuroscience *4*, 249-257 (1981).

Lee, S.L., Heinemann, S. and Taylor, P. Structural characterization of the asymmetric (17+13)S forms of acetylcholinesterase from *Torpedo*. I. Analysis of subunit composition : J. Biol. Chem. *257*, 12283-12291 (1982a).

Lee, S.L. and Taylor, P. Structural characterization of the asymmetric (17+13)S species of acetylcholinesterase from *Torpedo*. II. Component peptides obtained by selective proteolysis and disulfide bond reduction : J. Biol. Chem. *257*, 12292-12301 (1982).

Lee, S.L., Camp, S.J. and Taylor, P. Characterization of a hydrophobic, dimeric form of acetylcholinesterase from *Torpedo* : J. Biol. Chem. *257*, 12302-12309 (1982b).

Li, Z.Y. and Bon, C. Presence of a membrane-bound acetylcholinesterase form in a preparation of nerve endings from *Torpedo marmorata* electric organ : J. Neurochem. *40*, 338-349 (1983)

Lømo, T. and Slater, J.R. Control of junctional acetylcholinesterase by neural and muscular influences in the rat : J. Physiol. *303*, 191-202 (1980).

Massoulié, J. and Bon, S. The molecular forms of cholinesterase and acetylcholinesterase in vertebrates : Ann. Rev. Neurosci. *5*, 57-106 (1982).

Morel, N. and Dreyfus, P. Association of acetylcholinesterase with the external surface of the presynaptic plasma membrane in *Torpedo* electric organ : Neurochem. Int. *4*, 283-288 (1982).

Rosenberry, T.L. and Richardson, J.M. Structure of 18 S and 14 S acetylcholinesterase. Identification of collagen-like subunits that are linked by disulfide bonds to catalytic subunits :Biochemistry *16*, 135-148 (1977).

Rosenberry, T.L., Barnett, P. and Mays, C. The collagen-like subunits of acetylcholinesterase from the eel *Electrophorus electricus* : Neurochem. Int. *2*, 135-148 (1980).

Rotundo, R.L. and Fambrough, P.M. Synthesis, transport and fate of acetylcholinesterase in cultured chick embryos muscle cells. Cell *22* : 583-594 (1980a).

Rotundo, R.L. and Fambrough, D.M. Secretion of acetylcholinesterase. Relation to acetylcholine receptor metabolism : Cell *22*, 595-602 (1980b).

Rubin, L.L., Schuetze, S.M., Weill, C.L. and Fischbach, G.D. Regulation of acetylcholinesterase appearance of neuromuscular junctions *in vitro*: Nature *283*, 264-267 (1980).

Sanes, J.R. and Hall, Z.W. Antibodies that bond specifically to synaptic sites on muscle fiber basal lamina : J. Cell Biol. *83*, 357-370 (1979).

Silberstein, L., Inestrosa, N.C. and Hall, Z.W. Aneural muscle cells make synaptic basal lamina components : Nature *295*, 143-145 (1982).

Sørensen, K., Gentinetta, R. and Brodbeck, U. An amphiphile-dependent form of human brain caudate nucleus acetylcholinesterase : purification and properties : J. Neurochem. *39*, 1050-1060 (1982).

Sugiyama, H. Multiple forms of acetylcholinesterase in clonal muscle cells. FEBS Lett. *84*, 257-260 (1977).

Toutant, J.P., Toutant, M., Fiszman, M.Y. and Massoulié, J. Expression of the A_{12} form of acetylcholinesterase by developing avian leg muscle cells *in vivo* and during differentiation in primary cell cultures : Neurochem. Int. in press (1983).

Tsuji, S. Acetylcholinesterase positive electromotor neurons in the electric lobes of *Torpedo marmorata* : Brain. Res. *124*, 352-356 (1977).

Weinberg, C.G. and Hall, Z.W. Junctional form of acetylcholinesterase restored at nerve free endplate : Dev. Biol. *68*, 631-635 (1979).

White, N.K., Bonner, P.H., Nelson, D.R. and Hauschka, S.D. Clonal analysis of vertebrate myogenesis. IV. Medium-dependent classification of colony forming cells : Dev. Biol. *44*, 346-361 (1975).

Witzemann, V. and Boustead, C. Changes in acetylcholinesterase molecular forms during the embryonic development of *Torpedo marmorata* : J. Neurochem. *39*, 747-755 (1982).

Witzemann, V. and Boustead, C. Structural differences in the catalytic subunits of acetylcholinesterase forms from the electric organ of *Torpedo marmorata* : EMBO J. *2*, 873-878 (1983).

Younkin, S.G., Rosenstein, C., Collins, P.L. and Rosenberry, T.L. Cellular localization of the molecular forms of acetylcholinesterase in rat diaphragm : J. Biol. Chem. *257*, 13630-13637 (1982).

Zanetta, J.P., Rackonczay, Z., Reeber, A., Kása, P. and Vincendon, G. Antibodies againts the membrane-bound acetylcholinesterase from adult rat brain : FEBS lett. *129*, 293-296 (1981).

SOLUBILIZATION OF MEMBRANE-BOUND ACETYLCHOLINESTERASE BY A PHOSPHATIDYLINOSITOL-SPECIFIC PHOSPHOLIPASE C: ENZYMATIC AND PHYSICOCHEMICAL STUDIES

A.H. Futerman[1], R.M. Fiorini[1*], E. Roth[1], D.M. Michaelson[2], M.G. Low[3] and I. Silman[1].

[1]Dept. of Neurobiology, Weizmann Institute of Science, Rehovot 76100 (Israel), [2]Dept. of Biochemistry, Tel Aviv University, Ramat Aviv, Tel Aviv 69978 (Israel), and [3]Oklahoma Medical Research Foundation, Oklahoma City, OK 73104 (USA).

Introduction

AChE exists in a number of molecular forms which can be distinguished by their solubility characteristics and sedimentation coefficients (1). In *Torpedo* electric organ three major AChE fractions can be distinguished: 1) Low-salt-soluble AChE (LSSAChE); 2) Detergent-soluble AChE (DSAChE); and 3) High-salt-soluble AChE (HSSAChE) (2-4). HSSAChE resembles in quaternary structure the asymmetric forms purified from *Electrophorus* (5), in that it contains one, two or three tetramers of catalytic subunits attached to a collagen-like tail (6,7).

Much attention has recently been focused on the two other forms of AChE in *Torpedo*, LSSAChE and DSAChE (2-4,8,9). DSAChE appears to be a globular dimer in which the catalytic subunits are linked by disulphides (2-4). According to Bon and Massoulie (2), LSSAChE and DSAChE both consist of catalytic subunit dimers which are closely related but differ in their tendency to aggregate in the absence of detergent. However, substantial structural differences between these two classes have recently been suggested (9).

HSSAChE is believed to be attached to the extracellular basal lamina, primarily through ionic interactions (3,10). Much of the DSAChE

* Permanent address: Institute of Biochemistry, Faculty of Medicine, University of Ancona (Italy).

in Torpedo is associated with the presynaptic plasma membrane, where it is the only molecular form detected (11-13), presumably through hydrophobic interactions.

Several enzymes have been shown to be associated with the plasma membrane through a specific interaction involving phophatidylinositol (PI) (14). For instance, alkaline phosphatase is released from a wide range of mammalian tissues by phosphatidylinositol-specific phospholipase C (PIPLC) from Staphylococcus aureus (15). AChE is similarly released from erythrocytes (16,17) and from sheep basal ganglia (18).

We have recently shown that PIPLC is effective in specifically solubilizing DSAChE from Torpedo electric organ in the absence of detergent (19). In the following we present data relating to the specificity of release of DSAChE, and characterize PIPLC-solubilized AChE with respect to physicochemical behaviour and structural characteristics, as compared to other forms of Torpedo AChE.

Solubilization of AChE by PIPLC

On addition of PIPLC to homogenates of electric organ from Torpedo californica, a substantial portion of the AChE was solubilized in a concentration-dependent manner (Fig.1). Solubilization was completely inhibited by 1M NaCl and partially by 10mM $CaCl_2$ and 160mM KCl. Neither EDTA (10mM) nor phenylmethylsulphonyl fluoride (1mM) had any effect on the process. PIPLC from S.aureus was earlier shown to be independent of divalent cations and inhibited by high salt concentrations (20), and to be devoid of proteolytic activity (15). We have confirmed this by observing that PIPLC displays no detectable proteolytic activity towards either ^{125}I-casein or ^{3}H-Leu-enkephalin.

Several other phospholipases were tested for their ability to solubilize Torpedo AChE. Apart from PIPLC, none of those tested were able to solubilize AChE from purified synaptosomal membranes devoid of postsynaptic elements (21), prepared from freshly killed Torpedo ocellata (Table I). Likewise, none of them were able to release DSAChE from the particulate fraction of T.californica homogenates, even after

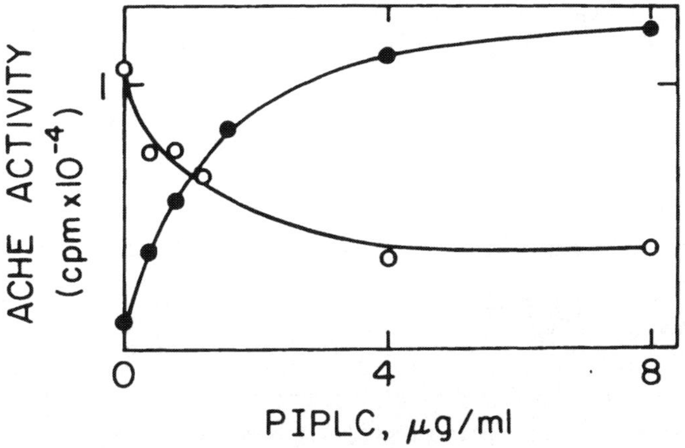

Figure 1. **Solubilization by PIPLC of AChE from T.californica electric organ.** Tissue (stored at -70°C) was homogenized in 10mM Tris, pH 7.5, to give a protein concentration of 5mg/ml. Aliquots of homogenate were incubated at 37°C with varying concentrations of PIPLC. After 30min, samples were centrifuged at 100,000g for 10min and AChE measured radiometrically (30) in pellet (o) and supernatant (•).

prolonged incubation (100μg/ml phospholipase, 37°C, 2h).

It was earlier shown that AChE was quantitatively solubilized by PIPLC from bovine and porcine erythrocytes but only to a limited extent (4.8%) from human erythrocytes (16). We have been able to show that AChE is also solubilized quantitatively from rat erythrocytes by PIPLC and to confirm that limited, but significant, solubilization occurs for human erythrocytes (Table II). In contrast to the complete solubilization of rat erythrocyte AChE by PIPLC, it had no effect on the solubilization of particulate AChE in four different regions of rat brain (Table II). Furthermore, none of the other phospholipases examined solubilized any significant amount of AChE from either rat brain or erythrocytes (not shown).

Fig.2A shows that the catalytic subunit of AChE is a major component of T.ocellata synaptosomal membranes, as revealed by sodium-dodecyl-sulphate-polyacrylamide-gel-electrophoresis (SDS-PAGE). This is in agreement with the earlier reports that a considerable proportion of the globular dimeric DSAChE is associated with the presynaptic membrane (11-13). Furthermore, this polypeptide is the only one visualized which is significantly solubilized by PIPLC (compare Fig.2D, the supernatant after PIPLC treatment, with Fig.2C, the corresponding control

Table I. Effect of various phospholipases on the solubilization of AChE from *T.ocellata* synaptosomal membranes.

Phospholipase	% of Triton-soluble AChE activity
Control	5.7
PLpase A_2 (*Naja naja* venom)	2.2
PLpase A_2 (Bee venom)	3.7
PLpase C (*Clostridium welchii*)	2.6
PLpase D (Cabbage)	2.3
PIPLC	95.6

Synaptosomal membranes (ca.1.2mg protein/ml) were incubated with the phospholipases (PLpases; final concentration 10µg/ml) at 37°C in 10mM Tris, pH 8.0. After 30min samples were centrifuged as described for Fig.1, and AChE measured in the supernatant. The results are the mean of two independent experiments, and express the percentage activity solubilized compared to the activity solubilized in the same buffer containing 1% Triton, taken as 100.

supernatant, and Fig.2F, a sample of purified *Torpedo* AChE).

It has been shown that *T.ocellata* synaptosomes release ACh in a K^+-evoked, Ca^{++}-dependent manner (21). In view of the quantitative solubilization by PIPLC of AChE from *T.ocellata* synaptosomal membranes

Table II. Effect of PIPLC on the solubilization of AChE from rat brain and from rat and human erythrocytes.

Tissue	% of Triton-soluble AChE activity	
	Control	PIPLC-treated
Rat erythrocytes	9.8	100.8
Rat cortex	24.1	19.1
Rat cerebellum	30.5	27.1
Rat striatum	48.3	39.4
Rat hypothalamus	28.5	26.5
Human erythrocytes	1.1	12.0

Erythrocytes were extensively washed so as to remove serum cholinesterase. Haemolysed erythrocytes and homogenates of rat brain were incubated with PIPLC (10µg/ml) and AChE activity was measured as in Table I.

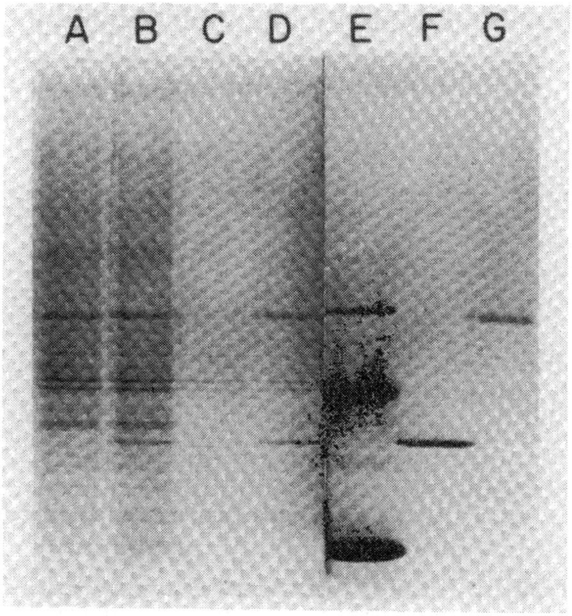

Figure 2. SDS-PAGE of synaptosomal membranes from *T.ocellata* before and after PIPLC treatment. Synaptosomal membranes (see ref.21) were incubated with PIPLC. A) Synaptosomal membranes, B) Synaptosomal membranes+PIPLC (5µg/ml, 37°C, 30min), C) 100,000g supernatant of A, D) 100,000g supernatant of B, E) Markers: Bovine serum albumin (69K), Ovalbumin (46K), Lysozyme (14K), F) Purified PIPLC (2.5µg), G) Purified DSAChE (2.2µg). 5-15% gradient gels were run in the presence of reducing agent.

(Table I), together with the apparent specificity of the effect (Fig.2), we examined whether PIPLC had any effect on K^+-evoked, Ca^{++}-dependent ACh-release from intact synaptosomes. Fig.3 shows that there is no difference in the amount of ACh released between control and PIPLC-treated synaptosomes, even though enzymatic assay showed that quantitative solubilization of AChE had been achieved by PIPLC treatment. These results support the notion that presynaptic AChE is not directly involved in regulating the amount of ACh released.

Characterization of PIPLC-solubilized AChE from *Torpedo*

Sucrose density centrifugation revealed that only one molecular form

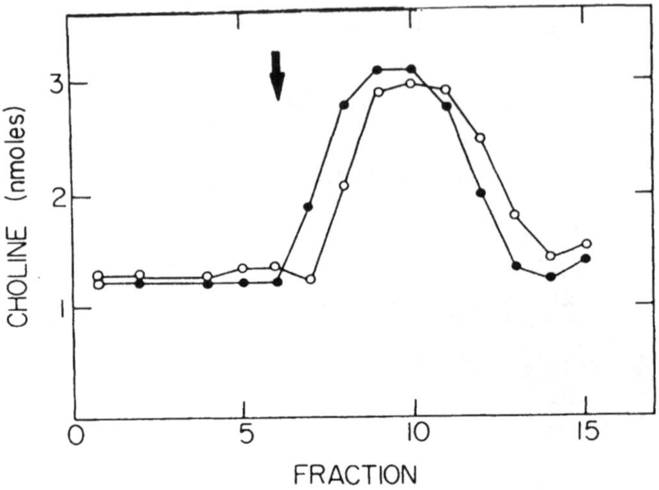

Figure 3. Ca^{++}-dependent, K^{+}-evoked ACh-release from T.ocellata synaptosomes. Synaptosomes (0.3mg protein) were preincubated with (•) or without (o) PIPLC (7µg/ml, 90min, 25°C). They were then loaded onto a continuous flow apparatus (31,32) and extensively washed (8ml) to remove soluble AChE. Addition of K^{+} (125mM, 3ml), in the presence of Ca^{++} (2mM), is indicated by the arrow. Choline, which is produced by hydrolysis of the released ACh by exogenous AChE added to the eluted fractions (700µl), was measured by the chemiluminescence method (33).

of AChE, of sedimentation coefficient 7.2S, was solubilized by PIPLC both from T.californica (19) and from T.ocellata (not shown). The enzyme released by PIPLC corresponds to DSAChE since no further extraction of AChE was possible with detergent following PIPLC treatment. However, the HSS forms could be extracted from the residual pellet subsequent to PIPLC treatment in T.californica (not shown). It should also be noted that AChE from Electrophorus electric organ was not significantly solubilized by PIPLC (19). This is to be expected, since Electrophorus contains almost exclusively HSS asymmetric forms which are believed to be associated with the basal lamina by ionic forces (3, 5), and there is no evidence for any substantial portion of the enzyme being associated with the plasma membrane through hydrophobic interactions. Preliminary data reveal that PIPLC-solubilized AChE from rat erythrocytes consists of a major 7.1S and a minor 11.7S form, presumably corresponding to dimer and tetramer.

In order to further examine the mode of interaction of DSAChE with the plasma membrane, we tested several agents for their ability to solubilize DSAChE from Torpedo homogenates. These included mannose, EDTA, inositol, and the chaotropic agents NaI, NaSCN and guanidine (22).

We also studied the effect of the acylating agents maleic anhydride and citraconic anhydride (see, e.g. ref.23), the former of which has been shown to solubilize HSS AChE from Electrophorus by modifying its electrical charge (10,24). None of these reagents solubilized any significant amount of active enzyme. Thus in terms of the forces involved in its interaction with the plasma membrane, DSAChE behaves like an integral membrane protein. Yet, as shown clearly in Fig.2, no other major protein species in Torpedo synaptosomes is significantly solubilized by PIPLC, nor is the nicotinic acetylcholine receptor (nAChR) solubilized from T.californica homogenates (19). Thus, although DSAChE and nAChR are both membrane-bound, detergent-soluble molecules, it appears that their mode of attachment to the plasma membrane is very different, and that the action of PIPLC is not a non-specific process leading to release of all membrane-bound molecules.

It was earlier reported that DSAChE had a sedimentation coefficient of 5.5-8S, depending on the detergent used for solubilization (2,3), and we have made similar observations (Table III). However, addition of various detergents to PIPLC-solubilized AChE did not modify its sedimentation coefficient. For example, under our conditions, AChE solubilized with Brij 96 had a sedimentation coefficient of 5.0S, whereas the enzyme solubilized with PIPLC had a sedimentation coefficient of 7.2S even in the presence of this detergent (Table III). The effect of PIPLC thus appears similar, in physicochemical terms, to that of Proteinase K (PK), which was shown earlier (2) to render DSAChE insensitive to detergent by this criterion, a finding which we have confirmed (Table III). These data suggest that the site of attachment to the membrane of DSAChE is identical to, or overlaps with the site of detergent-binding, and that detergent is not bound significantly after PIPLC solubilization.

We have purified DSAChE after solubilization with sodium cholate, essentially according to Viratelle and Bernhard (3). The sedimentation coefficient of DSAChE purified in cholate is 7.4S (Table III); if cholate is replaced by Brij 96, this value decreases to 5.4S (Fig.4A), i.e. to a value similar to that obtained by direct solubilization with Brij 96. However, if incubation of the cholate-purified AChE with either PIPLC (Fig.4B) or PK (Fig.4C) precedes replacement of cholate by Brij 96, no such decrease is observed. It is worth noting that none of the

Table III. Sedimentation coefficient of DSAChE from *Torpedo* in the presence of various detergents.

Mode of solubilization	Sedimentation coefficient			
	Buffer	Brij 96	Triton	Cholate
Brij 96		5.0+0.5(8)		
Brij 96/PK[1]		7.1+0.4(3)		
Triton X-100			6.3+0.4(8)	
PK	7.2+0.2(6)			
PIPLC	7.2+0.3(10)	7.3+0.1(3)	7.1+0.2(4)	7.0(1)
Cholate		5.3+0.2(4)		7.4+0.2(4)
Cholate/PK[1]		7.2(2)		
Cholate/PIPLC		7.4+0.2(5)		

DSAChE was solubilized from *Torpedo* electric organ with either the designated detergent (listed in the left-hand column), or by digestion with either PK or PIPLC. In some cases, detergent-solubilized enzyme was subsequently digested by either PK[1] or PIPLC[2]. If centrifugation was carried out in the same detergent used for solubilization, samples were layered directly onto the gradient. If the detergent was changed, samples were diluted 100-fold into the new detergent. The detergent employed for centrifugation is designated at the top of each column. The buffer in which the sucrose was dissolved was 40mM $MgCl_2$-100mM NaCl-10mM Tris, pH 8.0, in all cases.

other phospholipases tested in Table I could prevent the decrease in sedimentation coefficient produced by Brij 96 (data not shown). Our results suggest that one or more molecules of PI (or a PI derivative) is cosolubilized with DSAChE and is strongly attached to cholate-purified AChE. This adhering PI is presumably responsible for the detergent sensitivity of the enzyme; this property being eliminated by PIPLC treatment. Lack of detergent sensitivity after PK treatment could then be ascribed to removal of a small peptide to which PI might be strongly attached.

It was of interest to investigate the interaction of DSAChE with liposomes of defined lipid composition before and after treatment with PIPLC and PK. For this purpose, we used a flotation gradient technique for separation of bound and free AChE, in which liposomes (and adhering AChE) float to the top of the gradient whereas unbound AChE remains at the bottom (25,26). Upon mixing cholate-purified AChE with

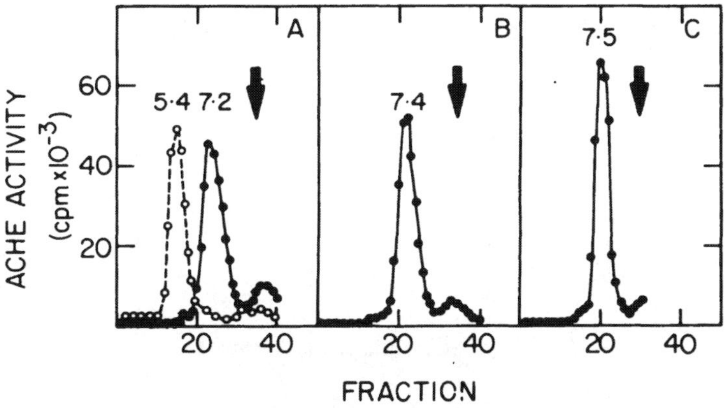

Figure 4. Sedimentation profiles of cholate-purified T.californica AChE in Brij 96 before and after PIPLC or PK treatment. 2µl of cholate-purified AChE was diluted into 200µl 1% sodium cholate or 200µl 1% Brij 96 and, after 1h at 25°C, layered on top of a 5-20% sucrose gradient containing the same detergent used for dilution in 40mM $MgCl_2$-0.1M NaCl-10mM Tris, pH 8.0. Centrifugation was for 16h at 39,000rpm in a Beckmann L8-70 ultracentrifuge using an SW40Ti rotor. A) Cholate-purified AChE diluted into cholate (●) and into Brij 96 (o). B) Cholate-purified AChE after incubation with PIPLC (16µg/ml, 37°C, 30min) diluted into Brij 96. C) Cholate-purified AChE after incubation with PK (100µg/ml, 25°C, 30min) diluted into Brij 96. The arrow denotes the position of catalase (11.4S).

phosphatidylcholine (PC), the enzyme moved to the top of the gradient along with the lipid (Fig.5A). However, prior incubation of cholate-purified AChE either with PIPLC (Fig.5B) or with PK (Fig.5C) rendered the enzyme incapable of binding to the liposomes, and thus the enzyme remained at the bottom of the gradient while the PC floated up. Prior incubation of cholate-purified AChE with PIPLC or PK also rendered it incapable of binding to mixed liposomes containing both PI and PC, whereas prior to such treatment the enzyme could bind to such liposomes.

The reconstitution data are in excellent agreement with the results concerning detergent-sensitivity. This is to be expected, since the results presented earlier (Table III; Fig.4), strongly suggested that the site of detergent binding corresponds to the site of lipid binding. Our results are also in agreement with those of Low and Zilversmit (27), who showed that alkaline phosphatase released from pig kidney microsomes by PIPLC did not bind to phospholipid vesicles, even if they contained PI.

The effects of PIPLC on the detergent-sensitivity of DSAChE and on reconstitution into liposomes suggest that PIPLC either eliminates a

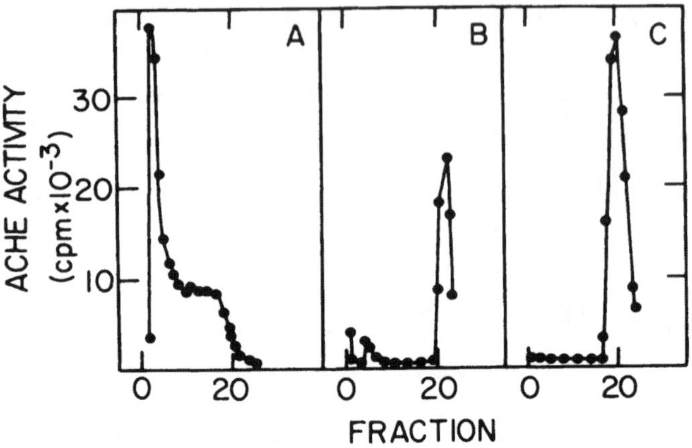

Figure 5. Interaction of cholate-purified AChE with phosphatidylcholine (PC) liposomes as demonstrated on a flotation gradient. 3µl of cholate-purified AChE was mixed with 280µl of sonicated PC (Sigma soybean L-α-phosphatidylcholine, Type IV-S). Step gradients consisted, from the bottom up, of 0.5ml of 2M sucrose; 0.7ml of the AChE-PC mixture in 1.2M sucrose, 3.1ml of 1M sucrose, 0.5ml buffer. The buffer, in which sucrose solutions were also made up, was 0.1M NaCl-0.01M phosphate, pH 7.0. Gradients were centrifuged for 3.5h at 45,000rpm in a SW50.1 rotor. A) Cholate-purified AChE+PC. B) Cholate-purified AChE after incubation with PIPLC (25µg/ml, 30min, 37°C)+PC. C) Cholate-purified AChE after incubation with PK (100µg/ml, 30min, 37°C)+PC. In all three gradients PC moved to the top of the gradient (i.e. to the left in the figure) as monitored by measuring turbidity at 300nm.

site responsible for binding of DSAChE to the plasma membrane or cleaves a phosphate-glycerol bond in such a manner as to leave a fragment of PI (or a derivative thereof) adhering to the enzyme, which blocks detergent binding and prevents reconstitution. The failure of PIPLC-released AChE and alkaline phosphatase to bind to liposomes containing PI favours this latter possibility.

2) Analysis by SDS-PAGE: It was of interest to use the technique of SDS-PAGE in order to investigate whether substantial differences exist in the size of the catalytic subunit of PIPLC-solubilized AChE as compared to intact DSAChE and to other forms of the enzyme. In order to accurately detect small differences in molecular weight (MW), we coelectrophoresed reduced samples of AChE, labeled with ^{3}H-DFP (28), with a mixture of ^{14}C-labeled proteins which served as internal standards, using 20cm long, 5-15% gradient gels so as to achieve high resolution.

Fig.6 shows that the catalytic subunit of the HSS fraction of T.californica AChE runs at approximately the same position as the ^{14}C-BSA marker, corresponding to a MW of 69,000. However, DSAChE, whether solubilized in Triton X-100, Brij 96 or sodium cholate (Fig.6C-E) runs with an apparent MW of 67,000, significantly lower than that of BSA, as does PIPLC-solubilized enzyme (Fig.6F).

PK-solubilized AChE also has a MW of 67,000 (data not shown) as does LSSAChE (Fig.6B). Thus neither PIPLC nor PK produce any detectable difference in MW of the catalytic subunit as compared to intact DSAChE. It thus seems that the putative peptide removed by PK, which we presume to bear the PIPLC-sensitive site, should be quite small (of the order of a few amino acids).

In the absence of reducing agent, SDS-PAGE revealed that PK-solubilized AChE and PIPLC-solubilized AChE consist, like intact DSAChE, of a single component of MW ca.135,000 (data not shown). All these forms thus seem to be disulphide-linked dimers of catalytic subunits.

Under the conditions employed for solubilization of DSAChE by PK and its subsequent purification, a product is obtained in which the catalytic subunit is not detectably smaller than that of intact DSAChE itself. DSAChE can, however, be further digested by the inclusion of PK

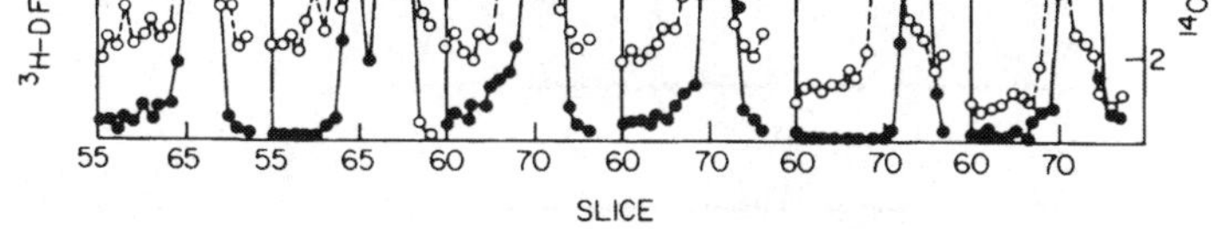

Figure 6. SDS-PAGE analysis of T.californica AChE in the presence of reducing agent. Aliquots (50µl) of AChE were incubated with 3µl of ^{3}H-DFP (5.2 Ci/mmol, NEN) for 1h at 25°C. A mixture of ^{14}C-methylated proteins (Amersham) was added to each sample. A) HSSAChE. B) LSSAChE. C) Triton-solubilized AChE. D) Brij 96-solubilized AChE. E) Cholate-solubilized AChE. F) PIPLC-solubilized AChE. Gel slices (1mm) were counted in a Packard Tri-Carb 4660 Scintillation counter using a double-labelling programme to process the data.

in the sample buffer before application to the gel, and this approach was pursued so as to produce subunit fragments of the various forms in order to seek structural differences. The catalytic subunit of PK-purified AChE (Fig.7A) can thus be further digested to yield ^{3}H-DFP-labelled fragments of apparent MW ca.32,000, 18,000 and 16,000 (Fig.7B). It should be noted that PK, itself a serine protease (29), is labelled by ^{3}H-DFP to yield a component of MW ca.35,000 (Fig.7E). This value is higher than the originally published MW value determined by gel filtration (29), but in good agreement with recent SDS-PAGE experiments (N.Hennrich, personal communication). Brij 96-purified DSAChE (Fig.7C) can likewise be further digested, by inclusion of PK in the sample buffer, to yield labelled components of MW similar to those obtained after digestion of PK-purified AChE. These breakdown products probably represent a protease-resistant core containing the active site after removal of peripheral regions which are probably responsible for interaction of the enzyme with the cellular environment, e.g. with the plasma membrane (cf.ref.11). We are currently performing experiments to determine the size of the protease-resistant core in the other forms

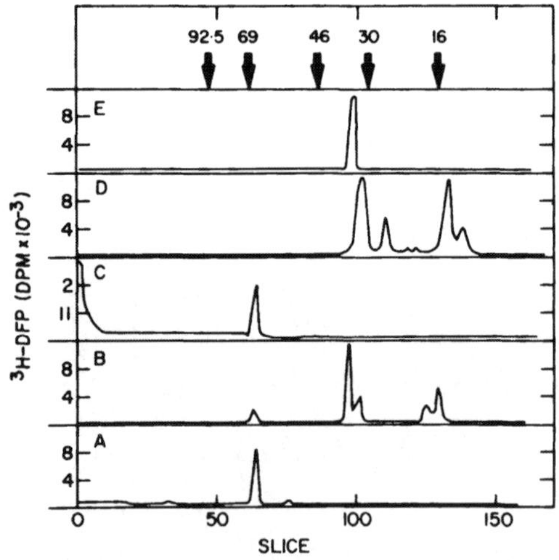

Figure 7. SDS-PAGE analysis of purified AChE before and after PK treatment. Aliquots of AChE were incubated with PK (100µg/ml, 30min, 25°C) in a final volume of 50µl, to which 25µl of sample buffer (containing β-mercaptoethanol as reducing agent) was added. Samples were then heated to 100°C for 5min. Control samples were similarly diluted and heated without PK. ^{3}H-DFP-labelled breakdown products of AChE were analysed in 5-15% gradient gel. A) PK-purified AChE. B) PK-purified AChE + PK. C) Brij 96-purified AChE. D) Brij 96-purified AChE+PK. E) PK alone. Arrows denote the position of ^{14}C-protein markers.

of AChE from Torpedo, in order to study the degree of homology of the various forms.

Conclusions

Our results provide evidence that DSAChE is associated with the plasma membrane of Torpedo electric organ through a strong and specific interaction which involves PI. We are currently investigating the nature of this interaction, and attempting to determine whether AChE is bound to PI by a covalent or a non-covalent linkage. The inability of PIPLC to solubilize DSAChE from a number of other sources suggests that DSAChE may be bound to the membrane by different mechanisms in different tissues, even in the same animal. The biosynthetic relationship between the various AChE forms in Torpedo, as well as between PIPLC-sensitive and insensitive forms in rat tissues, remains to be elucidated. PIPLC solubilization may further provide an alternative route for purification of Torpedo AChE. Finally, the specific solubilization of AChE from Torpedo synaptosomes by PIPLC offers a novel approach for examining the physiological role of AChE in synaptic transmission.

Acknowledgements

A.H.F. is supported by a studentship from the Science and Engeneering Research Council of Great Britain and R.M.F. by a fellowship from the Italian C.N.R.. Grants from the Muscular Dystrophy Association of America to I.S. and from the US-Israel Binational Science Foundation (BSF Grant No.2410) to D.M. are gratefully acknowledged. We thank Gordon McDowall for help with the ACh-release experiments.

References

1. Massoulie, J., Bon, S.: Ann. Rev. Neurosci. 5, 57-106 (1982).

2. Bon, S., Massoulie, J.: Proc. Natl. Acad. Sci. USA 77, 4464-4468 (1980).

3. Viratelle, O.M., Bernhard, S.A.: Biochem. 19, 4999-5007 (1980).

4. Witzemann, V.: Neurosci. Lett. 20, 277-282 (1980).

5. Anglister, L., Silman, I.: J. Mol. Biol. 125, 293-311 (1978).

6. Lee, S.L., Heinemann, S., Taylor, P.: J. Biol. Chem. 257, 12283-12291 (1982)

7. Lee, S.L., Taylor, P.: J. Biol. Chem. 257, 12292-12301 (1982).

8. Lee, S.L., Camp, S.J., Taylor, P.: J. Biol. Chem. 257, 12302-12309 (1982).

9. Witzemann, V., Boustead, C.: EMBO Journal 2, 873-878 (1983).

10. Dudai, Y., Herzberg, M., Silman, I.: Proc. Natl. Acad. Sci. USA 70, 2473-2476 (1973).

11. Witzemann, V., Boustead, C.: Neurosci. Lett. 26, 313-318 (1981).

12. Morel, N., Dreyfus, P.: Neurochem. Int. 4, 283-288 (1982).

13. Li, Z.Y., Bon, C.: J. Neurochem. 40, 338-349 (1983).

14. Shukla, S.D.: Life Sci. 30, 1323-1335 (1982).

15. Low, M.G., Finean, J.B.: Biochem. J. 167, 281-284 (1977).

16. Low, M.G., Finean, J.B.: FEBS Lett. 82, 143-146 (1977)

17. Ikezawa, H., Nakabayashi, T., Suzuki, K., Nakajima, M., Taguchi, T., Taguchi, R.: J. Biochem (Tokyo) 93, 1717-1719 (1983)

18. Majumdar, R., Balasubramanian, A.S.: FEBS Lett. 146, 335-338 (1982).

19. Futerman, A.H., Low, M.G., Silman, I.: Neurosci. Lett., in press.

20. Low, M.G., Finean, J.B.: Biochem. J. 154, 203-208 (1976).

21. Michaelson, D.M., Sokolovsky, M.: J. Neurochem. 30, 217-230 (1978).

22. Hatefi, Y., Hanstein, W.G.: Proc. Natl. Acad. Sci. USA 62, 1129-1136 (1969).

23. Eriksson, H., Liljeqvist, G., Heilbronn, E.: Biochim. Biophys. Acta 728, 449-454 (1983).

24. Dudai, Y., Silman, I.: J. Neurochem. 23, 1177-1187 (1974).

25. Watkins, M.S., Hitt, A.S., Bulger, J.E.: Biochem. Biophys. Res. Commun. 79, 640-647 (1977)

26. Kaufmann, K., Silman, I.: Neurochem. Int. 2, 205-207 (1980).

27. Low, M.G., Zilversmit, D.B.: Biochem. 19, 3913-3918 (1980).

28. Dudai, Y., Silman, I.: FEBS. Lett. 16, 324-328 (1971).

29. Ebeling, W., Hennrich, N., Klockow, M., Metz, H., Orth, H.D., Lang, H.: Eur. J. Biochem. 47, 91-97 (1974).

30. Johnson, C.D., Russell, R.L.: Analyt. Biochem. 64, 229-238 (1975).

31. Morel, N., Israel, M., Manaranche, R., Lesbats, B.: Prog. Brain Res. 49, 191-202 (1979).

32. Luz, S., Pinchasi, I., Michaelson, D.M., submitted.

33. Israel, M., Lesbats, B.: Neurochem. Int. 3, 81-90 (1981).

TWO CLASSES OF COLLAGEN-TAILED MOLECULAR FORMS OF ACETYLCHOLINESTERASE

Galo Ramírez, Javier Gómez-Barriocanal, Ana Barat and Corona Rodríguez-Borrajo

Centro de Biología Molecular, CSIC-UAM, Canto Blanco,
Madrid-34, Spain

Introduction

Among the AChE molecular forms, asymmetric, collagen-tailed species (A-forms) have attracted special interest due to their preferential association to synaptic sites, and their presynaptic regulation (1). Although these A-forms had been identified in fish brain and spinal cord (2,3) they were believed to be absent from the central nervous system (CNS) of higher vertebrates (4). Early work in our laboratory pointed out the existence of small amounts of collagenase-sensitive, asymmetric forms of AChE in several chick CNS areas (5, 6). We later found that the presence of a chelating agent (usually EDTA) in an extraction medium of high ionic strength resulted in the efficient solubilization of a fast-sedimenting (20S) collagen-tailed form of AChE from chick retina, a peripherally developed portion of the CNS (7). This collagen-tailed form, tentatively identified as the A_{12} molecular species (1), made up to 8-10% of the total retinal AChE activity. The existence of low amounts of fast-sedimenting AChE species in some chick, mouse and rat CNS tissues, without proof of their possible collagen-tailed nature, was also reported by Rieger and coworkers (8). Further work on chick retinal A_{12} led us to postulate the involvement of Ca^{++} in the attachment of the AChE tail to the cell membranes, and to suggest the existence of a tail-bound acidic lipid molecule mediating this interaction (9). By use of extraction solutions containing high salt (1M NaCl) and EDTA we have been able to show that collagen-tailed AChE species are actually present in different CNS areas of animal species encompassing all vertebrate classes (10,11) thus providing an experimental basis for an unified concept of the possible role of A-forms in cholinergic tissues. Some other recent papers have dealt with the localization and properties of collagen-tailed AChE in the vertebrate CNS (12-16).

The fact that in some tissues only a high salt concentration is required to solubilize collagen-tailed forms of AChE (e.g. electric organ and skeletal muscle (1), and CNS tissues of 'lower' vertebrates (2,3,11)), while EDTA (or EGTA) is additionally needed in some other cases (7,9,11) has led us to infer the existence of two different subpopulations or classes of collagen-tailed forms of AChE: one type of molecules, class I, would be linked to cell membranes by high ionic strength-sensitive forces, exclusively (17,18), while a second type, class II, would additionally establish tail-membrane bridges involving divalent cations (most likely Ca^{++}) thus explaining the concurrent need of high salt and chelating agents for their solubilization. In the present paper we give experimental proof of the existence of two such classes of asymmetric AChE molecular forms, and of their co-occurrence in most cholinergic tissues.

Methods

In some experiments, the tissues under study were repeatedly extracted with a solution containing 10mM Tris.HCl, pH 7, and 1M NaCl, supplemented at times with Triton X-100 and $CaCl_2$, followed by extractions with a second solution containing the same components plus EDTA (sequential extractions). In other series of experiments, equivalent samples of tissues were extracted with either 10mM Tris. HCl, pH 7/1M NaCl/1% Triton X-100/2mM $CaCl_2$ or 10mM Tris.HCl, pH 7/ 1M NaCl/1% Triton X-100/2mM EDTA (alternative extractions). The

AChE molecular forms contained in the different extracts (110,000g supernatants of the respective homogenates) were analyzed by velocity sedimentation in 5-20% linear sucrose gradients (prepared in the respective extraction solutions), calibrated with enzyme markers of known sedimentation coefficients (9). AChE peaks in the gradient were detected, and their activities measured as previously described (5,9). All samples from homogenates and extracts were corrected to equal composition before AChE assay.

Results and Discussion

Sequential extraction of skeletal muscle and electric organ samples. When a sample of chick skeletal muscle (mixed leg muscle) is repeatedly extracted with a 10mM Tris.HCl, pH 7/1M NaCl solution (Fig. 1A) the yield of solubilized A-forms decreases with further washes. If a chelating agent, such as EDTA, is then added to the above solution, and the pellet re-extracted,the new supernatant is again enriched in asymmetric AChE forms suggesting that the presence of EDTA in the homogenization medium causes the selective release of a different subpopulation of collagen-tailed AChE forms. The first pool of asymmetric AChE species (salt-extractable) has been tentatively termed class I, while the A-forms selectively extracted by EDTA, in the presence of high salt, have been included in class II. The muscle class II AChE molecules are most likely identical to those solubilized, under the same conditions, from CNS portions of higher vertebrates (9, 11). As seen in Fig. 1B, the presence of the non-ionic detergent Triton X-100 does not modify the overall results (see data in legend to Fig. 1). The same is true when small amounts of Ca^{++} (2mM) are present in the first four extractions (before EDTA)(Fig. 1C). The potential interest of this fact will be discussed later.

Fig. 2A shows the sedimentation profile of the molecular forms of AChE present in the pooled Tris/NaCl extracts of Fig. 1A, while Fig. 2C corresponds to the molecular species found in the pooled Tris/

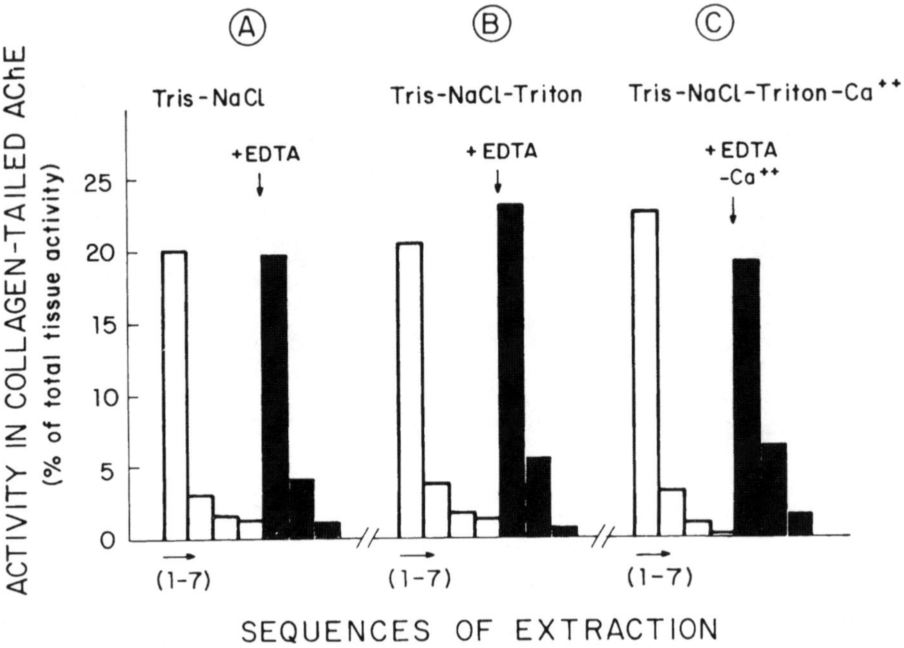

Fig. 1. Sequential extractions of chick skeletal muscle in different solutions: yield of collagen-tailed forms of AChE. Samples of mixed chick leg muscles were homogenized in the solutions indicated in the figure (concentrations: Tris.HCl, pH 7, 10mM; NaCl, 1M; Triton X-100, 1%(v/v); $CaCl_2$, 2mM) and centrifuged at 110,000g/2°C for 30 min. The supernatants were set aside and the pellets were re-homogenized as above. After four such cycles of extraction the differ ent solutions were supplemented with EDTA to a final concentration of 2mM (in series C, Ca^{++} was also discontinued, and 4mM EDTA was rather used to neutralize the previously added Ca^{++}) and the pellets extracted three more times under the new conditions. All seven supernatants of each series were analyzed by sucrose gradient centrifugation (154,000g/4°C/18-20 hours) to measure the activity in the peaks containing collagen-tailed forms. The activity of the A-forms in each extract has been expressed as % of the total tissue AChE activity, as measured in the initial homogenate. White (empty) bars: A-forms in EDTA-less extracts (class I). Black bars: A-forms in EDTA-containing extracts (class II). Total recovery of A-forms: A, 26/25; B, 28/31; C, 27/27 (class I/class II, respectively).

NaCl/EDTA extracts of Fig. 1A. That the A-forms (A_{12} and A_8) present in these two pools do not belong to the same class of collagen-tailed molecules, is further illustrated by their different behavior when Ca^{++} is added to the above extracts right after high

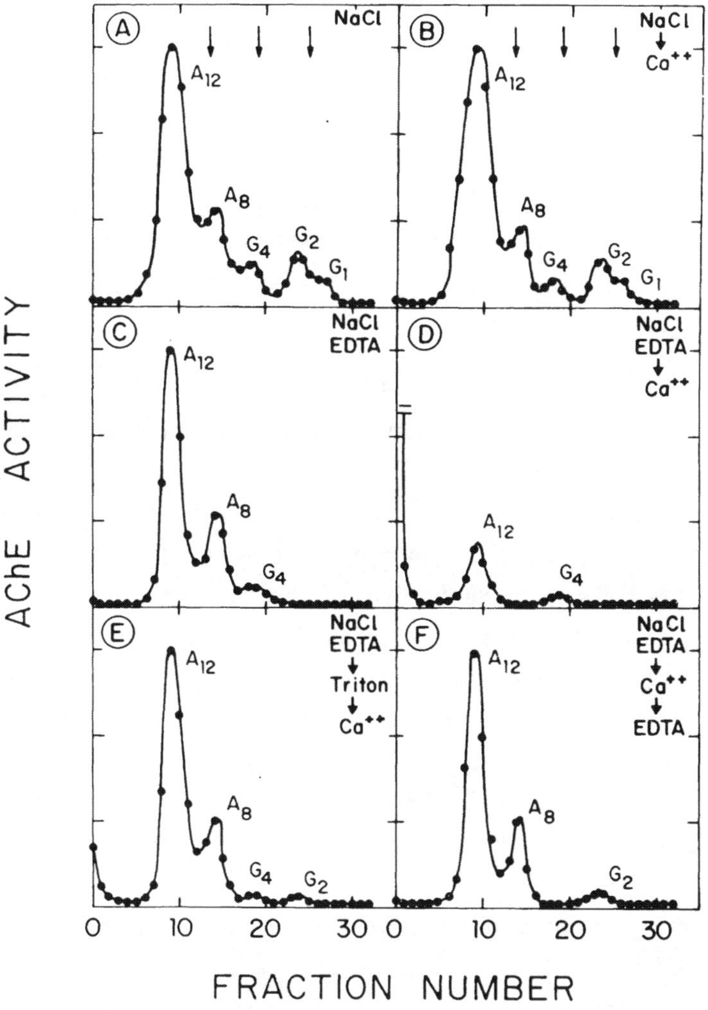

Fig. 2. Effects of Ca^{++} on class I and class II asymmetric molecular forms of chick skeletal muscle AChE. Samples of chick leg muscle were extracted sequentially as described in Fig. 1, series A. The first four extracts (no EDTA) were pooled, and the same was done with the three EDTA-containing extracts. The first pool, containing class I asymmetric forms, was divided in two portions: one was used as control (A), and $CaCl_2$ was added to the other one, to a final concentration of 2mM (B). The second pool, containing the class II asymmetric forms, was divided in four aliquots: the first (C) served as control; a second one (D) received $CaCl_2$ to a final concentration of 6mM (for a theoretical free Ca^{++} concentration of about 2mM after neutralization of EDTA present in the sample); the third one was made up to 1% (v/v) in Triton X-100 before adding

Ca^{++} as above (E); the last one (F) received $CaCl_2$ as in D and, after 5 min, was supplemented with EDTA up to 10mM. All six samples were analyzed by sucrose gradient centrifugation (in the modified media) and the fractions were assayed for AChE and marker enzyme activities (9). The different AChE peaks have been named according to Massoulié and coworkers (1). Actual sedimentation coefficients were: A_{12}, 19.8; A_8, 15.1; G_4, 11.6 (11.0 in E); G_2, 7.4 (6.5 in E); G_1, 5.2 (Svedberg units). No differences in sedimentation were observed between class I and class II A-forms. The arrows in the top of each panel point to the position of marker enzymes in the gradient, namely, from left to right, β-galactosidase (16S), catalase (11.3S) and alkaline phosphatase (6.1S).

---

speed centrifugation of the respective homogenates: while the profile of A-forms in the high salt extract (class I) remains unchanged (Fig. 2B), most of the A-forms in the high salt/EDTA extract (class II) aggregate in the presence of Ca^{++} and sediment to the bottom of the tube (Fig. 2D). This aggregation can be reversed by excess EDTA as shown in Fig. 2F. Also, as described in the case of retina (9), addition of Triton X-100 to the supernatant before adding Ca^{++} seems to counteract the effect of this cation (Fig. 2E). Actually, if after addition of Ca^{++} to the high salt/EDTA supernatant we centrifuge it at high speed, instead of layering it directly on top of a sucrose gradient, we find that, in the absence of Triton X-100, 93-100% of the class II A-forms are present in the pellet (vs. 54% recovered in the bottom of the gradient in Fig. 2D), and even when Ca^{++} is added after Triton X-100 the pellet contains close to 80% of them (while in the profile in Fig. 2E only 1-6% of the A-forms are found in the bottom of the tube). All this suggests that the Ca^{++} bridges hypothetically linking the tail of class II A-forms to the membrane do so by means of some anionic molecules (Fig. 3, X) hydrophobically bound to the collagen-like tail (9). These molecules seem to be slowly removed from the tail by Triton X-100, so that, in spite of the initial aggregation by Ca^{++} of class II A-forms in the presence of Triton (≈80%), most of them are finally released from the aggregates after the usual 20 hours of sedimentation (Fig. 2E). The association between the tail and these molecules is not completely stable even in the absence of detergent, as illustra-

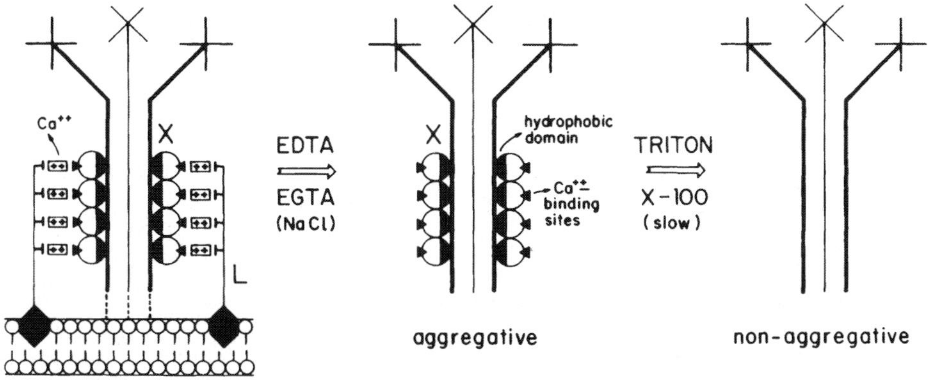

Fig. 3. Proposed working model for the attachment of class II AChE A-forms to membranes. In our hypothesis, the tail is coated with some unknown molecules (X) having both a hydrophobic domain (detergent-sensitive), interacting with the tail protein, and an anionic site neutralizing one of the Ca^{++} positive charges. The other charge is neutralized by L, a macromolecular complex (probably a chain of molecules) anchoring the enzyme to the membrane matrix. Chelating agents, such as EDTA and EGTA, release the tail from the membrane by dissociating Ca^{++} bridges. EDTA-dissociated A-forms (center) can be aggregated by excess Ca^{++} since the tails are still coated with the bifunctional molecule X. Exposure of the tail to non-ionic detergents, such as Triton X-100, slowly removes the X molecules from the tail thus giving rise to a non-aggregative A-form probably identical to class I forms (right). Other interactions between the A molecules and the membrane (for instance, the ionic strength-sensitive bonds) have not been considered in this model.

---

ted by the peak of A_{12} appearing in Fig. 2D, which corresponds to the difference between the initial precipitation by Ca^{++} of class II A-forms (almost 100%) and the 50-60% recovered in the bottom of the gradient in Fig. 2D. Fig. 3 summarizes this tentative model of attachment of class II collagen-tailed AChE to cholinergic membranes. As said before (9), the structural requirements for the tail-linked molecule bearing the Ca^{++}-binding anionic site could be met by a phospholipid. On the other hand, the slow effect of Triton X-100 is a likely explanation for the failure of the detergent to solubilize class II A-forms in the absence of EDTA (the solubilization of small amounts of A_{12} from chick retina by sodium cholate described in (6)

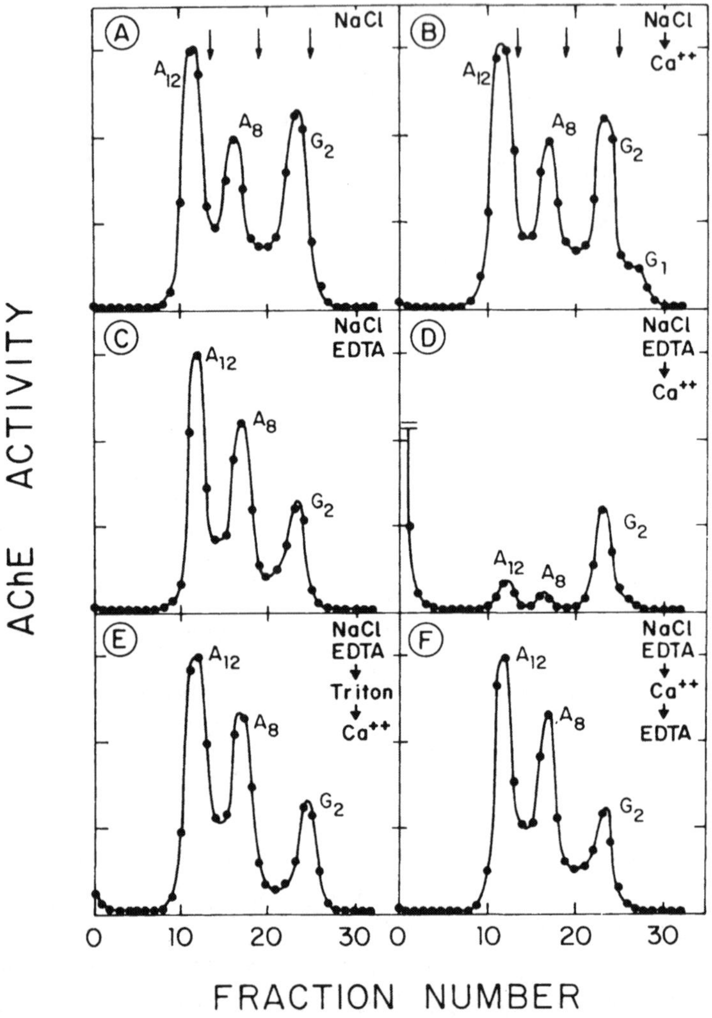

Fig. 4. Effects of Ca^{++} on class I and class II asymmetric molecular forms of *Torpedo marmorata* electric organ tissue. Electric organ tissue from young *Torpedo* fishes, kept previously frozen at -90°C, was processed exactly as described in Fig. 2. Sedimentation coefficients: A_{12}, 17.5; A_8, 13.5; G_4, 11.3; G_2, 7.5 (6.2 in E); G_1, 5.0. Other details as in Fig. 2.

---

should be attributed to the mild chelating properties of cholate rather than to a primary detergent effect). Thus, the three sequential extraction schedules illustrated in Fig. 1 give essentially the same results, EDTA being always necessary to release class II A-forms under the standard experimental conditions. Incidentally, we have shown that class II A-forms are degraded to globular forms, in the case of chick retina, if EDTA is not present in the first homogenization (19). This is not however the case in chick skeletal muscle and other tissues containing both classes of A-forms (Fig. 1, and our unpublished results).

Although Ca^{++} shows much more efficiency and specificity, Mg^{++},in concentrations over 40-50mM, produces the aggregation of class II A-forms and prevents their solubilization ((9), and our unpublished results). Thus, while class I A-forms can be efficiently extracted and solubilized by concentrated Mg^{++} solutions (20,21) this same cation blocks the release of class II molecules. Not surprisingly, it has been commonly held that EDTA increases the yield of A-forms, while Ca^{++} and Mg^{++} have been reported, in a few cases, to partially block the solubilization of erythrocyte or electric organ AChE (22,23). In Fig. 4 we present the results of an experiment similar to that of Fig. 2 but performed with electric organ tissue from *Torpedo marmorata*. All the conclusions derived from the results in Fig. 2 apply equally here. The properties of the two classes of A-forms in electric tissue explain the results previously reported by Dudai and Silman (23).

<u>Existence of two classes of asymmetric forms of AChE in different tissues and vertebrate species</u>. We have chosen skeletal muscle and electric organ samples for the experiments described so far in view of the extended use of both tissues as sources of AChE for structural studies (1). However, as we will presently show, the facts established in the first part of this paper seem to apply to practically all cholinergic structures and vertebrate species studied in our laboratory.

To achieve a reasonably fast but accurate screening of a wide variety of tissues we have adopted an alternative extraction procedure so that equivalent samples of the same tissue or area have been extracted with either 10mM Tris.HCl, pH 7/1M NaCl/1%(v/v) Triton

TABLE 1

AChE activity of class I and class II collagen-tailed forms in different tissues and vertebrate species.

Species	Tissue	Total	I	II	I/II
		(% of total tissue activity)			
Torpedo	Electric organ	46	32	14	2.3
Trout	Retina	5.5	4.5	1	4.5
	'Brain'	12	8	4	2.0
	Cerebellum	30	22	8	2.8
	Skeletal muscle	69	65	4	16.3
	Smooth muscle	15	9	6	1.5
	Heart	13	4	9	0.5
Frog	'Brain'	7	5.5	1.5	3.7
	Cerebellum	12	8.3	3.7	2.3
	Skeletal muscle	45	17	28	0.6
	Smooth muscle	5.4	1.2	4.2	0.3
Chick	Retina	9.2	0.8	8.4	0.1
	Skeletal muscle	55	27	28	1.0
	Smooth muscle	44	26	18	1.5
	Heart	5	0	5	0
Rat	Skeletal muscle	27	10	17	0.6
	Smooth muscle	23	6	17	0.4
	Heart	5	0	5	0
Rabbit	Cerebellum	5	2	3	0.7
	Skeletal muscle	55	30	25	1.2
	Smooth muscle	38	8	30	0.3

Equivalent samples of the different tissues were alternatively homogenized in 10mM Tris.HCl, pH 7/1M NaCl/1%(v/v) Triton X-100/2mM $CaCl_2$ or 10mM Tris.HCl, pH 7/1M NaCl/1% (v/v) Triton X-100/2mM EDTA. The homogenates were centrifuged at 110,000g/2°C for 30 min and the supernatants set aside. The pellets were re-extracted twice in the same media and the three supernatants of each kind were pooled. Aliquots of these pools were analyzed for molecular forms of AChE by su crose gradient centrifugation (9). Class I A-forms were taken as the A-forms present in the Ca^{++}-containing extracts. Class II A-forms were estimated as the difference between the A-forms present in EDTA-containing extracts (all tissue A-forms) and the class I A-forms. For a given type of sample, both classes of A-forms had identical sedimentation coefficients and responded equally to collagenase digestion. The term 'brain' refers to the cranial contents ex cept the cerebellum. Skeletal muscle samples are mixed muscle samples. Smooth muscle samples have been taken from the stomach wall (the gizzard in the case of chick). Heart samples are from the left ventricle. Values given are % of total tissue AChE activity, and are the mean of 2-9 experiments.

X-100/2mM $CaCl_2$ (class I A-forms) or 10mM Tris.HCl, pH 7/1M NaCl/ 1% (v/v) Triton X-100/2mM EDTA (all A-forms). The presence of small amounts of Ca^{++}, while not affecting the solubilization of class I collagen-tailed AChE, may prevent even minimal leakages of the class II A-forms after several washes (compare yields of the fourth extraction in series A, B and C of Fig. 1). Furthermore, the use of Triton X-100, which does not modify the recovery of class I and class II A-forms, helps to avoid trapping of collagen-tailed forms in tissue pellets, and leads to higher recoveries of AChE activity. In Table 1 we give some of the results of this screening procedure applied to representative tissues and animal species. Although a detailed analysis of these results is beyond the scope of the present report we see that, as a general rule, lower vertebrates have higher I/II ratios than higher vertebrates. CNS tissues of higher vertebrates contain almost exclusively class II A-forms, albeit in small proportions (11). We also notice that A-forms are usually present , in substantial proportions, in both smooth muscle and heart muscle. The fact that these A-forms are mostly class II, requiring EDTA for their solubilization, has probably hampered their previous identification (24). In any case, a correct interpretation of data in Table 1 has to wait until the distinctive physiological roles of class I and class II A-forms can be elucidated.

Physiological significance of the two classes of collagen-tailed AChE forms. The contrasting solubilization properties of class I and class II A-forms seem to reflect different mechanisms of attachment to cell membranes. We have chosen five criteria, including topographic and functional aspects, to look for associated differences in subcellular localization and/or function. Our results (not shown) can be summarized as follows. Concerning the synaptic/extrasynaptic alternative we have found, in the rat diaphragm, that both endplate and non-endplate regions contain the two classes of collagen-tailed forms. The same appears to be true when using the extracellular/intracellular criterion, also in the rat diaphragm, although there is a relative enrichment of class I forms in the intracellular pool, and of class II forms in the extracellular pool. We have also considered the alternative nicotinic/muscarinic; however, a close examination of data in Table 1 shows that typically nicotinic and muscarinic cholinergic tissues contain variable proportions of both classes of tailed enzyme. A fourth criterion, though limited in scope, has been, in the case of muscle, the possible preferential association of either class of A-forms to fast vs. slow fibers; however, both the *posterior latissimus dorsi* and the *anterior latissimus dorsi* muscles of the chick contain equal relative proportions of class I and class II A-forms. Finally, we have started to look for differential effects of denervation on both classes of enzyme forms in chick leg muscles with the preliminary conclusion that class I A-forms seem to disappear faster than class II after sciatic nerve section.

Our apparent failure to find clear-cut physiological differences between class I and class II A-forms, with the above criteria, does not rule out the possibility of more subtle differences in local regulation or catalytic activity *in situ*. This would be, perhaps, more in line with the loose evolutionary trend that can be appreciated in our previous (11) and present (Table 1) 'phylogenetic' studies.

Acknowledgements

This work was supported by grants from the Comisión Asesora de Investigación Científica y Técnica, Plan Nacional de Prevención de la Subnormalidad y Fondo de Investigaciones Sanitarias. C.R.-B. is a fellow of Caja de Ahorros y M. de P. de Madrid.

References

1. Massoulié, J., Bon, S.: Ann. Rev. Neurosci. 5, 57-106 (1982).
2. Rieger, F., Tsuji, S., Massoulié, J.: Eur. J. Biochem. 30, 73-80 (1972).
3. Guillon, G., Massoulié, J.: Biochimie 58, 465-471 (1976).
4. Massoulié, J.: Trends Biochem. Sci. 5, 160-164 (1980).
5. Villafruela, M.J., Barat, A., Villa, S., Ramírez, G.: FEBS Letters 110, 91-95 (1980).
6. Barat, A., Escudero, E., Gómez-Barriocanal, J., Ramírez, G.: Neurosci. Letters 20, 205-210 (1980).
7. Barat, A., Escudero, E., Gómez-Barriocanal, J., Ramírez, G.: Biochem. Biophys. Res. Commun. 96, 1421-1426 (1980).
8. Rieger, F., Chételat, R., Nicolet, M., Kamal, L., Poullet, M.: FEBS Letters 121, 169-174 (1980).
9. Gómez-Barriocanal, J., Barat, A., Escudero, E., Rodríguez-Borrajo, C., Ramírez, G.: J. Neurochem. 37, 1239-1249 (1981).
10. Ramírez, G., Rodríguez-Borrajo, C., Barat, A., Escudero, E., Gómez-Barriocanal, J.: Int. Soc. Neurochem. Abstr. 8, 366 (1981).
11. Rodríguez-Borrajo, C., Barat, A., Ramírez, G.: Neurochem. Int. 4, 563-568 (1982).
12. Witzemann, V., Boustead, C.: Neurosci. Letters 26, 313-318 (1981).
13. Nicolet, M., Rieger, F.: Neurosci. Letters 28, 67-73 (1982).
14. Barat, A., Escudero, E., Rodríguez-Borrajo, C., Ramírez, G.: Neurochem. Int. 5, 95-99 (1983).
15. Witzemann, V., Boustead, C.: J. Neurochem. 39, 747-755 (1982).
16. Bon, S.: Neurochem. Int. 4, 577-585 (1982).
17. Bon, S., Cartaud, J., Massoulié, J.: Eur. J. Biochem. 85, 1-14 (1978).
18. Bon, S., Vigny, M., Massoulié, J.: Proc. Natl. Acad. Sci. USA 76, 2546-2550 (1979).
19. Gómez-Barriocanal, J., Rodriguez-Borrajo, C., Barat, A., Ramírez, G.: Neurosci. Letters 38, 321-326 (1983).
20. Allemand, P., Bon, S., Massoulié, J., Vigny, M.: J. Neurochem. 36, 860-867 (1981).
21. Lee, S.L., Heinemann, S., Taylor, P.: J. Biol. Chem. 257, 12283-12291 (1982).

22. Burger, S.P., Fujii, T., Hanahan, D.J.: Biochemistry 7, 3682-3700 (1968).

23. Dudai, Y., Silman, I.: FEBS Letters 30, 49-52 (1973).

24. Skau, K., Brimijoin, S.: J. Neurochem. 35, 1151-1154 (1980)

TAILED, ASYMMETRIC ACETYLCHOLINESTERASE AND SKELETAL MUSCLE BASAL LAMINA IN VERTEBRATES -

Subcellular Location ; "Hydrophilic" and "Hydrophobic" Variants .

Marc Nicolet

Laboratoire de Physiologie Animale, Faculté des Sciences, Besançon, France.

François Rieger, Patrick Dreyfus, Martine Pinçon-Raymond and Lam Tran

Groupe de Biologie et Pathologie Neuromusculaires
INSERM U 153, Paris, France.

INTRODUCTION

Tailed, asymmetric acetylcholinesterase (AChE) has been detected all along vertebrate muscle fibers, and is often highly concentrated in muscle regions rich in motor end-plates (MEP), which has been demonstrated in both rat (1, 2, 3) or mouse (4) muscle. However, tailed, asymmetric AChE has been found to be equally distributed in MEP-free and -rich regions in muscle fibers, isolated from man (5), chick (6) or frog (7). The vertebrate neuromuscular junction is always characterized by a high cytochemically-demonstrated AChE accumulation (8). In frog muscle (9), part of this concentrated enzyme has been shown to be associated with the basal lamina sheaths (BLs). The discovery of the head-tail structure (10, 11) of asymmetric forms (12) of electric fish AChE and its structural (10, 11, 13) and chemical (14, 15, 16, 17) similarities with collagen, suggests that AChE may be specifically located in the muscle basal lamina.

In order to determine whether indeed tailed, asymmetric AChE is located in muscle basal lamina, we directly approached the problem of its subcellular location by studying 3 different biological systems : (i) a genetic condition, characterized by the lack of basal lamina in developing mouse muscle, the muscular dysgenesis (mdg) mutation (18, 19), (ii) the isolated mouse neuromuscular junction (20, 21)(iii) the frog muscle basal lamina sheaths preparation (9). We report here that tailed asymmetric AChE is indeed found in all muscle basal lamina studied. However, when basal lamina is absent, in the mdg/mdg mouse embryo, tailed asymmetric AChE is still partially present. We further found that tailed, asymmetric AChE is also associated to internal, microsomal membranes in adult mouse muscle. In frog, not only tailed but also globular forms of AChE were detected in the basal lamina. In addition, an hydrophobic variant of tailed AChE was found, that constitutes its major component in the mouse microsomal membranes and in the BLs of frog muscle.

MATERIAL AND METHODS

1 - Animals : the mdg mutation is propagated by brother-sister mating of heterozygote +/mdg mice (129 ReJ strain). Dated pregnancies were performed, day 0 being the day of vaginal plug discovery. Subcellular fractionation of mouse muscle and isolation of neuromuscular junctionswas performed with intercostal muscles dissected rib cages from 3 week old mice (C3H strain wild-type). Adult frogs (Rana temporaria L.) were kept in water tanks and experiments were performed during the winter period.

2 - Mdg tissues: Fore and hindlimbs or diaphragm from 13 to 19 day mouse embryos were dissected after caesarean delivery and further processed for electron microscopy or biochemistry as described below.

3 - Subcellular fractionation of mouse muscle : the intercostal muscles and ribs were homogenized, after dissection, in a Krebs medium as previously described (20, 21). Briefly, homogenization was performed in a Polytron (1 min) and the homogenate filtered and centrifuged at low

speed. The pellet was layered on a discontinuous sucrose gradient, after resuspension (layers : 1.8 M, 1.4 M, 1M and 0.6 M sucrose). After 2 hours of sedimentation (SW 27 rotor ; 10,000 g) the main fractions obtained were from the meniscus to the bottom : a soluble supernatant, and three bands (fraction A ; fraction B ; fractions C1 and C2) and a pellet. After dilution and centrifugation, the pellets were resuspended and will be refered to as the primary fractions.

4 - Biological preparation of frog basal lamina sheaths (BLs) :
The experimental procedure described by Mc Mahan et al (9) was performed on the cutaneus pectoris muscle, and contralateral muscle used as control muscle. On day 0, after MS 222 (Sandoz) anaesthesia, the nerve to the left cutaneus pectoris muscle was sectioned and a 4-7 mm nerve segment proximal to muscle excised. Two rectangular slabs were removed from the muscle, on each side of the main intramuscular nerve trunk, leaving a bridge, 1.5 mm wide of degenerating muscle (fig. 1).

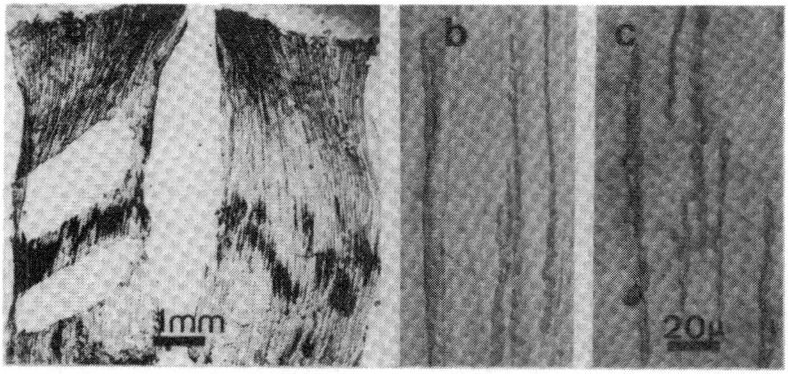

Fig. 1. Normal and operated cutaneus pectoris frog muscle. a. Whole intact muscle and bridge (BLs). b, c. AChE cytochemical staining of MEP-rich muscle fiber (b) and BLs (c).

On day 2, the experimental muscle was X-irradiated. Internal muscle cell components and nerve terminals degenerate, are phagocytized by macrophages and the bridge, after 2 weeks, is mainly composed of the BLs of the MEP-rich region of the muscle. Mild extraction by a detergent medium was sometimes performed to obtain pure BLs material.

5 - Light and electron microscopy (EM) : AChE cytochemistry was performed by a modification of the method of Koëlle and Friedenwald (22) and E.M. by conventional techniques (uranyl acetate ; osmium tetroxide) without or with prior AChE cytochemistry, following the method of Tsuji (23).

6 - AChE extraction : Primary fractions from the subcellular fractionation were either recentrifuged, or muscle samples from single mouse embryos or several frogs, were extracted in either a 1, 2 (mouse) or 3 (frog)-step procedure. In the 1-step procedure, AChE extraction was obtained by homogenizing the pellets or the muscle samples, in a minimal volume (200 µl) of either standard medium containing 1 M NaCl, 1 % Triton X-100, 0.001 M EGTA, 0.01 Tris-HCl pH 7.2 , high salt-only medium (NaCl, EGTA and Tris) or detergent-only medium (Triton, EGTA and Tris). In the 2-step procedure, we used detergent followed by high-salt. In the 3-step procedure (frog muscle), AChE was obtained by a mild extraction by simple incubation for 1 hour in the detergent medium, followed by homogenization in the presence of first detergent, then high salt medium.

7 - Analysis of AChE forms : extracts were layered on continuous 5-20 % sucrose gradients and the molecular forms of AChE were identified after sedimentation (Beckman L8 centrifuge ; SW 41 rotor ; 18 hours, 38,000 rpm, 4°C). Fractions were collected and assayed for AChE activity as previously described (19) by the method of Ellman et al (24). AChE peak areas were determined by computer curve analysis, with background substrate spontaneous hydrolysis subtraction.

8 - AChE inhibition by the methylphosphorothiolate derivative (MPT) and protection of extracellular AChE forms by BW 284 C 51 : MPT is a specific irreversible and cell permeant inhibitor of AChE (25, 26) ; BW 284 C 51 is a specific cell impermeant reversible AChE inhibitor. Both inhibitors were used simultaneously to determine the AChE forms which are in an extracellular location in mouse intercostal muscles. These forms were

protected by 5.10^{-6} M BW (27, 28) against irreversible inhibition by a 5 min exposure to $7.5\ 10^{-8}$ M MPT. MPT was also injected in experimental frogs (i.p. 100 µg/kg) in order to inhibit most of the preexisting enzyme in the intact cutaneus pectoris muscle or in the BLs bridge to study its recovery. All subsequent procedures in both types of experiments were performed as in sections 6 and 7.

RESULTS

1. Muscle basal lamina and tailed, asymmetric AChE in the developing normal and mutant (mdg/mdg) mouse embryo.

Tailed 16S AChE is induced in normal embryonic mouse muscle at day 12-13. As early as day 13-14, the 16S AChE induction in mdg/mdg is abnormally low (29) in both diaphragm and limb muscles, and this deficiency remains until the end of the gestation period (fig. 2), accompanied by a low induction of total AChE. The ultrastructural study of normal mdg/mdg myotubes shows that early mdg/mdg myotubes (day 14) lack a detectable basal lamina (fig. 3), which by contrast is easily identified on

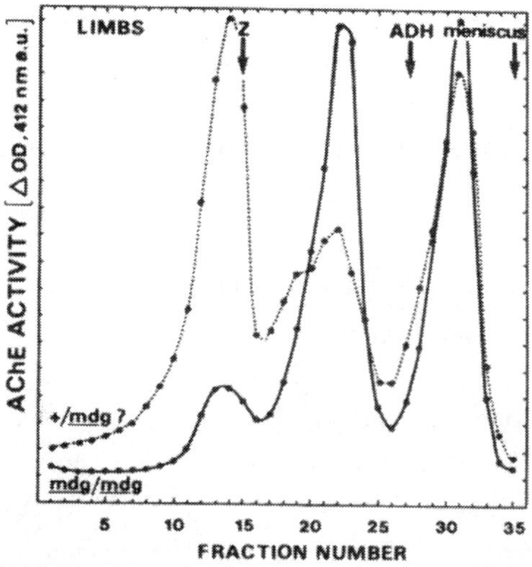

Fig. 2 : Comparison of 16S AChE in control and mdg/mdg limb muscles (end of gestation ; E 19).

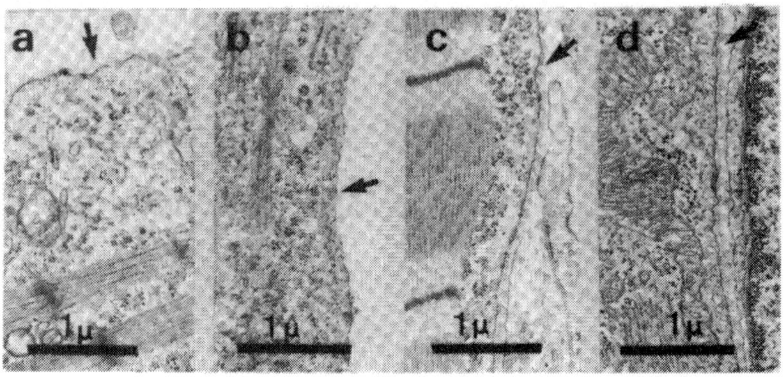

Fig. 3 : Extrasynaptic basal lamina (BL) in +/+ and mdg/mdg embryo myotubes. Embryonic day 14 (a : +/+ ; b : mdg/mdg) and 18 (c : +/+ ; d : mdg/mdg).

normal myotubes. Later in development, the basal lamina which accumulates on mdg/mdg myotubes is less electron dense than on normal myotubes. Most of normal or mutant tailed 16S AChE is extracted by the detergent medium, in both tissues. We thus compared the amount of tailed 16S AChE extracted by detergent only, to the amount extracted by detergent and high salt (single step ; standard medium). In +/+ new-born limb 9 % ± 2 (n = 4) of the detergent and high salt-extracted tailed 16S AChE can be extracted by detergent only ; in mdg/mdg, this proportion is increased to 29 % ± 9 (n = 4), demonstrating that the mutant limbs contain a rather high proportion of a "hydrophobic" tailed 16S AChE.

2. Tailed, asymmetric AChE in a subcellular fraction of mouse muscle enriched in neuromuscular junctions and a microsomal intracellular membrane fraction.

The subcellular fractionation of 3 week old mouse intercostal muscles leads to the separation of several membrane fractions. The total (per g of fresh tissue) and specific (per mg protein) contents in choline acetyltransferase (ChAT), acetylcholine receptor (AChR) and AChE are indicated in fig. 4.

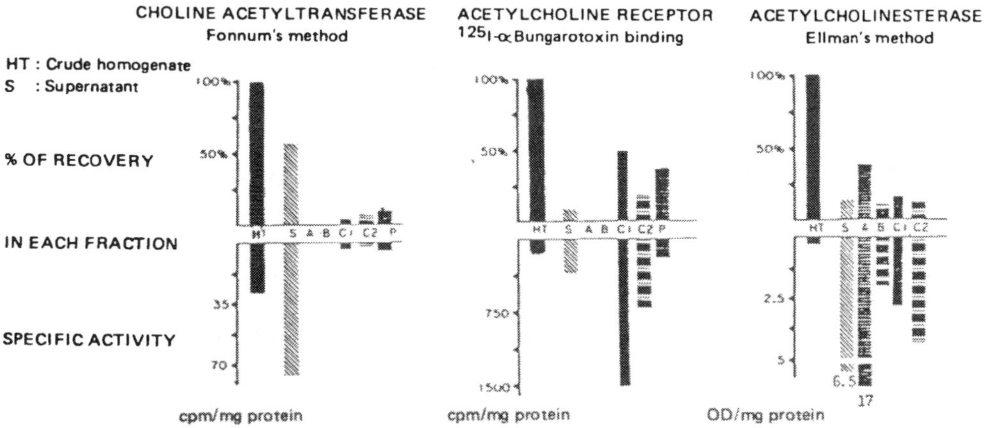

Fig. 4 : Pre- and post-synaptic elements of the mouse neuromuscular system in various subcellular fractions.

The two bands of great interest are the high density fraction C1, which contains about 50 % of all AChR, and the low density fraction A, which contains AChE at a very high specific activity. A light and electron microscopy study (20, 31) shows that fraction C1 contains mainly intact motor end-plates, with little presynaptic material (in agreement with the low ChAT recovery). An important proportion of the crude extract, tailed 16 AChE is recovered in fraction C1 but even more in fraction A (Table I).

Table I : Tailed, asymmetric 16S AChE recovery in the subcellular fractionation of mouse muscle.

	AChE activity*	Recovery (%)
Crude Homogenate	30.4 ± 2.0	100
Fraction A	14.9 ± 1.7	49
Fraction C	8.2 ± 0.3	27

* OD/hr/g fresh tissue ± SEM ; n = 3 .

We extracted AChE from the muscle crude homogenate and the primary fractions C1 and A in a sequential procedure : detergent followed by high salt. Tailed, asymmetric 16S AChE presents two different extraction characteristics in fraction C1 compared to fraction A. Most of 16S AChE is extracted by high salt in fraction C1 (85.6 ± 3.9 %) in contrast to only a minor proportion (20.4 ± 8.5 %) in fraction A, the crude homogenate showing a proportion of 74.6 ± 13.7 %. Thus, most of the tailed 16S AChE in fraction C1 (MEP-enriched) is "hydrophilic", and most of 16S AChE in the fraction A (microsomal membranes, as demonstrated by electron microscopy, data not shown) is "hydrophobic"(18, 19).

In order to further define the subcellular location of the AChE found in fraction A, we performed the BW-protection experiments of extracellular AChE on intact intercostal muscle and analyzed the fractions. Table II shows the percentage of protection of each group of AChE forms, "4S", "10S" and "16S" and average values from 3 independent experiments are indicated. It is clear that all AChE activity has been irreversibly inhibited in the fraction A, proving its intracellular location.

Table II : Protection of molecular forms of AChE by BW + MPT treated mouse muscle (% of control).

	Total AChE	"4S"	"10S"	"16S"
Crude homogenate	52.8	9.1	100	67
Fraction A	1.1	< 1	< 1	< 1

3. Presence of both "hydrophilic" and "hydrophobic" tailed, asymmetric AChE in the basal lamina sheaths (BLs) of frog muscle.

The procedure of Mc Mahan and associates (9) allows the biological preparation of myofiber ghosts, mainly composed of the BLs of the original myofiber. A light and electron microscope study shows empty BLs, with surrounding degenerating Schwann cells, nerve or muscle cellular debris, collagen fibrils and macrophages (fig. 5). The BLs have minor, although detectable, plasmic membrane remnants. AChE was extracted from control, MEP-rich regions and experimental BLs bridges, in a single step detergent and high salt procedure. Fig. 6 shows that all AChE forms are found in the BLs preparation and Table III gives the sedimentation coefficients of the various AChE forms of frog muscle. After irreversible inhi-

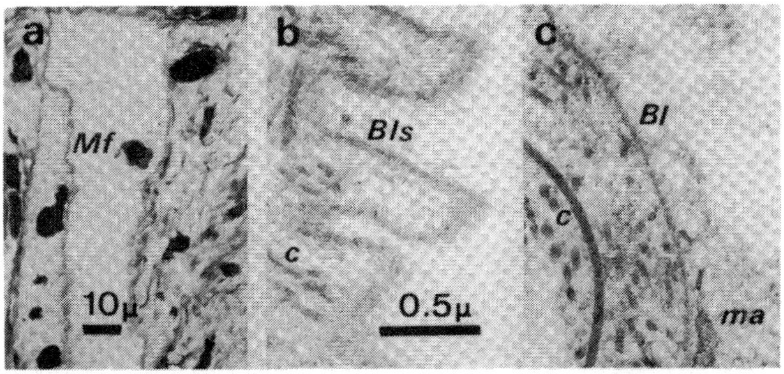

Fig. 5 : Basal lamina sheaths (BLs) preparation. a, semi-thin section (Mf. empty myofiber) ; b, c, EM (ma, macrophage ; c, collagen fibrils).

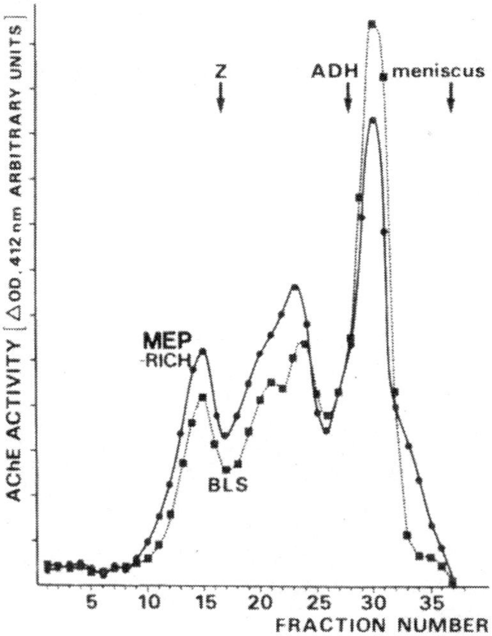

Fig. 6 : The BLs preparation of frog muscle contains the same AChE forms than the control MEP-rich region.

TABLE III : Major molecular forms of frog muscle AChE (S)

Collagenase insensitive (globular)	3.5 ± 0.11 6.1 ± 0.13 11.2 ± 0.25
	(n = 18)
Collagenase sensitive (tailed, asymmetric)	13.8 ± 0.31 18.5 ± 0.40

bition by MPT of all preexisting enzyme, AChE recovery was compared in control and BLs tissues, 52 hr and 216 hr later. All forms slowly recover in control muscle. Little (3.5 S, 6S and 11S) or no (14S and 18S) recovery are detected in the BLs (fig. 7). This experiment demonstrates that the AChE forms present in the BLs are not of an extraterritorial origin or synthesized by contaminating or invasive cells.

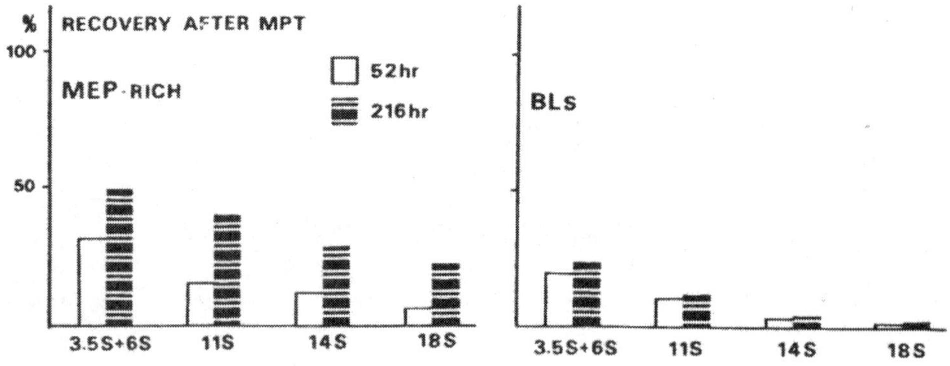

Fig. 7 : AChE recovery after MPT inhibition (% of control).

After a mild extraction of the BLs preparation by simple incubation in the detergent medium, the BLs preparation shows no cellular debris and the BLs are themselves structurally modified : the dense, centrally-located lamina has disappeared (fig. 8). These "pure" BLs were extracted by detergent and then high salt. Table IV shows that again tailed (18S) AChE is extracted in both steps, demonstrating the presence in frog muscle BLs of both "hydrophilic" and "hydrophobic" AChE, respectively as minor and major components.

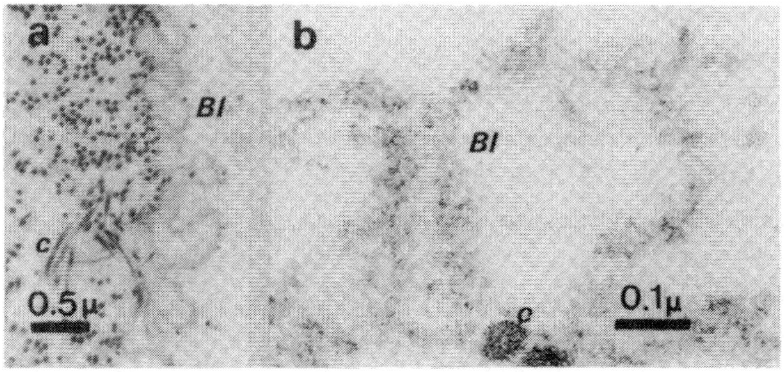

Fig. 8 : Pure BLs preparation after mild detergent extraction.

Table IV : High salt (hydrophilic) versus total* extracted tailed (18S) frog AChE.

	Hydrophilic 18S AChE (% total)	Total 18S AChE specific activity**
Control MEP-rich region (contralateral)	42.3 ± 0.99	42.6 ± 3.28
BLs (15 days)	32.1 ± 0.71	275.6 ± 6.78 (purification factor : 6.5)

* : Total 18S AChE is all 18S AChE extracted in the 3 step-procedure, from 4-8 bridges or control MEP-rich regions.

** : OD/hr/mg of protein.

DISCUSSION

Three experimental approaches, the mdg mouse mutation, the subcellular fractionation of 3 week old mouse muscle and the preparation of basal lamina in frog muscle were used to determine the location of tailed, asymmetric AChE. Our present findings demonstrate that tailed, asymmetric AChE is not only associated to the muscle basal lamina, but also to plasmic and sarcoplasmic membranes.

The mdg mutation is characterized by a lack of muscle basal lamina during early embryogenesis (29) and a low level of tailed AChE (21, 29). The paucity of tailed AChE cannot be simply due to the absence of any spontaneous or nerve-triggered contractile activity observed in mdg/mdg muscle, since we recently gathered evidence for normal nerve-triggered muscle electrical activity in mdg/mdg muscle in vivo (30, 31). Also, the levels of tailed asymmetric AChE are regulated by action potential generation which are normal, in mdg/mdg muscle,and not by contractile activity (32). Thus, the lack or immaturity of BL is probably the cause of the tailed 16S deficiency in muscular dysgenesis. However, some tailed 16S AChE is present, and has a more pronounced "hydrophobic" character. Thus, its location must be either the plasmic membrane or the sarcoplasmic reticulum.

The subcellular fractionation of 3 week old mouse muscle gives two fractions possessing very different properties. The fraction C1 is a high-density fraction, enriched in neuromuscular junctions, in which most of the tailed 16S AChE is high salt-soluble and not extracted by detergent. This 16S AChE is thus BL associated and "hydrophobic" in nature (18, 19). The fraction A is a low density fraction, rich in microsomal membranes of an intracellular origin, as demonstrated by permeant-non permeant inhibitor protection experiments. The existence of a small internal pool of 16S AChE has recently been reported in rat diaphragm (33), which is in agreement with our present findings. In fraction A, tailed 16S AChE is essentially extracted by detergent, is "hydrophobic" in nature

(20, 21) and is thus tightly incorporated into membranes, probably sarcoplasmic membranes.

The BLs preparation of frog muscle gives the most direct information on the association of AChE with the muscle extracellular matrix material. The preparation obtained is almost exclusively composed of BLs elements, with a mild extraction of the BLs bridges by detergent. In frog BLs, not only tailed, asymmetric AChE is present, but also all other forms, in almost the same proportions than in intact MEP-rich regions of muscle. Moreover, both "hydrophilic" <u>and</u> "hydrophobic" tailed 18S AChE are found in the BLs, suggesting the presence of hydrophilic and hydrophobic domains in the basal lamina. At the EM level, we observed that the mild detergent extraction eliminates the dense, central BL sheath, suggesting a high concentration of hydrophobic constituents in the central region.

Therefore, each of our 3 different approaches to the problem of the localization of tailed, asymmetric AChE at the subcellular level bring complementary information and stress the diversity of the associations of tailed, asymmetric AChE with many cellular structures, namely the basal lamina, the plasmic and the sarcoplasmic reticulum membranes. In conclusion, there is no such simple situation as generally hypothesized previously : the original suggestion that hydrophilic, tailed AChE is preferentially or exclusively associated with the muscle basal lamina needs to be modified in light of the present findings. In fact, both hydrophobic and hydrophilic tailed AChE probably coexist in BL. Also, tailed AChE is found intracellularly, suggesting an internal processing of these complex lipoglycoproteic structures.

ACKNOWLEDGEMENTS : This work was partially supported by research grants from DRET (81-399 § 82-282) and AMF (1983- to M.N).

REFERENCES

1. Hall Z.W., J. Neurobiol. <u>4</u>, 343-361 (1973).

2. Rieger F. and Vigny., J. Neurochem. 27, 121-129 (1976).
3. Vigny M., Koenig J. and Rieger F., J. Neurochem. 27, 1347-1353 (1976).
4. Rieger F., Goudou D. and Tran L.H., J. Neurochem. in press (1983).
5. Carson S., Bon S., Vigny M., Massoulie J. and Fardeau M., FEBS Lett. 97, 348-352 (1979).
6. Koenig J. and Vigny M., C.R.Soc. Biol. 172, 1069-1074 (1978).
7. Nicolet M. and Rieger F., C.R. Soc. Biol. 175, 316-322 (1981).
8. Couteaux R., Intern. Rev. Cytol. 4, 355-375 (1975).
9. Mc Mahan U.J., Sanes J.R. and Marshall L.M., Nature 271, 172-174 (1978).
10. Rieger F., Bon S., Massoulie J. and Cartaud J., Eur. J. Biochem. 34, 539-547 (1973).
11. Dudaī Y., Herzberg M. and Silman I., Proc. Natl. Acad. Sci. USA, 70, 2473-2476 (1973).
12. Bon S., Rieger F. and Massoulie J., Eur. J. Biochem. 35, 372-379 (1973).
13. Cartaud J., Rieger F., Bon S. and Massoulie J., Brain Res. 88, 127-130 (1975).
14. Lwebuga-Mukasa J.S., Lappi S. and Taylor P., Biochem. 15, 1425-1434 (1976).
15. Anglister L. and Silman I., J. Mol. Biol. 125, 292-293 (1978).
16. Johnson C.D., Smith S.P. and Russell R.L., J. Neurochem. 28, 617-624 (1977).
17. Rieger F., Ruberg M. and Shelanski M.L., Brain Res. 170, 568-571 (1979).
18. Gluecksohn-Waelsch S., Science 142, 1269-1279 (1963).
19. Rieger F. and Pinçon-Raymond M., Dev. Biol. 87, 85-101 (1981).
20. Dreyfus P. and Rieger F., in "Cholinesterases", Raven Press New-York (1983).
21. Dreyfus P., Rieger F. and Pinçon-Raymond M., Proc. Natl. Acad. Sci. USA, in press (1983).
22. Koelle G.B. and Friedenwald J.S., Proc. Soc. Exp. Med. 70, 617-622 (1949).
23. Tsuji S., Histochem. 42, 99-105 (1974).
24. Ellman G.L., Courtney M.D., Andres V. Jr and Featherstone R.M., Biochem. Pharm. 7, 88-95 (1961).
25. Vigny M., Bon S., Massoulie J. and Leterrier F., Eur. J. Biochem. 85, 317-323 (1978).

26. Goudou D. and Rieger F., Biol. Cell. in press, 1983.
27. Mc Isaac R.J. and Koelle G.B., J. Pharmacol. Exp. Ther. 126, 9-20 (1959).
28. Taylor P.B., Rieger F., Shelanski M. and Greene L.A., J. Biol. Chem. 256, 3827-3830 (1981).
29. Rieger F., Powell J.P. and Pinçon-Raymond M., Dev. Biol. in press, 1983.
30. Bournaud R., Int. Soc. Dev. Neurosci. Strasbourg, p. 190 (1980).
31. Rieger F., Bournaud R., Pinçon-Raymond M., Dreyfus P., Blondet B. and Tran L.H., Am. Soc. Neurosci., Cincinatti, p. 743 (1980).
32. Powell J.P., Rieger F. and Holmes N., Nature submitted (1983).
33. Younkin S.G., Rosenstein C., Collins P.L. and Rosenberry R.L., J. Biol. Chem. 257, 13630-13637 (1982).

Key-words : **Tailed, asymmetric AChE ; muscle basal lamina ; intracellular AChE ; Hydrophilic and hydrophobic variants.**

Subject Index : Subcellular location of tailed, asymmetric AChE.

MOLECULAR ASPECTS OF THE BIOSYNTHESIS AND DISPOSITION OF THE MULTIPLE FORMS OF ACETYLCHOLINESTERASE[1]

Palmer Taylor, Shelley Camp, Stephanie Lee, Gabriel Amitai, Susan S. Taylor, and B.P. Doctor[2]

Division of Pharmacology, M-013 H
University of California, San Diego
La Jolla, California 92093

Abstract

In the *Torpedo* electric organ both the elongated species of acetylcholinesterase which is confined to the basal lamina and the hydrophobic, dimeric species which associates with plasma membranes are present in sufficient abundance to obtain comparative information on the primary structures of the catalytic subunits. Although high pressure liquid chromatography of the corresponding tryptic peptides reveals substantial homology between the two forms, at least two of the non-oligosaccharide-containing tryptic peptides appear unique to each enzyme. Chromatographic separation of the tryptic and cyanogen bromide peptides has allowed us to identify the active site peptide, the oligosaccharide-containing peptides and surface peptides of the peripheral anionic site which react with the photoaffinity label, azidopropidium. Monoclonal antibodies have been prepared to both forms of the enzyme and while the majority show nearly equivalent reactivity with both forms of the enzyme, one shows a 100-fold selectivity for the catalytic subunit of the hydrophobic, dimeric species. Thus structural studies and the immunologic reactivity suggest that the acetylcholinesterase forms arise either as separate gene products or from distinct RNA translation products.

---

1 Supported in part by USPHS grant GM18360 and a grant from the Muscular Dystrophy Association.

2 Division of Biochemistry, Walter Reed Army Institute of Research, Washington, D.C. 20012

Introduction

Acetylcholinesterase is known to be present in two distinct classes of molecular forms: elongated species which contain several catalytic subunits disulfide-linked to a collagen-like tail unit and globular species primarily existing as simple dimers or tetramers (1). The elongated species are localized within the basal laminal of the synapse (2,3,4), whereas the globular forms are sufficiently hydrophobic to expect that they are associated with the plasma membrane (5,6). In Torpedo, both forms of the enzyme have been identified and are present in near-equal quantities (6-8). The elongated forms from Torpedo exist primarily as 17S and 13S species (2,9,10) and contain a noncollagenous structural subunit of 100,000 daltons in addition to the multiple catalytic subunits of 80,000 daltons and the smaller collagen-containing subunits (9,10). The catalytic and structural subunits are linked by disulfide bonds. The simpler globular form in Torpedo is a dimer of subunits with a sedimentation constant of 5.6S. It aggregates in the absence of detergent (6).

Characterization of the catalytic subunits from the two classes of acetylcholinesterase

If the elongated and dimeric forms of acetylcholinesterase were the result of a single gene product and m-RNA transcript, structural differences between the forms would arise from post-translational changes involving either oligosaccharide addition to the nascent protein, or the assembly of the catalytic subunits with structural subunits. Alternatively, the catalytic subunits could be encoded for by separate genes or differ in primary sequence due to alternate RNA processing. To examine these alternatives we have purified the catalytic subunits from the elongated (17S + 13S) form of Torpedo acetylcholinesterase and compared them with the purified hydrophobic dimer or 5.6S species. Selective proteolytic cleavage with trypsin removes the structural subunits from the (17 + 13)S enzyme yielding an 11S species (3,9). Gel electrophoresis indicates that the catalytic subunits remain intact during this procedure. Since the structural subunits are disulfide-linked to the catalytic subunits (3,9),

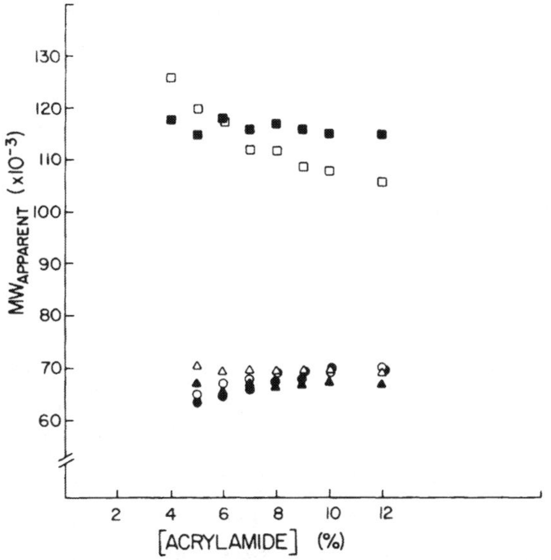

Figure 1. Electrophoretic Migration of the Catalytic Subunits from 5.6S and 11S Acetylcholinesterase as a Function of Acrylamide Concentration.

Details of the procedure are given in ref. 6. The 5.6S and 11S forms of acetylcholinesterase were purified, reduced where specified, and electrophoresed on polyacrylamide gels in the presence of sodium dodecyl sulfate. ■, 5.6S acetylcholinesterase, dimer, nonreduced; ●, 5.6S acetylcholinesterase, monomer, nonreduced; ▲, 5.6 S monomer, reduced (1% β-mercaptoethanol); □, 11S acetylcholinesterase, dimer, nonreduced; ○, 11S acetylcholinesterase, monomer, nonreduced; △, 11S acetylcholinesterase, monomer, reduced (1% β-mercaptoethanol).

small residual fragments of the structural subunits may remain linked to the catalytic subunit (11), but they can be removed following denaturation, disulfide bond reduction and dialysis.

The catalytic subunits of the two forms show different migration rates upon electrophoresis in the presence of SDS (Fig. 1). The differences are largest for the dimer of catalytic subunits where we observe that at low acrylamide concentrations, catalytic subunits from the 5.6S species migrate more rapidly than those of the 11S species, while the order of migration is reversed at high acrylamide concentrations (6). Intermediate concentrations can be selected where the catalytic subunits show indistinguishable migration rates. Since this behavior is most notable in the dimers and the carbohydrate content is very similar in the 5.6S and 11S species (6), it is likely that secondary structure contributes substantially, but not solely, to the divergent migration rates.

Following reduction of the catalytic subunits with dithiothreitol, carboxymethylation and digestion with trypsin, the tryptic peptides were separated by high pressure liquid chromatography (Fig. 2). Remarkably similar profiles for the two enzyme species are found (6). The active site peptide was identified by [^{3}H]DFP labeling of the native enzyme followed by aging to remove one of the isopropoxy groups. This peptide is found at position 36 in both catalytic subunits. Each enzyme contains seven carboxymethylcysteine-containing peptides in their catalytic subunits which appear at comparable positions. However, the profiles show a few peptides which differ in the two cases. Peptides #10 and #42 appear to be unique to the 11S species while #45 and 47 are found only in the 5.6S enzyme. Qualitative differences are also apparent in several other peptides, but their isolation would be necessary to establish them as unique peptides.

Identification of tryptic peptides in functional and surface regions of acetylcholinesterase

We have also attempted to identify the peptides which form the surface of the peripheral anionic site. Previous work has indicated that this site is unique to the acetylcholinesterases and in the native structure is greater than 20Å removed from the catalytic serine in the active center (12). To label the peripheral site we have prepared a monoazido analogue of [^{3}H]propidium and examined the profile of labeled peptides following light activation. Most of the labeling occurs in three modified peptides, migrating near positions 8, 18 and 32, with the predominate peak being near position 18. Labeling of more than a single peptide is to be anticipated for the peripheral site since the azido group is highly reactive.

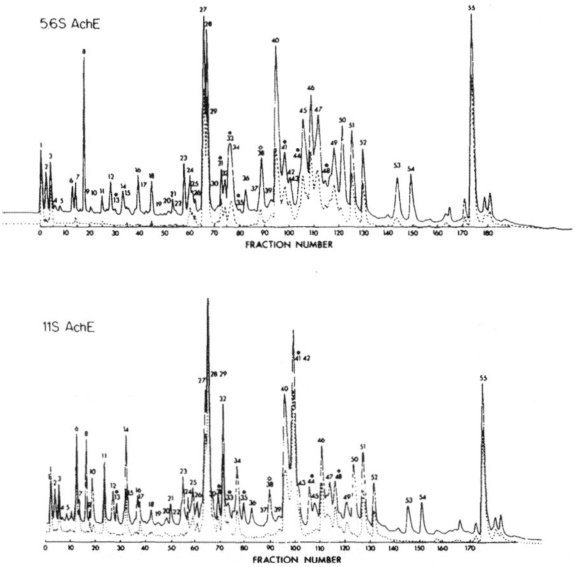

Figure 2. High Pressure Liquid Chromatography of Tryptic Peptides from Top: 5.6S (hydrophobic dimer) and Bottom: 11S Forms of Acetylcholinesterase.

Tryptic peptides were prepared from the reduced, denatured and $[^{14}C]$iodoacetate alkylated enzyme. Prior to reduction the enzymes were inhibited with $[^{3}H]$DFP and allowed to age by incubation at 25° for 18-24 hours. The tryptic hydrolyzate was placed on a reverse phase microbondapack C_{18} column and eluted with a programmed 0-50% acetonitrile gradient in 0.1% TFA/H_2O. ___, Absorbance 219 nm; ---, Absorbance 280 nm; ●, $[^{14}C]$carboxymethyl peptides; ◇, $[^{3}H]$diisopropylphosphoryl peptides. The peptides labeled with $[^{3}H]$monoazidopropidium were identified in a separate chromatographic run and found to run near positions 8, 18, and 32. Complete details of the digestion and chromatographic procedures are given in reference 14.

Secondly, multiple orientations of the ligand should be possible since previous work on competition of monovalent and divalent inorganic cations with propidium binding to the peripheral site suggests that a matrix of anionic loci may constitute this site (13). Of significance is that the same peptide(s) are not labeled by [^{3}H]DFP and [^{3}H]azidopropidium. Since an active site peptide containing more than 45 residues (>5,000 daltons) can be isolated after cyanogen bromide cleavage, a more rigorous test of the non-identity of the active center and peripheral site surfaces should come from CNBr peptide isolation.

The catalytic subunits from the hydrophobic dimer and the elongated species of acetylcholinesterase contain 5-7% carbohydrate and the overall composition would indicate that the oligosaccharides are asparagine N-linked rather than O-linked sugars. To identify the oligosaccharide-containing peptides, we have adsorbed the tryptic peptides on to columns of wheat germ agglutinin, ricin-I and pea lectin linked to Sepharose. Seven peptides have been tentatively identified as oligosaccharide-containing. We might expect that this number is incomplete since oligosaccharide-containing peptides of low absorbance at 230 nm may go undetected in these profiles. Differences in the profiles of tryptic peptides appear in regions where we have been unable to detect oligosaccharides. A more complete analysis of the oligosaccharide-containing peptides is underway (A. Drotar, A.N. Miller and P. Taylor) since elucidation of the post-translational modifications of acetylcholinesterase will be critical to future considerations on the structure and biosynthesis of the enzyme.

Antigenic differences in the molecular forms of acetylcholinesterase

Our early studies with polyclonal antibodies did not uncover a significant antibody titer which was selective for the structural subunits of the asymmetric (17 + 13S) species of acetylcholinesterase (2). In contrast, monoclonal antibody production has yielded clones with the requisite specificity for studies on the localization and structure of the various acetylcholinesterase forms (14). Although most of the antibodies showed little difference in reactivity, one denoted as 4F-3 was selective for the asymmetric (17 + 13S) species (Fig. 3) and its reactivity was lost following treatment of the enzyme with collagenase or trypsin. Western blots show slight reactivity with the position of the tail subunits (~48,000 daltons), although the antibody also reacts with a lower molecular weight fraction.

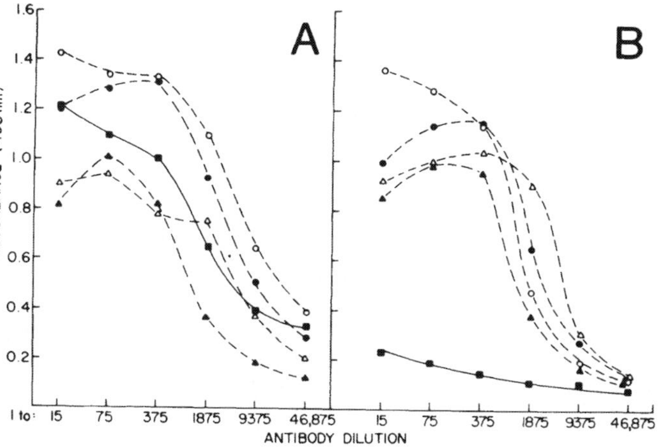

Figure 3. Specificity of Five Monoclonal Antibodies Raised against a Mixture of (17 + 13)S and 5.6S Acetylcholinesterase:

The monoclonal antibodies were obtained from the culture supernatant of the hybridoma cell lines and partially purified by $(NH_4)_2SO_4$ precipitation. Assay was done by the enzyme-linked immunoadsorbent method using peroxidase coupled rabbit antimouse IgG + IgM as the second antibody. Panel A: Reaction with (17 + 13)S acetylcholinesterase. Panel B: Reaction with 5.6S acetylcholinesterase: o, 4E7; •, 4D1, Δ, 4G1; ▲, 2C8; ■, 4F3. Note that 4F3 shows a selectivity for the asymmetric forms of acetylcholinesterase. See reference 14 for details on the isolation of the antibodies.

A second antibody, 4E-7, exhibits a 100-fold selectivity for the catalytic subunits of the hydrophobic, dimeric (5.6S) species (Fig. 4). Immunoblots also show reactivity with the migration positions of the 5.6S enzyme. Since the specificity of the antibody for the 5.6S enzyme is also retained after denaturation, the monoclonal antibodies should prove useful in the identification of domains of primary structure within the catalytic subunits that differ between the two forms.

Structural differences between the molecular forms of acetylcholinesterase

Our studies with antibody selectivity and peptide mapping indicate that the various molecular forms of acetylcholinesterase do not arise solely from different assembly processes for identical catalytic subunits. Rather, we should consider regulatory steps occurring at levels of transcription and translation. The forms of acetylcholinesterase could arise

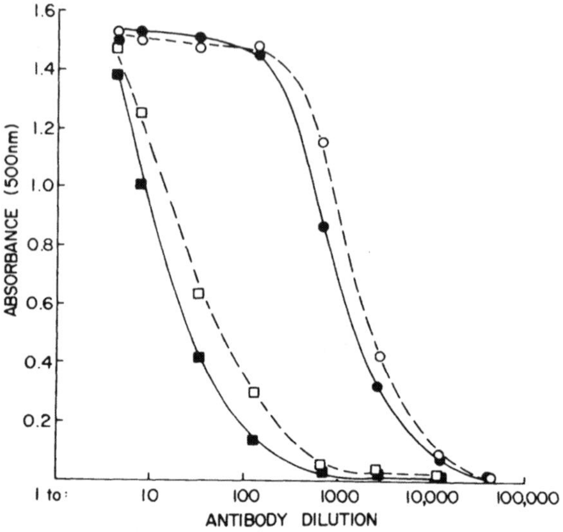

Figure 4. Specificity of Monoclonal Antibody, 4E7 for the 5.6S (hydrophobic dimer) and 11S (lytic form derived from the elongated species) Acetylcholinesterase.

Denaturation of acetylcholinesterase was carried out in 6 M guanidine HCl and the sample dialyzed: ■, native 11S; □, denatured 11S; ○, native 5.6S; ●, denatured 5.6S. The assay procedure was identical to that in Fig. 3.

as separate gene products. Alternatively, through message processing a single mRNA could give rise to acetylcholinesterase species with distinct, but closely homologous, sequences (15). Isolation of the m-RNA and c-DNA species should enable one to distinguish between these alternatives.

The study of the biosynthesis and assembly of acetylcholinesterase

Future studies on the biosynthesis of acetylcholinesterase can be expected to include two complementary approaches. The first would employ cell culture systems that secrete acetylcholinesterase where precursor-labeled amino acids can be followed through formation of the nascent chains, the post-translational processing steps and export from the cell. The chief advantage of this approach is that it employs an intact cellular system. However, since acetylcholinesterase is in low abundance in the known cell lines and primary cultures, characterization of the enzyme forms and isolation of the appropriate m-RNA's will provide formidable obstacles.

Alternatively, biosynthesis could be examined in the electric organ where quantities of the enzyme are large and the gene products can be characterized. Since these electrocyte cells have not been maintained in cultures, the examination of precursor-product relationships will be limited by cell viability. However, biosynthesis and post-translational processing can still be approached using an _in vitro_ protein synthesis system. With acetylcholinesterase in high abundance, both the gene products and the corresponding m-RNA's should be amenable to characterization. Torpedo provides an ideal system for _in vitro_ protein synthesis work since both forms of the enzyme are present in substantial quantities and in near equal abundance.

Over the past decade, the multiple forms of acetylcholinesterase have been characterized and their location in various tissues documented. Moreover, their dispositions are under precise regulatory control and factors such as synapse formation, denervation, muscle activity and development all affect the disposition and relative abundance of the enzyme forms. In the coming years, we can expect that the tools of molecular biology and protein chemistry will enable us to examine the mechanism of regulation of biosynthesis and cellular disposition of this enzyme.

References

1. Massoulie, J. and Bon, S.: Ann. Rev. Neurosciences _5_, 57-106 (1982).
2. Lwebuga-Mukasa, J., Lappi, S. and Taylor, P.: Biochemistry _15_, 1425-1434 (1976).
3. Rosenberry, T.L. and Richardson, J.M. Biochemistry _16_, 3550-3558 (1977).
4. Anglister, L. and Silman, I. J. Mol. Biol. _125_, 293-311 (1978).
5. Ott, P. and Brodbeck, U. Eur. J. Biochem. 88, 119-125 (1978).

6. Lee, S.L., Camp, S.J. and Taylor, P.: J. Biol. Chem. 257, 12302-12309 (1982).

7. Viratelli, O.M. and Bernhard, S.A.: Biochemistry 19, 4999-5007 (1980).

8. Bon, S. and Massoulie, J. Proc. Natl. Acad. Sci. USA 77, 4464-4468 (1980).

9. Lee, S.L., Heinemann, S., and Taylor, P.: J. Biol. Chem. 257, 12283-12291 (1982).

10. Lee, S.L. and Taylor, P.: J. Biol. Chem. 25, 12292-12301 (1982).

11. Mays, C. and Rosenberry, T.L. Biochemistry 20, 2810-2817 (1981).

12. Berman, H.A., Yguerabide, J. and Taylor, P. Biochemistry 19, 2226-2235 (1980).

13. Taylor, P. and Lappi, S. Biochemistry 14, 1989-1997 (1975).

14. Doctor, B.P., Camp, S., Gentry, M.K., Taylor, S.S. and Taylor, P. Proc. Natl. Acad. Sci. USA, in press (1983).

15. Early, P., Rogers, J., Davis, M., Calame, K., Bond, M., Wall, R. and Hood, L.: Cell 20, 313-319 (1980).

HUMAN ERYTHROCYTE ACETYLCHOLINESTERASE IS AN AMPHIPATHIC FORM

Terrone L. Rosenberry, David M. Scoggin,
Tapu Ashis Dutta-Choudhury, and Robert Haas

Department of Pharmacology, Case Western Reserve University
Cleveland, Ohio 44106

Introduction

AChE (EC 3.1.1.7) occurs in several forms in vertebrate tissues. These forms are classified either as asymmetric if they include a collagen-like tail structure or as globular if they are devoid of such a structure (see 1, 2). The globular class includes AChE forms with a hydrophobic domain that interact with nonionic detergents following extraction. The term amphipathic has been applied to proteins with distinct hydrophilic and hydrophobic domains that can be separated by protease cleavage (3, 4, 5). The hydrophobic domain is presumed to anchor these proteins as integral membrane proteins in situ, while the hydrophilic domain generally retains any enzymatic activity associated with the intact protein. Bon and Massoulié (6) first reported that protease digestion could abolish the detergent interactions of an AChE form. They noted that pronase and proteinase K digestion blocked the aggregation and prevented the binding of nonionic detergents by hydrodynamic criteria to a G_2 form from torpedo electric organ. Pronase had a similar action on the detergent-binding G_4 AChE in crude extracts from bovine brain (7). In this paper we examine human erythrocyte AChE (RBC AChE) as an example of the detergent-binding AChE forms and show that it meets several criteria for an amphipathic membrane protein.

Materials and Methods

Proteins and protease resin. RBC AChE was extracted with 1% Triton X-100, purified by affinity chromatography on acridinium resins, and depleted of Triton X-100 by chromatography on hydroxyapatite as described in (8). Lyophilized trypsin and aqueous crystalline suspensions of catalase (100 mg/ml) and papain (25-28 mg/ml) were from Sigma. Lyophilized pronase was from Boehringer-Mannheim, and lyophilized carboxypeptidase Y, from Worthington. Protease resins were prepared by coupling the protease to N-(Sepharose CL-4B)-6-aminocaproic acid by a N-hydroxysuccinimide ester activation procedure (9). Papain resins were sometimes taken through a cysteine activation cycle in which they were incubated in an assay solvent for benzoyl arginine-p-nitroanilide (BAPA; 10) minus BAPA for 15 min and washed extensively in 5 mM sodium phosphate, pH 7. Washed resin was then assayed in BAPA assay solvent minus cysteine, in which it retained cysteine-stimulated activity for a few hours. Cysteine activation increased papain resin activity with BAPA 10-fold and with azoalbumin (11), 3-fold.

Analytical procedures. AChE assays, AChE protein determination, polyacrylamide gel electrophoresis (PAGE) in sodium dodecylsulfate (SDS), active site labeling with [^{3}H]DFP, gel slicing, amino acid analysis, molecular weight estimation, sucrose gradient centrifugation, and Stokes radius determination were conducted as outlined elsewhere (8).

Digestion with carboxypeptidase Y. Carboxypeptidase Y was prepared for digestion by dissolving the lyophilized stock (1.7 mg/ml) in 50 mM sodium phosphate (pH 6.5) and dialyzing 48 hr against this buffer. Frozen aliquots (20-50 µl) were stored until use, and their initial activity was confirmed by spectrophotometric assay with N-acetyl-L-tyrosine ethyl ester

(12). RBC AChE was dialyzed 30 hr against 10 mM sodium phosphate (pH 7), concentrated 5-fold, and 150-350 µl aliquots (100-500 µg) were incubated with carboxypeptidase Y (50 µg/ml) and norleucine (10 nmol; an internal control) for 4 hr at 25° C unless otherwise noted. Controls minus carboxypeptidase Y or RBC AChE were prepared in parallel. Digestion was terminated by addition of an equal volume of 20% trichloroacetic acid, and the supernatant of a low speed centrifugation was combined with a 20% trichloroacetic acid wash (200 µl) of the pellet and dried extensively on a Speedvac concentrator. Dried samples were suspended in 500 µl buffer and run on a three buffer amino acid analysis system (8). The following recoveries of C-terminal amino acids (mol/mol 67 kDa protein) from bovine serum albumin (700 µg) were obtained with this procedure: ALA, 1.58 ± 0.09 (positions 1 and 3); LEU, 1.06 ± 0.06 (position 2); THR, 0.36 ± 0.05 (positions 4 and 6); and smaller amounts of all other amino acids (average of 4 determinations with 3 carboxypeptidase Y stocks).

Results

Purification of dimeric (G_2) RBC AChE and its conversion to monomers (G_1) by disulfide reduction. Enzyme was purified from erythrocyte membrane extracts by affinity chromatography with an acridinium resin that was modified slightly from the resin used to purify eel electric organ AChE (8). When combined with high volume molecular filtration of large quantitites of erythrocyte membranes, the purification procedure permitted the routine isolation of about 5 mg of enzyme from 10 liters of outdated erythrocytes. The purified and detergent-depleted enzyme was obtained with an overall 48% yield and had a specific activity of 5000-5800 units per mg protein. The purity of our isolated RBC AChE was confirmed by PAGE in SDS as indicated in Fig. 1. The heavily loaded cylindrical

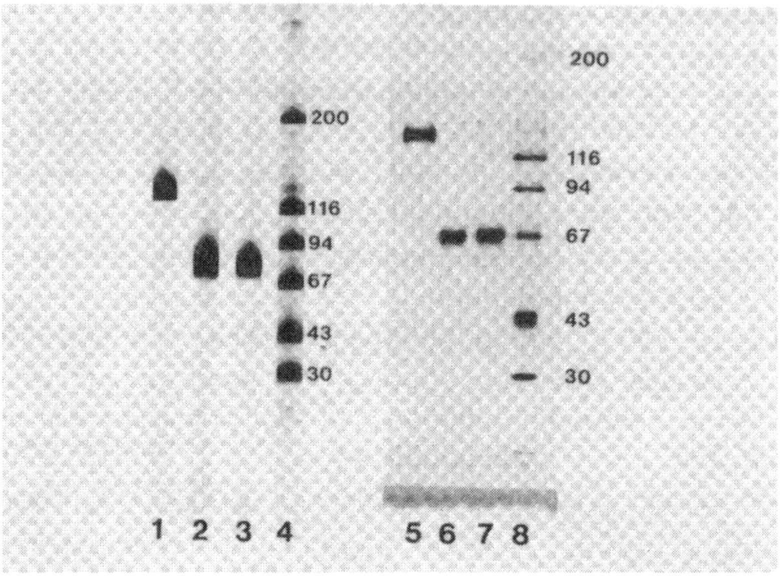

Fig. 1. SDS-PAGE gels of purified RBC AChE before and after disulfide reduction. Cylindrical 3.5% gels (1-4) were stained with Coomassie Blue, and the 5-13% gradient slab gel (5-8) was stained with silver. Gels 1-3 contained 18 µg RBC AChE; gels 5-7, 0.15 µg RBC AChE; gels 4 and 8, polypeptide standards with the indicated molecular masses in kDa. Samples in gels 1 and 5 were not reduced; those in gels 2 and 6 were reduced under nondenaturing conditions; and those in gels 3 and 7 were fully reduced with dithiothreitol in 1% SDS. Details in (8).

gels establish that no apparent contaminants were copurified with RBC AChE. Prior to disulfide reduction the enzyme existed as a disulfide-linked dimer, and the dimer was converted to monomers of about 75 kDa by complete reduction in SDS. These observations are consistent with previous reports for RBC AChE (13, 14, 15, 16). Conversion to monomers also occurred during reduction with 5-20 mM dithiothreitol at pH 8-8.5 under nondenaturing conditions, an indication that intersubunit disulfide(s) were relatively accessible to solvent. This reduction procedure resulted in some loss of enzyme activity (50-70%); but this loss could be decreased to 40-50% by inclusion of edrophonium chloride (0.1-1 mM), a competitive inhibitor of RBC AChE, in the reduction mixture. Monomers produced under these conditions could be radiolabeled with [^{14}C]N-ethylmaleimide. Label incorporation levels of 1.7 mols per mol of monomer were interpreted as indicating a single intersubunit disulfide bond in the dimer (8). No free sulfhydryl groups were detected prior to reduction.

Sucrose gradient sedimentation of purified RBC AChE in the presence of 1% Triton X-100 revealed a single peak with an apparent sedimentation coefficient of 6 S consistent with a G_2 form, while in the absence of detergent the enzyme formed a mixture of aggregated oligomers (8). Similar observations have been reported previously for RBC AChE (14, 15) and for the amphipathic G_2 torpedo AChE (18). Disulfide reduction under nondenaturing conditions had little effect on the aggregated sedimentation pattern but shifted the peak in the presence of 1% Triton X-100 to an apparent 4 S value (8; similar observations following reduction of the torpedo G_2 form in 6, 18). Precise determinations of the sedimentation coefficients required quantitative estimates of the amount of bound detergent in Table I below. The aggregation of the G_1 enzyme in the absence of detergent indicated that the hydrophobic domain responsible for aggregation remained associated with the monomers. Since the only sulfhydryl groups that could be radiolabeled in this preparation were on the catalytic subunit polypeptides themselves, no intervening peptide like that in G_4 AChE from eel electric organ was involved in the intersubunit disulfide linkage (8). This is a strong argument that the hydrophobic domain is part of the catalytic subunit polypeptide itself.

Molecular weight estimates for G_2 and G_1 RBC AChE. In the absence of nonionic detergents, both the G_2 and the G_1 enzymes formed aggregates with average Stokes radii of 10 nm on

Table I

Hydrodynamic and Detergent-binding Properties of RBC AChE[a]

Form	$S_{20,w}$	R_s nm	detergent binding g per g protein	protein MW
G_2	6.5 ± 0.2	7.4 ± 0.2	0.63 ± 0.04	160,000 ± 8,000
G_1	4.3 ± 0.1	6.2 ± 0.1	0.75 ± 0.07	85,000 ± 6,000
G_2 by papain	6.8 ± 0.2	5.8 ± 0.1	-	157,000 ± 5,000

[a]Purified RBC AChE was obtained as a G_2 form, and samples were converted to G_1 by reduction under nondenaturing conditions. G_2 by papain corresponds to enzyme disaggregated by papain as outlined in the Methods. Triton X-100 (1.0%) was included in measurements of sedimentation coefficients ($S_{20,w}$) and Stokes radii (R_s) with the nondigested enzymes. $S_{20,w}$ values were corrected for detergent binding. Triton X-100 was deleted in the $S_{20,w}$ and R_s estimates for the papain-disaggregated enzyme, but these estimates did not differ significantly from those obtained in the presence of 1% Triton X-100 ($S_{20,w}$ = 6.8, R_s = 5.9 ± 0.1). Tabulated means were averages of 3-5 determinations and are listed with standard errors.

Bound detergent was determined by affinity chromatography. The estimate for G_2 was an average of 3 experiments with 2-10 mM tetrapropylammonium iodide elution, and the estimate for G_1 used this G_2 value plus the average ratio of binding to G_1 and G_2 for 5 experiments involving elution with either 2 mM tetrapropylammonium iodide or 10 mM decamethonium bromide.

Molecular weights (MW) were estimated from the Svedberg equation assuming a partial specific volume for protein of 0.715 (19) and do not include bound detergent. Details in (8, 9).

Sepharose CL-4B in 20 mM sodium phosphate (8). Introduction of Triton X-100 above its critical micelle concentration gave enzyme-detergent complexes, and the amount of detergent bound was determined with [^{3}H]Triton X-100 by affinity chromatography. Decamethonium bromide, our standard elution ligand in affinity chromatography, was found to decrease the [^{3}H]Triton X-100 binding, perhaps by partitioning into the micelle phase and reducing the amount of detergent per micelle. Tetrapropylammonium iodide appeared to have no effect on detergent binding when used as the elution ligand. Estimates of [^{3}H]Triton X-100 bound to the G_2 and G_1 forms of RBC AChE are given in Table I. Each G_2 molecule bound about 140 detergent molecules and each G_1, about 80. Thus each <u>subunit</u> in G_2 and G_1 bound 70-80 detergent molecules, an amount typical of a single Triton X-100 micelle when bound to other amphipathic proteins (see 8). [^{3}H]Triton X-100 below its critical micelle concentration of 0.016% neither bound in significant amounts nor disaggregated RBC AChE (8), a further indication that the enzyme interacted only with detergent micelles as suggested previously (20). Since each subunit in G_2 can interact independently with a Triton X-100 micelle of about 45 kDa, the hydrophobic domains on each subunit must be well separated.

Molecular weight estimates for the glycoprotein components of the G_2- and G_1-detergent complexes were obtained from an analysis of their sedimentation coefficients, Stokes radii, and detergent binding as outlined in Table I and corresponded to 160,000 and 85,000 respectively. This estimate for G_2 is in reasonable agreement with the value of 151,000 reported by Ott et al. (1982) from sedimentation equilibrium measurements in the presence of a detergent isopycnic with water.

<u>Papain was the protease most efficient in cleaving the hydrophobic domain from RBC AChE.</u> Since the aggregation of RBC AChE in the absence of detergent is presumed to be mediated by

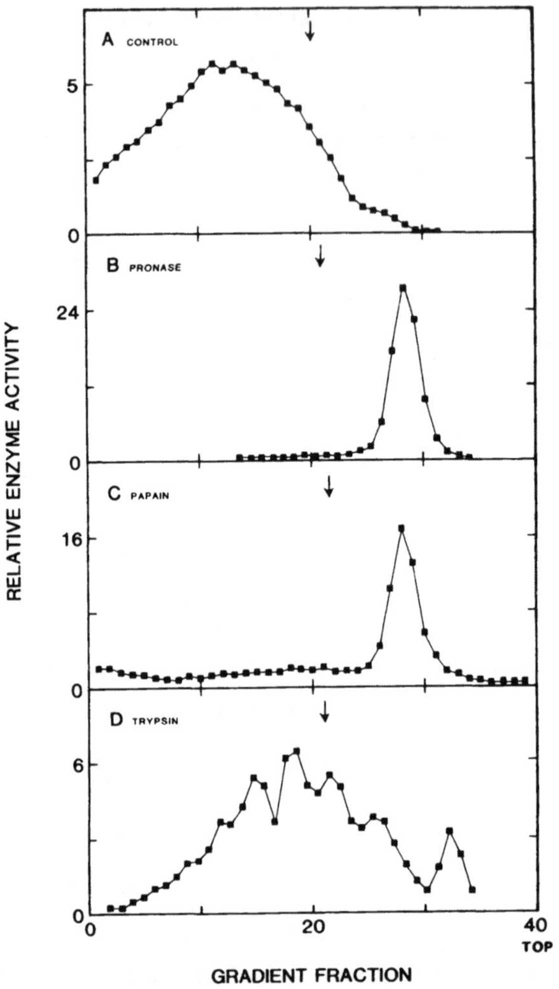

Fig. 2. Sucrose gradient centrifugation of a control RBC AChE sample (A) and of samples digested with pronase (B), papain (C), and trypsin (D). RBC AChE (2 µg/ml) was incubated with 100 µg/ml protease (protease was deleted in the control) in 20 mM Tris-HCl, 0.1 mM edrophonium chloride (pH 7) for 24 hr at 4° C, after which 30 µl of incubation mix and 20 µl of stock catalase were applied to gradients that contained no detergent. RBC AChE activities are expressed as the percentage of total activity recovered from the gradient. Enzyme activities in the gradient onputs following digestion were 50%, 65% and 100% of the control for pronase, papain, and trypsin, respectively. Arrows mark the position of catalase migration (11.4 S) in each gradient. See (9) for details.

its hydrophobic domain, we evaluated the ability of proteases to cleave this domain by the extent to which they disaggregated the enzyme activity on detergent-free sucrose gradients. A variety of protease effects were observed: for example, papain gave considerable disaggregation; pronase gave nearly complete inactivation; and carboxypeptidase Y neither disaggregated nor inactivated RBC AChE (9). The introduction of edrophonium chloride to the digests significantly improved the ratio of disaggregation to inactivation for all the proteases tested. The percent inactivation was particularly decreased for pronase and proteinase K. Digestion with either papain or pronase in the presence of edrophonium chloride resulted in nearly complete disaggregation of RBC AChE to a 7 S peak, as shown in Fig. 2B, C. Trypsin produced a different sedimentation pattern that is considered further in the Discussion.

Size and location of the hydrophobic domain cleaved by papain. When amounts of RBC AChE significantly larger than those in Fig. 2 were digested, the ratio of disaggregation to inactivation decreased. Furthermore, residual protease severely degraded RBC AChE gel bands during analysis by PAGE in SDS, even after fractionation of the digests by gel exclusion chromatography. To minimize such degradation, proteases were covalently attached to Sepharose CL-4B. Papain resin was particularly useful in producing larger amounts of disaggregated RBC AChE, because its efficiency was increased by prior activation with cysteine, a reducing agent. Reducing agents were not added to the digest directly because the G_2 RBC AChE would be converted to less stable G_1 enzyme. Two pools arising from papain resin digestion could be separated by gel exclusion chromatography on Sepharose CL-4B in the absence of detergent, as shown in Fig. 3. An activity peak corresponding to a Stokes radius (R_s) of 5.8 nm appeared in the digests and was eluted after the 9.8 nm R_s peak that corresponded to

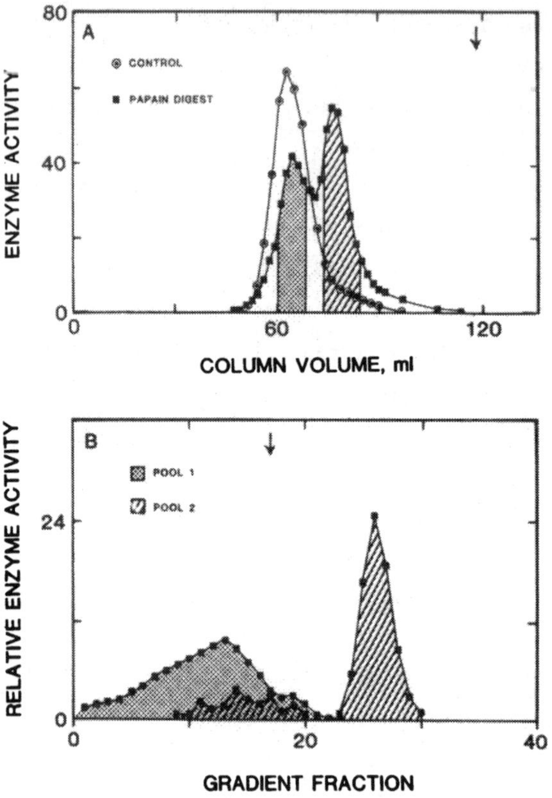

Fig. 3. Separation of aggregated and disaggregated RBC AChE from a papain digest by gel exclusion chromatography on Sepharose CL-4B. RBC AChE (400 µg) was digested with papain resin (0.4 ml with 1.0 mg papain; not activated with cysteine) in 2.0 ml of 50 mM sodium phosphate, 1.0 mM edrophonium chloride (pH 7) for 4 hr at 4° C. Digestion was terminated by briefly centrifuging the mixture at low speed and removing the supernatant. A. Supernatant from the digest (■) was applied to a 120 ml Sepharose CL-4B column (1.5 x 70 cm) equilibrated at 4° in 20 mM sodium phosphate, pH 7. Fractions (1.7 ml) were collected, and those corresponding to Pool 1 (stippled area) or Pool 2 (crosshatched area), respectively, were combined. Control RBC AChE (depleted of detergent) was applied as a separate sample under identical conditions (O). Activity recoveries from both column runs were about 70%. Arrow marks elution position of $K_2Cr_2O_7$. B. Pools 1 and 2 from A were concentrated 3-4 fold, and 50 µl aliquots (0.3-0.7 µg) and catalase were applied to sucrose gradients and centrifuged as in Fig. 2.

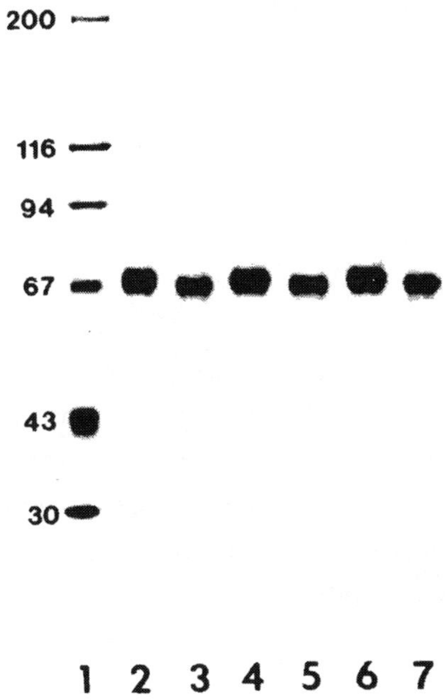

Fig. 4. PAGE analysis in SDS of control nondigested and papain-disaggregated RBC AChE following complete disulfide reduction. A gradient slab gel was run and stained with silver as indicated in (8). RBC AChE (2.9 mg) was digested with papain resin (1.0 ml with 2.0 mg papain; activated with cysteine as described in the Methods) in 10.5 ml of 5 mM sodium phosphate (pH 7) for 45 min as outlined in Fig. 3. The digestion supernatant was concentrated, and disaggregated Pool 2 was collected as in Fig. 3. About 90% of the recovered RBC AChE was disaggregated. Samples were fully reduced (Fig. 1) and aliquots (0.2 µg protein) were applied to gel lanes in triplicate. Lane 1, polypeptide standards as in Fig. 1. Lanes 2, 4 and 6, control nondigested RBC AChE. Lanes 2, 5 and 7, disaggregated Pool 2 RBC AChE. Apparent molecular masses were 72 kDa for the control nondigested and 70 kDa for the papain-disaggregated enzymes, but to conform to estimates from both cylidrical and slab gels we refer to the control mass as 75 kDa (8). Pool 1 (Fig. 3) and nondigested control samples had identical mobilities, and comparison of [^{3}H]DFP-labeled Pool 1 and Pool 2 samples confirmed that the disaggregated RBC AChE quantitatively retained nearly full length catalytic subunit polypeptides (9).

control G_2 RBC AChE aggregate (Fig. 3A). Sucrose gradient sedimentation analyses in Fig. 3B of samples from the two pools revealed that the earlier pool was residual aggregated RBC AChE while the later pool was almost completely disaggregated. The molecular weight of the papain-disaggregated Pool 2 was estimated from its hydrodynamic properties as outlined in Table I. The estimate of 157,000 for disaggregated enzyme appeared slightly smaller than the 160,000 molecular weight estimated for nondigested control G_2 enzyme associated with Triton X-100, but the difference was within the errors of the estimates. The sedimentation coefficient and Stokes radius of the papain-disaggregated enzyme were not altered in the presence of 1% Triton X-100 within experimental error, confirming that digestion had removed the hydrophobic domain. The small molecular weight change accompanying this cleavage indicates that the hydrophobic domain itself must be quite small.

Analysis of papain-disaggregated RBC AChE by PAGE in SDS is shown in Fig. 4. Control catalytic subunits of about 75 kDa migrated slightly more rapidly than disaggregated Pool 2 samples, and the difference corresponded to about 2 kDa. Fig. 4 further confirmed the small size of hydrophobic domain cleaved by papain, but it also indicated that this domain corresponded to the N- or C-terminus of the catalytic subunit polypeptide: A mass decrease of just 2 kDa in the papain-disaggregated catalytic subunit polypeptides in which all internal disulfide linkages are broken can occur only if the 2 kDa mass is removed from one end of the 75 kDa species.

<u>Carboxypeptidase Y digestion of RBC AChE.</u> If papain cleaved a C-terminal segment of the catalytic subunit polypeptides, an altered amino acid release pattern by carboxypeptidase Y would be expected (4, 22). Although the procedure for determining C-terminal amino acids in the Methods worked well for both bovine serum albumin and a CNBr fragment CB-2 from avian

retrovirus pp12 nucleocapsid protein (23), results obtained for control and papain-disaggregated RBC AChE could not be interpreted. Relatively reproducible recoveries of released amino acids (mol/70,000 g protein) were obtained with nondigested control RBC AChE (LEU, 1.1 ± 0.2 and VAL, 0.7 ± 0.1 were highest over 4 preparations, but several other amino acids were between 0.3 and 0.6), and the release pattern for papain-disaggregated RBC AChE was not significantly different. However, the mole percentages of released amino acids remained relatively constant as the digestion temperature was increased to 50° C despite about a 12-fold increase in total released amino acids (to nearly 15% of the total RBC AChE amino acid residues). In contrast, digestion of bovine serum albumin at 50° C gave nearly stoichiometric release of the first 21 C-terminal amino acids. These observations suggested that amino acid release from RBC AChE during the digestion arose not from the C-terminus of the intact catalytic subunit polypeptides but instead arose from slow polypeptide fragmentation followed by rapid release of amino acids from the fragments.

Discussion

The hydrophobic domain of RBC AChE. Integral membrane proteins that have been termed amphipathic exhibit several common characteristics that can serve as criteria for this class of proteins. 1) The intact protein requires detergent for extraction from membranes, binds to detergent micelles only, aggregates but does not generally precipitate when detergent is removed, and can be reconstituted into liposomes. 2) The larger hydrophilic domain is oriented on one side of the membrane only, is solubilized by protease cleavage generally with full retention of associated enzymatic activities, and following protease cleavage shows no aggregation or detergent- or liposome-binding properties. 3) The hydrophobic domain is quite small (generally < 10 kDa) and is located at the N- or C-terminus of the primary sequence. RBC AChE meets all of these criteria except possibly one: Proteases solubilized it only poorly from intact erythrocytes (< 10%), although the efficiency of protease solubilization appeared to parallel the efficiency of disaggregation of the purified RBC AChE (9). Of several proteases investigated, papain appeared to be most efficient in removing the hydrophobic detergent-binding domain from RBC AChE (9). The hydrodynamic data in Table I for the papain-disaggregated RBC AChE is remarkably similar to that reported for pronase-treated G_2 AChE from torpedo electric organ (6). This similarity suggests that the hydrophobic domains cleaved by proteases from both of these AChE sources are of comparable size and derive from the same region of catalytic subunit primary sequence. The apparent 2 kDa size of the hydrophobic domain cleaved from RBC AChE by papain is even smaller than that of hydrophobic domains in other amphipathic proteins (see 9), and a small size estimate was supported by our inability to detect differences between nondigested control and papain-disaggregated RBC AChE in amino acid composition, specific activity, or subunit equivalent weight within experimental error (9). Our best evidence that this domain in fact anchors RBC AChE in phospholipid membranes is the observation that papain-disaggregated RBC AChE, in contrast to nondigested control RBC AChE, could not be reconstituted into liposomes prepared with crude egg phospholipid (24).

Trypsin digestion of RBC AChE. Trypsin generated a sedimentation pattern different from those of papain and pronase, and we digress here briefly to consider the action of trypsin. Little discrete 7 S G_2 form could be detected in Fig. 2D, but aggregation was reduced and several other peaks were apparent, including ones at 11 S and 9 S and one at 4.5 S suggestive of a G_1 monomer. Trypsin also failed to cleave the hydrophobic domain from the G_2 torpedo AChE, although it did alter the sedimentation pattern of the aggregate (6). Active G_1 monomers were produced by trypsin from G_2 and G_4 AChE forms from bovine superior cervical ganglion (25), and trypsin also generated active monomers from tetrameric human serum ChE (26). Tryptic production of monomers from these oligomeric enzyme forms implies that the catalytic subunit segments containing the intersubunit disulfide bond (see 8) have been proteolytically removed. Loss of this disulfide linkage segment can be directly observed on PAGE on SDS, and this loss resulted in a very small change in the apparent molecular weight of the fully reduced catalytic subunits of serum ChE (26). Trypsin also degraded the disulfide-linked catalytic subunits of G_4 eel AChE to monomers both by cleaving residual tail subunit fragments (27) and by apparently cleaving the catalytic subunit primary sequence itself, again without significant change in the apparent molecular weight of the fully reduced cleaved subunits (28). As Lockridge and La Du (26) have noted, these observations imply that trypsin can remove small segments containing the intersubunit disulfide linkage from either the N- or C-terminus of the catalytic subunits. We make precisely the same argument in the Results to account for the site of papain cleavage of RBC AChE. The qualitatively different digestion patterns obtained with papain and trypsin from a number of AChE forms could be reconciled if papain and trypsin cleave at _opposite_ ends of the catalytic subunit polypeptides.

The hydrophobic domain appears to correspond to the C-terminus of RBC AChE. To determine which end of the intact catalytic subunit polypeptides are cleaved by papain digestion, we have investigated both N-terminal radiolabeling by reductive methylation and C-terminal digestion with carboxypeptidase Y. The N-terminal amino acid of nondigested control RBC AChE was radiolabeled with [^{3}H]HCHO and $NaCNBH_3$ and identified as GLU by a modified amino acid analysis system (29). Papain digestion of the labeled enzyme resulted in the same pattern of aggregated and disaggregated RBC AChE shown in Fig. 3, and amino acid analysis revealed virtually the same relative stoichiometry of N,N-[^{3}H]dimethylated GLU in both pools (29). Thus we conclude that papain does not cleave a segment at the N-terminus of the catalytic subunit and presume that cleavage occurs at a C-terminal segment. However, we indicate in the Results that we have been unable to confirm a C-terminal cleavage by digestion with carboxypeptidase Y. No significant difference in the pattern of amino acids released by carboxypeptidase Y between nondigested control and papain-disaggregated RBC AChE was observed, but this result was inconclusive. Our data suggested that nonspecific release of amino acids occurred following slow fragmentation of RBC AChE during our carboxypeptidase Y digestion procedure. No fragmentation could be observed with PAGE in SDS, but discrete fragments would not be detected if the fragmentation was nonselective or highly cooperative. The similar amino acid release patterns for control and disaggregated enzyme could arise entirely from this nonspecific process if carboxypeptidase Y digestion at the C-terminus of both polypeptides was blocked. A blockade of digestion of a C-terminal hydrophobic domain would be consistent with the total failure of carboxypeptidase Y to disaggregate RBC AChE. The digestion pattern of control RBC AChE at 25° C could not be altered by preincubating RBC AChE at 50° C for 1 hr or by including SDS (30 mM) in the digestion.

Recently we have been able to specifically label the hydrophobic domain of RBC AChE (30) with the photoactivatable probe [^{125}I]TID (31). This reagent partitions selectively into the hydrophobic phase of membranes, liposomes, and protein-detergent micelle complexes and, on photoactivation, covalently reacts with molecules in the hydrophobic phase. Papain digestion quantitatively cleaves the [^{125}I]TID label from RBC AChE, and isolation of the labeled hydrophobic domain is currently in progress. Characterization of the this domain and of the position of [^{125}I]TID label in the primary sequence of the catalytic subunits of RBC AChE prior to papain digestion should permit confirmation both of the small size of this domain and of its location in a C-terminal segment.

This investigation was supported by Grant NS-16577 from the National Institutes of Health and by grants from the Muscular Dystrophy Association U.S.A.

References

1. Massoulié, J., Bon, S.: Ann. Rev. Neurosci. 5, 57-106 (1982).

2. Rosenberry, T.L.: in The Enzymes of Biological Membranes, Volume IV, Second edition, Martonosi, A. (editor), Plenum Press, New York 1983, in press.

3. Fleming, P.J., Dailey, H.A., Corcoran, D., Strittmatter, P.: J. Biol. Chem. 253, 5369-5372 (1978).

4. Macnair, R.D.C., Kenny, A.J.: Biochem. J. 179, 379-395 (1979).

5. Frielle, T., Brunner, J., Curthoys, N.P.: J. Biol. Chem. 257, 14979-14982 (1982).

6. Bon, S., Massoulié, J.: Proc. Nat. Acad. Sci. U.S.A. 77, 4464-4468 (1980).

7. Grassi, J., Vigny, M., Massoulié, J.: J. Neurochem. 38, 457-469 (1982).

8. Rosenberry, T.L., Scoggin, D.M.: J. Biol. Chem., in press (1984).

9. Dutta-Choudhury, T.A., Rosenberry, T.L.: J. Biol. Chem., in press (1984).

10. Arnon, R.: Methods Enzymol. 19, 226-244 (1970).

11. Tomarelli, R.M., Charney, J.,, Harding, M.L.: J. Lab. Clin. Med. 34, 428-433 (1949).

12. Hayashi, R.: Methods Enzymol. 47, 84-93 (1977).

13. Bellhorn, M.B., Blumenfeld, O.O., Gallop, P.M.: Biochem. Biophys. Res. Commun. 39, 267-273 (1970).

14. Ott, P., Jenny, B., Brodbeck, U.: Eur. J. Biochem. 57, 469-480 (1975).

15. Grossmann, H., Liefländer, M.: Hoppe-Seyler's Z. Physiol. Chem. 356, 663-669 (1975).

16. Niday, E., Wang, C.S., Alaupovic, P.: Biochim. Biophys. Acta 469, 180-193 (1977).

17. Ott, P., Brodbeck, U.: Eur. J. Biochem. 88, 119-125 (1978).

18. Lee, S.L., Camp, S.J., Taylor, P.: J. Biol. Chem. 257, 12302-12309 (1982).

19. Bon, S., Huet, M., Lemonnier, M., Rieger, F. , Massoulié, J.: Eur. J. Biochem. 68, 523-530 (1976).

20. Wiedmer, T., Di Francesco, C., Brodbeck, U.: Eur. J. Biochem. 102, 59-64 (1979).

21. Ott, P., Lustig, A., Brodbeck, U., Rosenbusch, J.P.: FEBS Lett. 138, 187-189 (1982).

22. Brunner, J., Hauser, H., Braun, H., Wilson, K.J., Wacker, H., O'Neill, B., Semenza, G.: J. Biol. Chem. 254, 1821-1828 (1979).

23. Leis, J., Johnson, S., Collins, L., Traugh, J.: J. Biol. Chem., in press (1984).

24. Kim, B.H., Rosenberry, T.L.: to be published.

25. Vigny, M., Bon, S., Massoulié, J., Gisiger, V.: J. Neurochem. 33, 559-565 (1979).

26. Lockridge, O., La Du, B.N.: J. Biol. Chem. 257, 12012-12018 (1982).

27. Rosenberry, T.L., Barnett, P., Mays, C.: Neurochem. Int. 2, 135-147 (1980).

28. Rosenberry, T.L., Barnett, P., Mays, C.: unpublished observations.

29. Haas, R., Rosenberry, T.L.: Biochemistry, submitted (1984).

30. Roberts, W.L., Rosenberry, T.L.: to be published.

31. Brunner, J., Semenza, G.: Biochemistry 20, 7174-7182 (1981).

STUDIES ON MEMBRANE-BOUND AND SOLUBILIZED ACETYLCHOLINESTERASE

D.T. Plummer, M.S.Y. Chai, C.J. Vidal

Biochemistry Department, Chelsea College (University of London), Manresa Road, London SW3 6LX, U.K.

Introduction

Acetylcholinesterase from a variety of sources is associated with membrane structures and in many cases the binding of the enzyme to the membrane is very strong (1). Most workers have therefore sought to bring the acetylcholinesterase (AChE) into solution prior to investigation and various methods of solubilization have been used depending on the source of the enzyme. For example, the relatively mild procedure of extraction with high ionic strength media will solubilize the enzyme from electric tissue (2). However, more severe methods are usually needed and extraction with detergent is now a routine procedure for many tissues (3, 4, 5). Most of the work on AChE has been carried out on the solubilized enzyme in which the membrane structures associated with the AChE have been destroyed.

In general membrane lipids have a modulating effect on the proteins with which they are associated. For example, the active site of a membrane-bound enzyme is likely to be influenced by the nature of the phospholipids in the immediate vicinity of the protein, and indeed the activity of AChE is known to be affected by membrane lipids (6, 7, 8, 9).

In view of this it was decided to look at some of the properties of membrane-bound AChE and see how these may be changed when solubilized with detergent. Extraction of these tissues with a simple aqueous medium does bring a small amount of AChE into solution (3, 10, 11, 12) and so the properties of this 'naturally soluble' form of the enzyme have also been examined and compared with the Triton-solubilized form of acetylcholinesterase.

Experimental

The details of the methods used in this investigation are given in previous publications as set out below. Assay of AChE, extraction of tissues and gradient-gel electrophoresis (13); starch-block electrophoresis and density gradient centrifugation (14), preparation of red cell ghosts (4). The inhibition of AChE by a range of organophosphorous compounds was determined both in the absence and presence of substrate at 25°C (15).

Results

Michaelis constants

The Michaelis constants (Km values) of membrane-bound AChE from a number of sources are very similar and these are hardly changed when the enzyme is brought into solution with detergent. The Km values of the naturally soluble enzyme preparations however are higher than those for the membrane-bound and detergent-soluble enzymes and again the values are virtually the same for the different preparations studied. These results are given in Table I.

Arrhenius plots

Arrhenius plots of the acetylcholinesterase preparations were determined between 5°C and 50°C using the pH-stat. The V_{max} was obtained from a plot of s/v against s using a computer and log V_{max} plotted against the reciprocal of the absolute temperature. The membrane preparations were obtained by resuspending the erythrocyte ghosts or the 100,000 g pellet of the muscle homogenate (20%

Table I. The Michaelis constants of acetylcholinesterase preparations

Enzyme source	Michaelis constant (μM acetylcholine)		
	Membrane-bound	Naturally soluble	Detergent soluble
Pig brain (grey matter)	76 ± 3.1	118 ± 6.2	62 ± 2.0
Pig brain (white matter)	70 ± 2.9	106 ± 5.6	64 ± 1.5
Rat skeletal muscle	84 ± 1.7	110 ± 5.3	72 ± 1.3

The Michaelis constants were measured at 30°C and pH 7.9 by means of a pH-stat. The results shown are the mean ± S.E.M. of 4 experiments.

w/v) in 30 mM sodium phosphate buffer, at pH 7.0.
The Arrhenius plots of the membrane-bound AChE from human erythrocytes gave two straight lines with a discontinuity in the region of 26°C (Fig. 1). Similar results were obtained for the AChE from rat skeletal muscle which also showed a linear plot for the naturally soluble enzyme (Fig. 2).

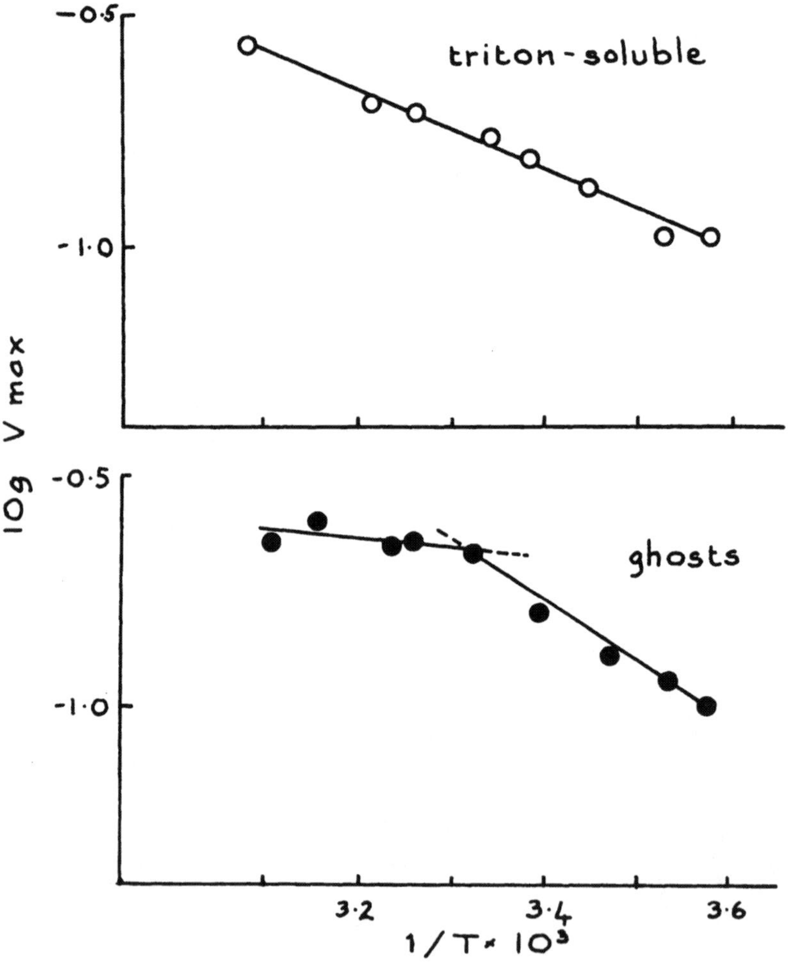

Fig. 1. Arrhenius plots of acetylcholinesterase from human erythrocytes
(a) Triton soluble enzyme ○
(b) Membrane-bound enzyme ●

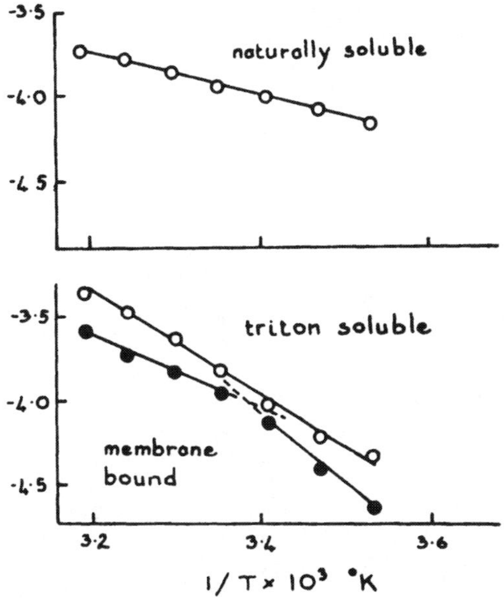

Fig. 2. Arrhenius plots of acetylcholinesterase preparation from rat skeletal muscle
(a) Naturally soluble enzyme
(b) Triton soluble enzyme (○) and membrane-bound enzyme (●)

Substrate specificity

The specificity of the naturally soluble and detergent soluble forms of AChE from rat muscle was investigated for a number of substrates. The relative rates of hydrolysis of each substrate at 1 mM concentration shows that both preparations were very similar in terms of their substrate specificity (Table II).

Electrophoresis

Electrophoresis of the naturally soluble enzyme on a starch-block gave two peaks of activity and a similar result was obtained with the Triton soluble enzyme (Fig. 3). However in the latter case, Triton X-100 (1% w/v) had to be present in the block and

Table II. Hydrolysis of choline esters by muscle acetylcholinesterase

Substrate	% Relative rate (acetylcholine iodide = 100%)	
	Naturally soluble enzyme	Triton soluble enzyme
Acetylcholine iodide	100	100
Propionylcholine iodide	90	84.1
Butyrylcholine iodide	3	2.5
Acetyl-β-methylcholine bromide	21.0	20.7
Tributyrin	15.0	13.8

The rate is expressed as a percentage of that with acetylcholine iodide. The activity was determined at 30°, pH 7.6 and 1 mM substrate using a pH-stat. The values given above are the mean of four experiments.

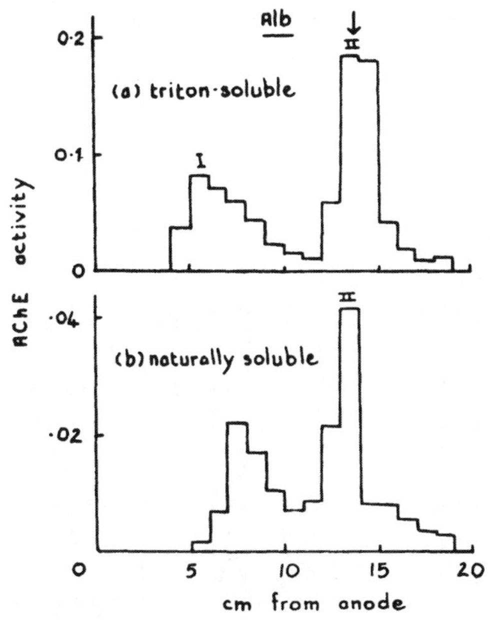

Fig. 3. Starch-block electrophoresis of acetylcholinesterase from rat skeletal muscle

(a) Naturally soluble enzyme

(b) Triton soluble enzyme

The arrow denotes the point of application of the sample while Alb marks the position of the albumin marker.

electrophoresis buffer to obtain the two peaks. If detergent was excluded from the block then the Triton solubilized enzyme showed only one peak with a low negative mobility close to the origin (peak II).

Electrophoresis of the preparations in gradient slabs of polyacrylamide (4%-24%) showed a large number of enzymatically active species covering a wide range of molecular weights.

Peak II from the starch-block electrophoresis of the Triton solubilized or the naturally soluble acetylcholinesterase had a species of high molecular weight which just entered the gel. Peak

I from both preparations gave a very similar pattern of staining to the extracts before they were separated on the starch-block, with only a few minor differences in the staining intensity of some bands. These findings are summarized in Fig. 4.

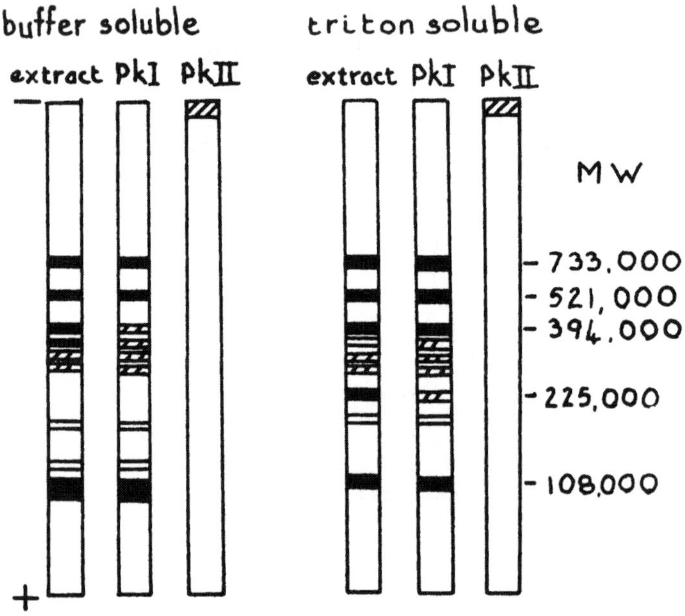

Fig. 4. Electrophoresis of acetylcholinesterase from rat skeletal muscle on a gradient of polyacrylamide. Depth of staining: strong, ■ ; moderate, ▨ ; light, □ . Experimental details as in the text.

The incorporation of eserine (10 μM) into the staining system abolished the bands showing that the enzymes detected are cholinesterase while ethopropazine (30 μM) had no effect on the staining pattern, suggesting that the bands are true and not pseudocholinesterases.

Density-gradient centrifugation

The peaks of activity obtained by starch-block electrophoresis were concentrated and also centrifuged on a sucrose gradient. Peak II from both preparations sedimented to the bottom of the tube and thus appears to be an aggregated form of the enzyme. In contrast to this, peak I from both preparations gave a single peak of enzyme activity with a sedimentation constant of 11 S.

The effect of organophosphorus compounds

The bimolecular rate constants (k_i) for the inhibition of the soluble preparations of the enzyme were determined as described in the methods section, in the absence and presence of substrate. The k_i values shown by the naturally soluble enzyme were lower than those of the detergent solubilized acetylcholinesterase for all the inhibitors studied. The Triton soluble enzyme was twice as sensitive to inhibition by malaoxon and four times as sensitive to methyl paraoxon. The enzyme preparations were also sensitive to different inhibitors. The naturally soluble enzyme was most strongly inhibited by ethyl malaoxon while the Triton soluble acetylcholinesterase was most strongly inhibited by methyl paraoxon.

The bimolecular rate constants were the same whether or not substrate was present during inhibition of the acetylcholinesterase. These results are summarized in Fig. 5.

Discussion

The Michaelis constants of acetylcholinesterase were very similar for all the membrane-bound preparations studied. Solubilization of the AChE with detergent caused little change in the enzyme-substrate affinity so that loss of the membrane matrix has little effect on the conformation of the enzyme protein at least in the region close to the active site. The naturally soluble

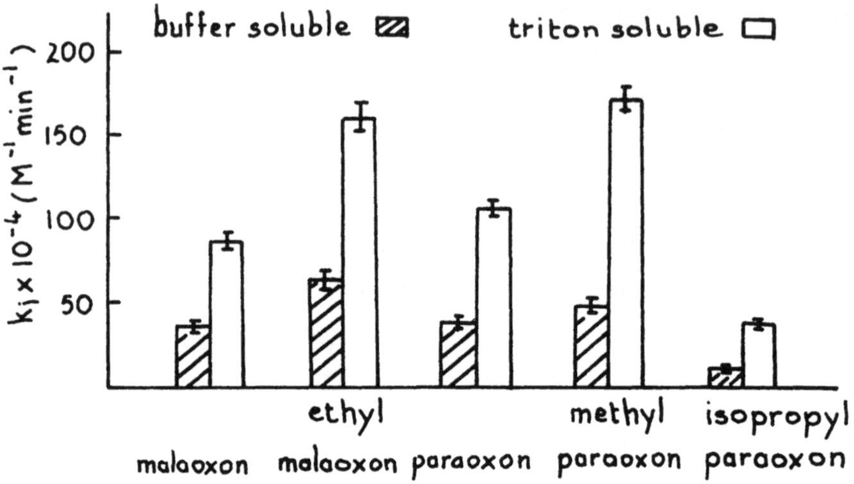

Fig. 5. The inhibition of acetylcholinesterase from rat skeletal muscle by organophosphorus compounds
Naturally soluble enzyme, ▨
Triton soluble enzyme, □

enzymes however all had higher Km values possibly indicating a small difference in their structures compared with the corresponding membrane-bound and Triton solubilized enzymes. Differences between the membrane-bound and solubilized AChE were most clearly seen with Arrhenius plots where the membrane enzymes showed a discontinuity in the region of 26°C whereas the Triton soluble preparation gave a linear plot with no break. This was seen for both human erythrocytes and rat muscle AChE (Figs. 1 and 2). Very similar results have been reported for the membrane-bound AChE from pig cerebral cortex which gave a break in the Arrhenius plot at 27°C. This discontinuity was abolished by the addition of Triton X-100 and again the naturally soluble enzyme gave a linear plot with no break (16). Such a discontinuity in the Arrhenius plot of membrane-bound enzymes has often been considered to represent a phase transition of the membrane lipid in the immediate vicinity of the enzyme (17, 18), and when the Triton soluble enzyme from pig brain was purified by affinity chromatography and incorporated into liposomes, a break was introduced into the Arrhenius plot that reflected the lipid composition of the liposomes (7). This demonstrates the influence of lipid on the AChE, an observation supported by other workers (8, 19, 20, 21). The discontinuity seen in preparations of membrane-bound AChE could well be due to a phase change in the membrane lipids although other explanations cannot be ruled out (22, 23). The results so far indicate only minor differences between the membrane AChE solubilized with Triton X-100 and the naturally soluble enzyme. These observations are largely confirmed by the more detailed studies made of the soluble preparations from rat muscle. Starch-block electrophoresis for example shows that the two preparations are very similar (Fig. 3). Almost identical patterns were obtained for the naturally soluble and Triton soluble enzymes although in the latter case the detergent had to be present in the block and electrophoresis tank. If the detergent was absent then only one peak of activity was obtained corresponding to peak II. This slow peak appeared to be an aggregated form of the enzyme since it sedimented to the bottom of the tube during density gradient centrifugation and failed to enter the polyacrylamide gel during electrophoresis. Both enzyme preparations therefore show a strong tendency to aggregate judging by the relative size of peak II. However in the absence of Triton X-100 complete aggregation of the detergent soluble enzyme occurs and Triton X-100 is needed to keep the enzyme extracted from the membrane in solution. In contrast to this, electrophoretic and sedimentation studies clearly showed that peak I was not an aggregated form of the enzyme.

Sedimentation of peak I on a sucrose gradient showed the presence of a single species of 11 S. This was the same whether peak I was obtained from the naturally soluble or the Triton soluble enzyme . Identical results were obtained when peak I from the starch-block electrophoresis of pig brain acetylcholinesterase was centrifuged on a sucrose gradient (14). This 11 S form probably corresponds to the globular G_4 species found in a number of tissues (24). It appears therefore that the molecular forms of acetylcholinesterase are the same in the membrane and the soluble parts of the cell and this suggestion is supported by the results of the gradient gel electrophoresis which showed virtually identical patterns for the naturally soluble and Triton soluble forms of the enzyme (Fig. 4). This electrophoretic technique however, showed a multiplicity of bands rather than the single species found by sedimentation analysis. The range of smaller molecules may have arisen by partial proteolysis but this is unlikely to be the sole explanation of the number of molecular entities detected since a multiplicity of bands is obtained whether electrophoresis is carried out at 40°C, 25°C or 4°C (25). Another possibility is that electrophoresis removes an aggregating factor (26) leading to the development of smaller forms and possibly some rearrangement of the enzyme molecule. A similar multiplicity of bands has been reported by other workers (27). Whatever the final explanation, the results clearly show that there is little difference between the molecular forms present in the buffer and detergent extracts of rat muscle.

There were also similarities between the two preparations in their response to inhibition by organophosphorus compounds. The bimolecular rate constants (k_i) were the same whether or not substrate was present during the inhibition in agreement with other workers (11, 28). However, the bimolecular rate constants suggest that the naturally soluble enzyme is generally less susceptible to inhibition by organophosphates than the Triton soluble enzyme. Differences are also seen in the response to particular organophosphorus compounds. Ethyl malaoxon is the best inhibitor for the naturally soluble enzyme while methyl paraoxon is the best inhibitor for the Triton solubilized acetylcholinesterase (Fig. 5). The properties of the naturally soluble and Triton soluble acetylcholinesterase from rat skeletal muscle are not identical but the two forms appear to be very similar and are therefore probably closely related in vivo.

Acknowledgment

C.J.V. wishes to thank the Spanish Fundacion Cultural-Privada 'Esteban Romero' for their financial support.

References

1. Nachmansohn, D.: Handbook of Sensory Physiology (ed. Lowenstein, W.R.) Vol. 1 pp. 18-102, Springer-Verlag, New York 1971
2. Silman, I., Karlin, A.: Proc. Natl. Acad. Sci. U.S.A. 58, 1664-1668 (1967).
3. Ho, I.K., Ellman, G.L.: J. Neurochem. 16, 1505-1513 (1969).
4. Wright, D.L., Plummer, D.T.: Biochim. Biophys. Acta 261, 398-401 (1972).
5. Vigny, M., Koenig, J., Rieger, F.: J. Neurochem. 27, 1347-1353 (1976).
6. Sihotang, K.: Eur. J. Biochem. 63, 519-524 (1976).
7. Reavill, C.A., Wooster, M.S., Plummer, D.T.: Biochem. J. 173, 851-856 (1978).
8. Frenkel, E.J., Roelofen, B., Brodbeck, U., Van Deenan, L.L.M., Ott, P.: Eur. J. Biochem. 109, 377-382 (1980).
9. Chialing, C., Devonshire, A.L.: Pest. Sci. 13, 156-160 (1982).
10. McIntosh, C.H.S., Plummer, D.T.: Biochem. J. 133, 655-665 (1973).
11. Devonshire, A.L.: Biochem. J. 149, 463-469 (1975).
12. Oderfeld-Nowak, B., Skangiel-Kramska, J.: J. Neurochem. 27, 1241-1244 (1976).
13. McIntosh, C.H.S., Plummer, D.T.: J. Neurochem. 27, 449-457 (1976).

14. Chai, M.S.Y., Reavill, C.A., Vidal, C.J., Plummer, D.T.: Neurochem. Int. 3, 311-321 (1981).

15. Ellman, G.L., Courtney, K.D., Andres, V. Jnr., Featherstone, R.M.: Biochem. Pharmac. 7, 88-95 (1961).

16. Plummer, D.T., Reavill, C.A., McIntosh, C.H.S.: Croat. Chem. Acta 47, 211-223 (1975).

17. Raison, J.K.: J. Bioenerg. 4, 285-309 (1973).

18. McMurchie, E.J., Raison, J.K.: Biochim. Biophys. Acta 554, 364-374 (1979).

19. Farias, R.N., Bloj, B., Morero, R.D., Sineriz, F., Trucco, R.E.: Biochim. Biophys. Acta 415, 231-251 (1975).

20. Beauregard, G., Roufogalis, B.D.: Biochem. J. 179, 109-117 (1979a).

21. Beauregard, G., Roufogalis, B.D.: Biochim. Biophys. Acta 557, 102-111 (1979b).

22. Dixon, M., Webb, E.C.: Enzymes. Longmans, London 1979

23. Londesborough, J.: Eur. J. Biochem. 105, 211-215 (1980).

24. Massoulie, J., Bon, S., Vigny, M.: Neurochem. Int. 2, 161-184 (1980).

25. Vidal, C.J., Chai, M.S.Y., Plummer, D.T.: Neurochem. Int. 3, 229-238 (1981).

26. Kremzner, L.T., Fei, S.C.: Fed. Proc. 30, 1193 (1971).

27. Rakonczay, Z., Mallol, T., Schenk, H., Vincendon, G., Zanetto, J.P.: Biochim. Biophys. Acta 657, 243-256 (1981).

28. Main, A.R., Dauterman, W.C.: Nature 198, 551-553 (1963).

Acknowledgment: D.T.P. wishes to thank the Royal Society for the award of a travel grant to enable him to attend the Meeting on cholinesterases.

AMPHIPHILE DEPENDENCY AND AMPHIPHILIC STRUCTURE OF DETERGENT SOLUBLE ACETYLCHOLINESTERASE

Urs Brodbeck and Peter Ott
Medizinisch-chemisches Institut der Universität,
Postfach
CH-3000 Bern 9

Introduction

In most tissues several forms of AChE occur side by side and their classification is operationally based on criteria of solubility (for a recent review see reference 1). The two main classes are the salt-soluble (SS-AChE) and the detergent-soluble enzyme (DS-AChE). The former comprises the collagen tailed, asymmetric forms A of AChE that are soluble under high ionic strength conditions (i. e. the high salt soluble = HSS-AChE) and the globular forms G of the enzyme that are soluble in conditions of low ionic strength (i. e. the low salt soluble = LSS-AChE). Further distinction can be made with respect to localization and occurrence of the different forms, their structure and subunit assembly as well as the detergent-binding properties. Table 1 relates the classification based on solubility properties to that based on molecular shape. Whereas a wealth of information exists on SS-AChE (2, 3), much less is known about the properties of DS-AChE because, up to date, purification

Table 1: CLASSIFICATION AND PROPERTIES OF DIFFERENT CLASSES OF ACETYLCHOLINESTERASE

Classification	salt soluble AChE		detergent soluble
	HSS-AChE	LSS-AChE	DS-AChE
Molecular characteristics	Asymetric protein with collagen-like tail	Globular protein	Amphiphilic protein with hydrophobic anchor
Classification according to shape	A	G	-
Condition in which enzyme is soluble	High ionic strength e.g. 1 M NaCl, 50 mM $MgCl_2$ in 10 mM Tris pH 7.4	Low ionic strength e.g. 100 mM NaCl in 10 mM Tris pH 7.4	Detergents > CMC[1)] e. g. 100 mM NaCl, 1 % Triton X-100 in 10 mM Tris pH 7.4
Interactions with detergents	weak (if any)	weak (if any)	strong
Amphiphile dependence of enzyme activity	no	no	yes

1) CMC = critical micelle concentration (for Triton X-100 CMC ≈ 0.016 %)

Table 2: PURIFICATION OF DS-ACHE BY AFFINITY CHROMATOGRAPHY

The table comprises those references that list a specific activity and give evidence for the homogeneity of the purified enzyme preparation

Enzyme Source	Affinity ligand 1)	Detergent used 2)	Specific activity (IU/mg protein)	Ref.
Torpedo california and Torpedo marmorata				
electric organ	m-PTA Sepharose	Cholate	200	4
	Acridinium Sepharose	TX-100	3750	5
	m-PTA Sepharose	TX-100	4500	20
Brain				
bovine	m-PTA Sepharose	TX-100	4250	6
rat	m-DMAEBA Sepharose	TX-100	3100	8
human	m-PTA Sepharose	TX-100	4500	9
Erythrocytes				
human	m-PTA Sepharose	TX-100	4270 3)	10
human	m-PTA Sepharose	TX-100	5700 3)	11
human	p-PTA Sepharose	TX-100/DOC	418	12
bovine	m-PTA Sepharose	TX-100	4130	13

1) PTA: Phenyltrimethylammonium; DMAEBA: dimethylaminoethyl-benzoic acid;

2) TX-100: Triton X-100; DOC: sodium deoxycholate; cholate: sodium cholate

3) Purification deploying two consecutive affinity chromatography steps

to homogeneity has been achieved in few cases only. These include the electric organ of Torpedo (4, 5), brain tissue of various origins (6-9) and red cell membranes (10-13). In those cases where a homogeneous enzyme preparation was obtained the specific activities of the pure products are comparable (table 2) and range between 3100 and 5700 IU/mg protein. On the other hand, when sodium cholate (4) or sodium deoxycholate (12) were used to solubilize and/or for purification much lower specific activities were obtained albeit the final product did appear as a single band on sodium dodecylsulfate gel electrophoresis. Such large differences in specific activities may be explained in terms of the requirement of native DS-AChE for an amphiphilic molecule that provides the hydrophobic interactions necessary to express catalytic activity.

Amphiphile Dependency of DS-AChE

The original suggestion that the activity of DS-AChE is sensitive to the hydrophobic environment of the enzyme came frome the studies of Farias et al. (14), Sihotang (15) and from Beauregard and Roufogalis (16). Wiedmer et al. (17) however were first to clearly establish the amphiphile dependency of pure native DS-AChE, namely the enzyme from human red cell membranes. Meanwhile this fact was corroborated by our further studies on this enzyme (18, 19) as well as on DS-AChE from human brain (9) and from the electric organ of Torpedo marmorata (20). As shown by Landauer et al. (21, 22) DS-AChE from bovine caudate nucleus is also sensitive to suitable hydrophobic interactions.

The experimental approach we used to establish the amphiphile dependency is as follows: Pure native DS-AChE is kept in solution by micellar concentrations of a detergent that is able to fully sustain catalytic activity (see table 3 for typical examples). The enzyme is then diluted at least 1000 fold into buffer that does not contain detergents and the activity is monitored as a function of time. In these conditions DS-AChE rapidly looses enzyme activity due to the dissociation of the stabilizing amphiphile (i. e. the detergent molecules) from the hydrophobic part of the molecule. The loss of activity is at least a two step process in which the enzyme first becomes reversibly inactivated. At this stage the readdition of a suitable amphiphile restores enzymes activity. The second, somewhat slower process is characterized by an irreversible loss of enzyme activity i. e. the readdition of any amphiphilic molecule does not restore enzyme activity. It is clear from our studies (9, 19) that even monomeric detergent molecules are able to interact with DS-AChE in such a way that the catalytic activity is preserved as the concentration of detergent needed to express full enzyme activity is well below the critical micellar concentration (CMC) of the detergent. Furthermore this concentration is also well below that needed to solubilize DS-AChE from its natural surroundings.

There exists a great variety of detergents but not all of them are able to warrant enzyme activity of DS-AChE. The effect of β-D-octylglucoside on the activity of DS-AChE

Table 3

ACTIVITY OF DS-AChE FROM TORPEDO MARMORATA IN DIFFERENT DETERGENTS

ACTIVE	PARTIALLY ACTIVE	VIRTUALLY INACTIVE
TRITON X-100	CHAPS	LDAO
TRITON X-114	OCTYL-POE	OCTYL-GP
TWEEN 40, 60, 80	NONYL-GP+	ZWITTERGENTS
BRIJ 35	DECYL-GP	
DODECYLMALTOSIDE	NA-CHOLATE	

Enzyme was preincubated for 30 minutes in detergents at twice their CMC and then activity measured by addition of AThCh and Ellman's reagent

+GP = Glucopyranoside

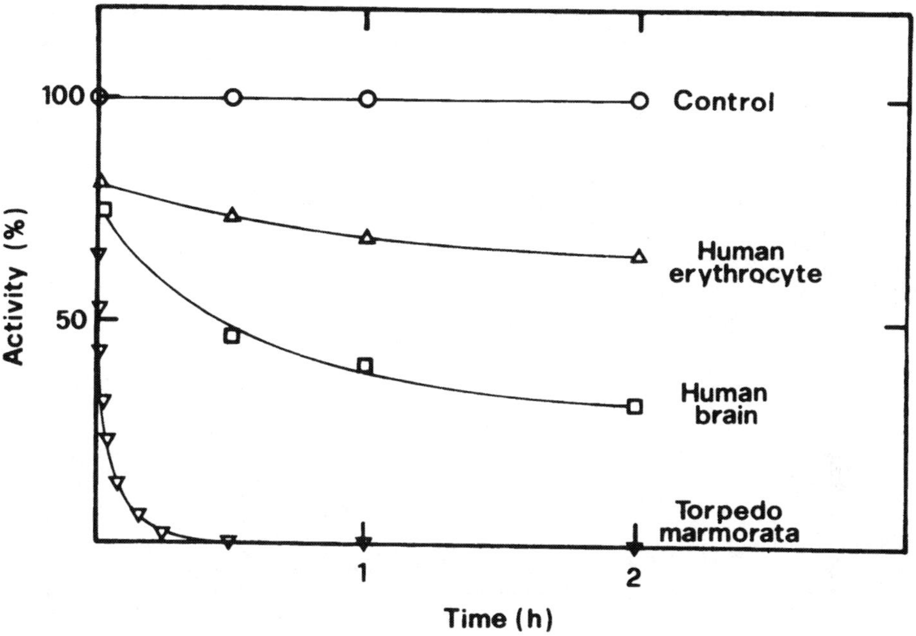

Figure 1: Effect of β-D-octylglucoside on DS-AChE from different sources. Enzyme (1 μl in Triton X-100 above CMC) was diluted 3000-fold into incubation medium containing 10 mM Tris-HCl, pH 7.4 and 0.1 % TX-100 (control) or 0.74 % (=CMC) β-D-octylglucoside. At times inidcated ATCh and Ellmans reagent were added and the enzyme activity recorded.

from three different sources is shown in Figure 1. It is obvious that the enzyme from human red cell membranes is the most stable one whereas the Torpedo marmorata enzyme rapidly looses activity. The rate of decay depends on the concentration of the detergent and does not obey first order kinetics. The decay is faster at detergent concen-

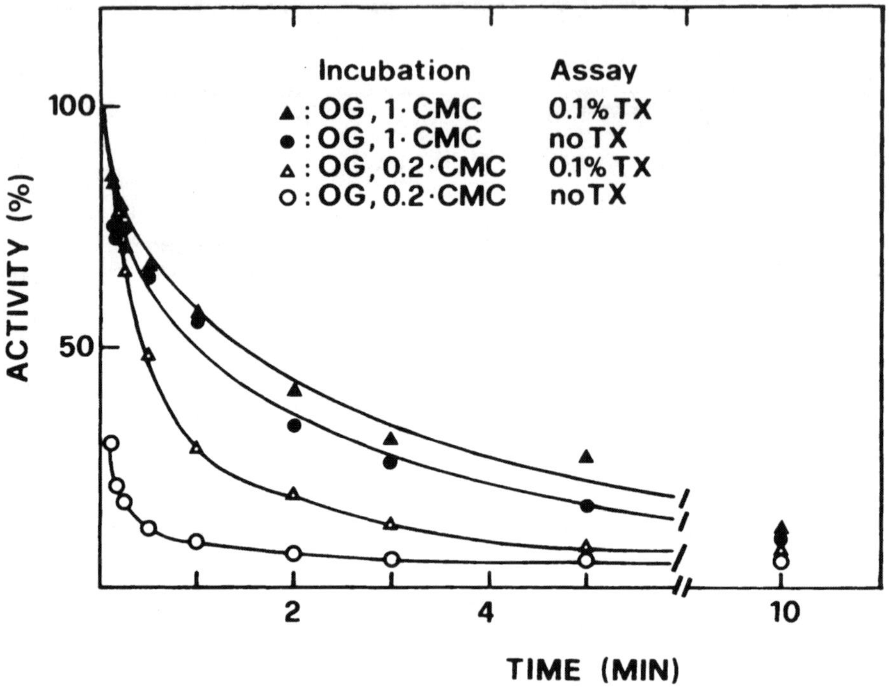

Figure 2: Inactivation of DS-AChE from Torpedo marmorata in presence of β-D-octylglucoside. Enzyme (1 μl containing 0.13 IU) in 0.05 % Triton X-100 was diluted 3000 fold into incubation medium containing 10 mM Tris-HCl, pH 7.4 and β-D-octylglucoside at 1 times CMC (=0.74 %; closed symbols) or 0.2 times CMC (=0.15 %; open symbols). At times indicated ATCh and Ellmans reagent were added and enzyme activity was mesured in absence and presence of 0.1% Triton X-100.

trations below CMC and slower at concentrations equal to, or above CMC (Fig. 2). The enzyme from Torpedo marmorata is particularly interesting as its requirement is rather specific for detergents from the polyoxyethylene-series. With the exception of dodecylmaltoside, the alkylglycosides are less satisfactory and in zwitterionic detergents the enzyme was inactive (Table 3). In this context an (unpublished) result of Sörensen is of importance. He showed that DS-AChE from human brain is irreversibly inactivated by β-D-octylglucoside which corroborates the finding of Landauer et al. (21) who noted a similar behavior for the enzyme from bovine caudate nuclei. It is interesting to note, however, that in conditions where enzyme activity decreased by more than 90 % the immuno-chemical reactivty decreased by less than 7 % (Fig. 3). This indicates that the enzyme assumes

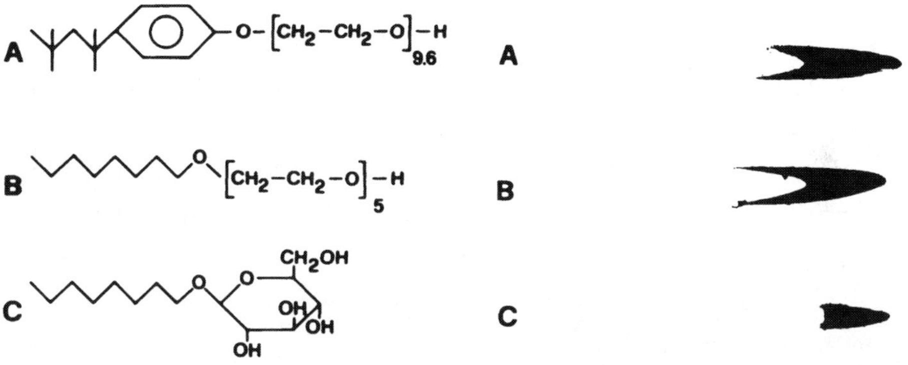

Figure 3: Immunochemical reactivity of DS-AChE from human brain. Left: Chemical formulas of Triton X-100 (A), octylpolyoxyethylene (B) and β-D-octylglcoside (C). Right: Activity stain after rocket immunoelectrophoresis carried out in presence of the respective detergents. Position of wells (start of electrophoresis) is indicated by position of letters.

subtilely different conformations in stabilizing or non-stabilizing detergents which are large enough to significantly influence its catalytical activity but are too small to be detected by the binding of (polyclonal) antibodies.

Amphiphilic Structure of DS-AChE

DS-AChE is a typical representative of those membrane bound enzymes that are firmly anchored into the lipid bilayer by a hydrophobic peptide sequence. Such anchoring sequences are well established in a number of membrane proteins (23) but to date only circumstantial evidence is available for it in DS-AChE. At protein concentrations high enough to allow rapid hydrophobic interactions the enzyme forms aggregates by self-micellarization (5, 9, 13, 20, 24, 25). Those protein micelles can be dissociated to protomeric DS-AChE in the presence of detergents above their CMC. Furthermore DS-AChE, in presence of lipids, is readily reconstituted into artificial lipid vesicles by either one of several methods of detergent depletion (7, 18, 20, 26) or by the addition of the enzymes to preformed lipid vesicles (19). The hydrophobic nature of membrane proteins is further corroborated by charge shift and by hydrophobic interactions crossed immunoelectrophoresis according to the method of Bhakdi et al. (27). By these criteria DS-AChE from human caudate nucleus (9), human red blood cells (28) and from Torpedo marmorata (20) behave like typical integral membrane proteins.

Furthermore all these enzymes are oligomeric proteins with their subunits pairwise interlinked by disulfide bridges. In situ, DS-AChE in the electric organ of Torpedoes and in red cell membranes most likely are dimers (5, 11, 20, 29) composed of identical subunits that both are catalytically active. DS-AChE from brain of different origins appears to be a tetramer (8, 9, 13). An interesting question pertains to the anchoring of the subunit assembly into the lipid bilayer. Does each subunit contain a hydrophobic peptide sequence or is there one anchor per pair of subunits? Again circumstantial evidence only is presently available to answer this question. As shown by Ott et al. (30) pure DS-AChE from human red cell may be converted to a monomeric enzyme with almost no loss in specific activity that fully retained its detergent binding properties as well as its amphiphile dependency (Ott, unpublished). This indicates that each of the two subunits contain a hydrophobic peptide sequence and that each subunit penetrates into the lipid bilayer.

DS-AChE belongs to those membrane enzymes that function in a non-vectorial way and that direct their catalytic activity entirely towards one side of the lipid bilayer. According to current views (23) such enzymes need an intact lipid bilayer only for anchoring purposes and not for biological function. Often cited examples of non-vectorial enzymes are the brush border hydrolases (aminopeptdases and glycosidases) which can be detached from the membrane by proteolytic digestion without affecting the catalytic activity. Bon and Massoulié (31) and more recently Li and Bon (32) described conditions in which DS-AChE could be solubilized from nerve endings by treatment with proteinase K or pronase. Our findings with DS-AChE from Torpedo (20) sustain their results and show that proteolytic digestion detaches the presumed hydrophobic peptide sequence. The product of digestion is smaller by about 1000 Daltons than native DS-AChE, it does no more undergo a charge shift nor is it amphiphile dependent (20). DS-AChE is thus converted by proteolysis to a low salt soluble presumably globular enzyme. It must, however be emphasized, that native DS-AChE is an integral membrane protein, embeded into the lipid bilayer via hydrophobic interactions between its hydrophobic anchor and neighbouring hydrophobic molecules. It is most likely that these molecules are the (phospho-) lipids of the membrane as their composition can modulate enzyme activity (8, 14, 18). On the other hand neighbouring hydrophobic proteins could also provide the hydrophobic environment necessary for DS-AChE to be catalytically active. A model which summarizes our current views on structure and amphiphile dependency of DS-AChE is shown in Fig. 4.

Conclusion

Basically, there are two different types of AChE. Their main difference lies not in molecular shape but in their mode of attachment to subcellular structures. One type is the integral, membrane bound, detergent soluble and amphiphile dependent DS-AChE, the other comprises the

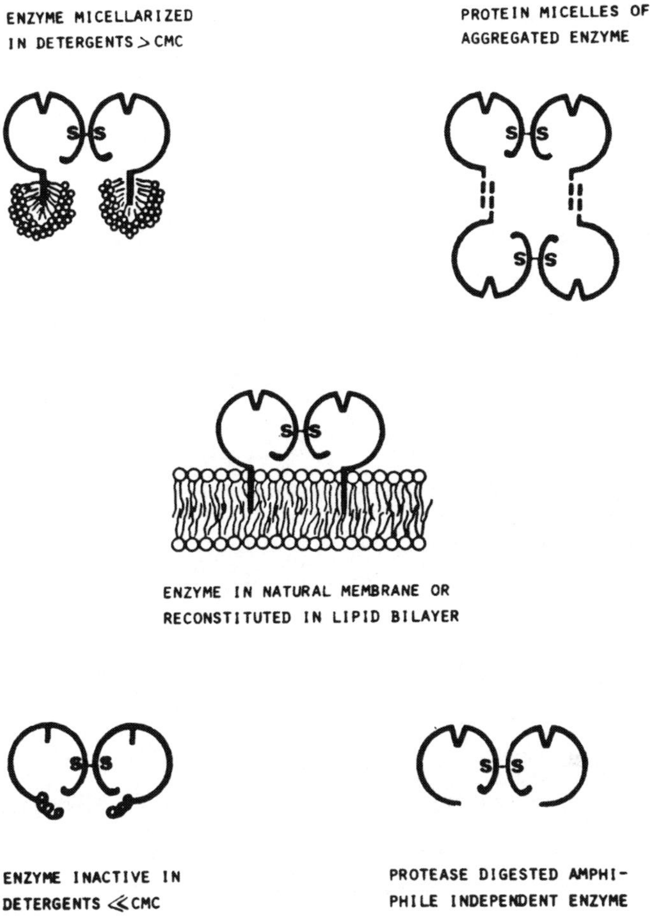

Figure 4: Proposed model for structure-function relationship of DS-AChE.

intra- and extracellular, low and high-salt soluble SS-AChE which occur either as globular or asymmetric forms. The designation of forms A and G bases on molecular shape only. In connection with DS-AChE this designation is incomplete and we therefore suggest that the designation "D" is used in connection with detergent soluble, amphiphile dependent AChE.

Acknowledgements

The authors are indebted to the Swiss National Science Foundation for financial support (Grant No. 3.300-0.82).

References

1. Massoulié, J. and Bon, S.: Ann. Rev. Neurosci. 5, 57-106 (1982).
2. Rosenberry, T. L., Barnett, Ph. and Mays, C.: Methods Enzymol. 82, 325-339 (1980).
3. Schofeniels, E. and Neumann E. (eds.): Molecular Aspects of Bioelectricity, Neurochem. Internatl. 2, (1980).
4. Viratelle, O. M. and Bernhard, S. A.: Biochemistry 19, 4999-5007 (1980).
5. Lee, S.L., Camp, S. J. and Taylor, P.: J. Biol. Chem. 257,12302-12309 (1982).
6. Ruess, K. P., Weinert, M. and Liefländer, M.: Hoppe-Seyler's Z. Physiol. Chem.: 357,783-793 (1976).
7. Reavill C. A., Wooster, M. S. and Plummer, D.T.: Biochem. J. 173, 851-856 (1978).
8. Rakonczay, Z., Mallol, J., Schenk, H., Vincendon, G. and Zanetta, J.-P.: Biochim. Biophys. Acta 657, 243-256 (1981).

9. Sörensen, K., Gentinetta, R. and Brodbeck, U.: J. Neurochem. 39, 1050-1060 (1982).
10. Ott, P., Jenny, B. and Brodbeck, U.: Eur. J. Biochem. 57, 469-480 (1975).
11. Ott, P., Lustig, A., Brodbeck, U. and Rosenbusch, J.-P.: FEBS Lett. 138, 187-189 (1982).
12. Niday, E., Wang, C. S. and Alaupovic, P.: Biochim. Biophys. Acta 469, 180-193 (1977).
13. Grossmann, H. and Liefländer, M.: Z. Naturforsch. 34c, 721-725 (1979).
14. Farias, R. N., Bloj, B., Morero, R. D., Sineriz, F. and Trucco, R. E.: Biochim. Biophys. Acta 415, 231-251 (1975).
15. Sihotang, K.: Eur. J. Biochem. 63, 519-524 (1976).
16. Beauregard, G. and Roufogalis, B. D.: Biochem. Biophys. Res. Commun. 77, 211-219 (1977).
17. Wiedmer, T., Di Francesco, Ch. and Brodbeck, U.: Eur. J. Biochem. 102, 59-64 (1979).
18. Frenkel, E. J., Roelofsen, B., Brodbeck, U., van Deenen, L. L. M. and Ott, P.: Eur. J. Biochem. 109, 277-382 (1980).
19. Di Francesco, Ch. and Brodbeck, U.: Biochim. Biophys. Acta 640, 359-364 (1981).
20. Stieger, S. and Brodbeck, U.: Abstr. Second Meeting on Cholinesterases, Bled (1983).
21. Landauer, P., Ruess, K.-P. and Liefländer, M.: Biochem. Biophys. Res. Commun. 106, 848-855 (1982).
22. Landauer, P., Ruess, K.-P. and Liefländer, M.: Hoppe-Seyler's Z. Physiol. Chem. 364 433-437 (1983).

23. Warren, G., in "Membrane Structure", J.B. Finean and R. H. Michell, (eds.), Elsevier/North Holland Biomedical Press, 215-257 (1981).
24. Ott, P. and Brodbeck, U.: Eur. J. Biochem. 88, 119-125 (1978).
25. Rakonczay, Z., Vincendon, G. and Zanetta, J.-P.: J. Neurochem. 37, 662-669 (1981).
26. Hall, E. R. and Brodbeck, U.: Eur. J. Biochem. 89, 159-167 (1978).
27. Bhakdi, S., Bhakdi-Lehnen, B. and Bjerrum, O. J.: Biochim. Biophys. Acta 470, 35-44 (1977).
28. Weitz, M., Bjerrum, O. J., Ott, P. and Brodbeck, U.: J. Cell. Biochem. 19, 179-191 (1982).
29. Römer-Lüthi, C., Ott, P. and Brodbeck, U.: Biochim. Biophys Acta 601, 123-133 (1980).
30. Ott, P., Ariano, B. H., Binggeli, Y. and Brodbeck, U.: Biochim. Biophys. Acta 729, 193-199 (1983).
31. Bon, S. and Massoulié, J.: Proc. Natl. Acad. Sci. USA 77, 4464-4468 (1980).
32. Li, Z.-Y. and Bon, C.: J. Neurochem. 40, 338-349 (1983).

SYNTHESIS, ASSEMBLY, AND PROCESSING OF AChE IN TISSUE CULTURED MUSCLE

Richard L. Rotundo

Carnegie Institution of Washington, Department of Embryology, Baltimore, Maryland 21210

Introduction

Since the initial findings of Massoulié and colleagues showing that cholinesterases consist of families of structurally related oligomeric forms (1,2,), and the concerted efforts of several laboratories to elucidate their structure (2-6), considerable research has been devoted to understanding how these complex molecules are assembled, localized, and regulated in eucaryotic cells. For the most part, interest has focused on electrically excitable cells such as muscle and nerves where AChE plays an important role in terminating the actions of the neurotransmitter acetylcholine. Furthermore, the localization of this enzyme at synapses, and its apparent regulation by cell-cell interactions and/or the electrical activity of cells (7-13) has provided strong impetus for neurobiologists to study this enzyme. Rather than provide a detailed review of AChE metabolism, what I would like to do in this chapter is simply summarize some of the recent work from my laboratory. Most of our studies have employed tissue cultured avian muscle obtained from chicken and quail embryos. These two systems are very similar with respect to the synthesis and metabolism of AChE molecules, the major exception being that quail muscle cells synthesize much greater amounts of the collagen-tailed AChE form. Although I will discuss experiments on either one or the other system, with minor exceptions so far the results apply equally to both cell types.

Molecular Forms of AChE in Chicken and Quail Muscle Cultures

The major forms of AChE in chicken muscle cultures are the 7S dimer and the 11S tetramer, in the ratio of about 4:1 (14). Under appropriate conditions, small amounts of the 19S asymmetric form are also apparent, although usually it is difficult to detect (15). The monomeric 5.5S AChE is present at very low levels. The pattern of AChE forms found in cultured quail muscle is quite different; all molecular forms are present and sufficient asymmetric AChE is synthesized to make direct studies on its assembly feasible. The patterns of AChE forms in these two systems are presented in Figures 1 and 2. Details of these systems have been published (14-15).

We have recently purified the membrane-bound hydrophobic form of AChE from adult chicken brain for both structural and biochemical studies as well as for use as an antigen. Using the purified protein we have raised highly specific antisera as well as produced monoclonal antibodies to the AChE molecule (Rotundo, submitted for publication). Both types of antibodies are specific for AChE, do not cross react with BuChE, do not cross react with mammalian AChEs, but recognize all the molecular forms of AChE found in chicken and quail. We have used these antibodies extensively to study the synthesis, assembly, and metabolic fate of this enzyme in tissue cultured muscle. An example of the specificity of these antibodies is illustrated in Figure 3. In this example, the polyclonal antibodies were used to label the neuromuscular junction on teased fibers from adult chicken ALD or to immunoprecipitate ^{35}S-methionine labeled AChE and analyze the labeled proteins by SDS gel electrophoresis and fluorography. Identical specificity is obtained using the monoclonal anti-AChE (Rotundo, in preparation).

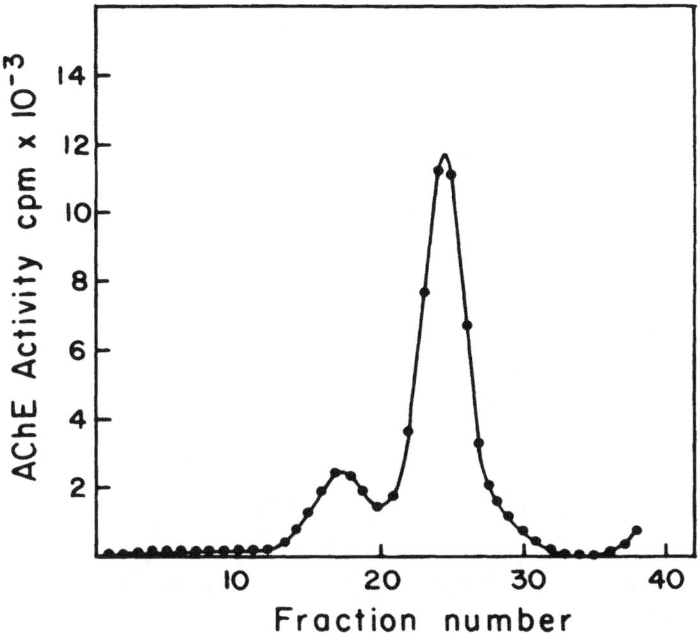

Figure 1: Molecular Forms of AChE in Chicken Embryo Muscle Cultures. Five day old muscle cultures were rinsed with Hank's Balanced Salt Solution (HBSS), extracted, and analyzed by velocity sedimentation as previously described (14). Under our standard culture conditions chick embryo skeletal muscle contains about 20% G4 AChE and 80% G2 AChE. A small amount of the G1 monomer appears as a slight shoulder on the G2 peak. When the cultures are incubated in serum-free media about 3-5% of the total AChE activity occurs as the A12 asymmetric AChE form.

Synthesis of AChE

Evidence for multiple polypeptide chains

Our initial studies using polyclonal or monoclonal antibodies to immunoprecipitate isotopically labeled AChE molecules from tissue cultured muscle showed that the enzyme migrated as a broad band on SDS polyacrylamide gels. This is due to the fact that AChE is a glycoprotein containing approximately 10-15% carbohydrate by

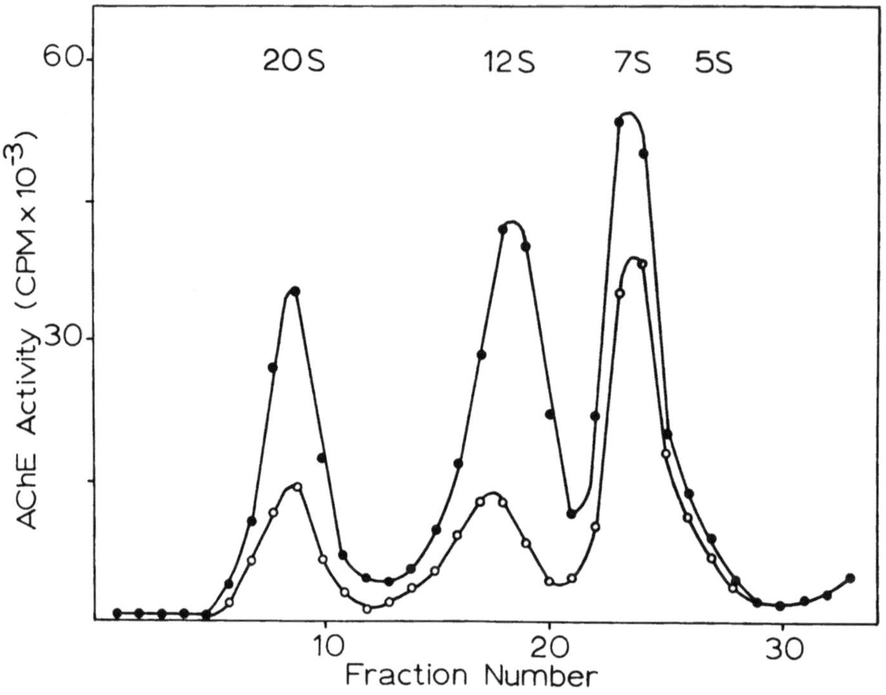

Figure 2: Molecular Forms of AChE in Quail Embryo Muscle Cultures. Quail muscle cultures were washed and incubated for 15 minutes on ice with either HBSS alone or containing 10^{-5} M ecothiophate iodide (phospholine) to inhibite cell surface AChE. After extensive washing the cells were extracted and analyzed by velocity sedimentation. Solid circles: AChE molecular forms in untreated cultures. Open circles: intracellular AChE forms in cultures treated with the membrane impermeant inhibitor echothiophate. Copyright PNAS, with permission.

weight (see below) and that it consists of at least two distinct polypeptide chains (Figure 4). When the newly synthesized AChE molecules are treated with endoglycosidase-H, an enzyme which cleaves asparagine-linked oligosaccharides of the high mannose type, the α and β AChE polypeptides are readily discernible (Figure 4). Pulse-chase studies, with labeling times as short as five or ten minutes, show that the two polypeptides are synthesized independently, that one is not a degradation product of the other, nor do they have a precursor product relationship. In the presence of

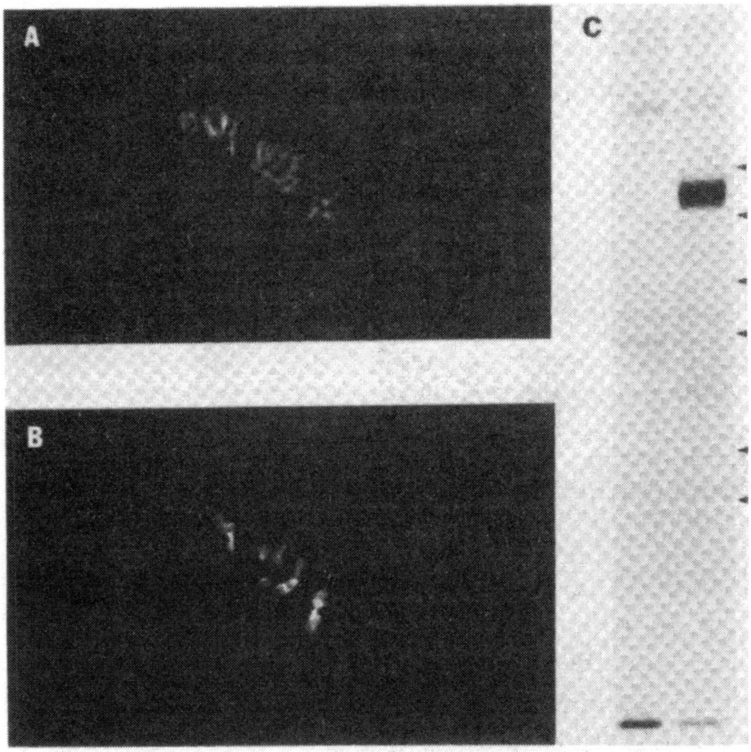

Figure 3: Specificity of Polyclonal anti-AChE Antibodies.
The tetrameric form of AChE from adult chicken brain was purified to homogeneity and used to immunize rabbits after obtaining pre-immune serum (Rotundo, submitted for publication). The sera were then fractionated by ammonium sulfate precipitation and DEAE-cellulose chromatography to obtain purified IgG. A) Endplate of adult chicken ALD muscle fiber visualized by indirect immunofluorescence using the polyclonal anti-AChE antibody and fluorescein labeled second antibody. B) Same endplate stained with rhodamine labeled alpha-bungarotoxin to visualize the distribution of acetylcholine receptors. C) Immunoprecipitation of ^{35}S-methionine labeled AChE from chicken embryo muscle cultures. Left lane: precipitation with pre-immune IgG. Right lane: precipitation with anti-AChE IgG. In both cases the immunoprecipitates were dissolved in SDS sample buffer and reduced with beta-mercaptoethanol before running on 10% polyacrylamide gels and fluorographed. Similar results are obtained with monoclonal anti-chicken AChE antibodies.

tunicamycin, a drug that inhibits the addition of asparagine-linked oligosaccharides to nascent polypeptide chains, both the α and β

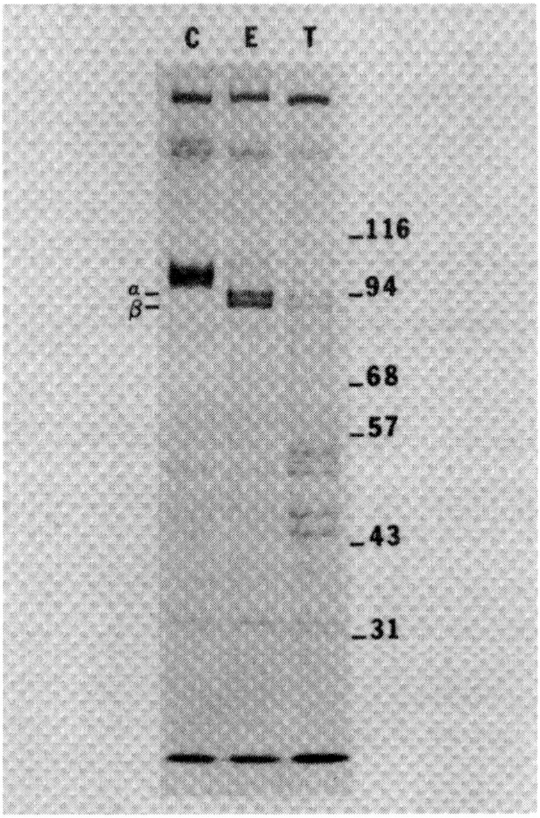

Figure 4. Resolution of the α and β AChE Polypeptide Chains of Chicken Muscle AChE.
Primary cultures of chicken embryo muscle were labeled with ^{35}S-methionine in the presence and absence of 1 μg/ml tunicamycin, a drug that blocks the addition of asparagine-linked oligosaccharides. The cultures were then washed, extracted in detergent containing buffer, and the labeled AChE immunoprecipitated using the polyclonal anti-AChE IgG. The immunoprecipitate from control cultures was divided into two aliquots and incubated in the presence or absence of endoglycosidase-H, an enzyme which removes asparagine-linked oligosaccharides of the high mannose type. The samples were then electrophoresed on 7.5% polyacrylamide gels and fluorographed. The numbers indicate the positions of molecular weight markers (in kilodaltons).

AChE polypeptides are still synthesized, however in reduced amounts (Figure 4). By SDS gel electrophoresis the apparent molecular weights of the two polypeptides synthesized in the presence of tunicamycin are approximately the same as for the endoglycosidase-H treated protein. During chases of isotopically labeled AChE we find that the ratio of the α and β polypeptides remains constant, providing further evidence against a precursor-product relationship. Furthermore, analysis of the AChE molecular forms synthesized in culture, including the cell associated and secreted forms indicates that all AChE oligomers consist of equal ratios of the two polypeptide chains.

Assembly of AChE

Because we have found considerable differences in the time and place of assembly of the globular and asymmetric AChE forms I will discuss the two separately. Like most membrane and secreted proteins, the AChE molecule is a glycoproetin and hence is synthesized on the RER. The addition of about 10,000 daltons of asparagine-linked oligosaccharides occurs co-translationally in the case of AChE. Several lines of evidence indicate that the globular forms of AChE are assembled in the RER. First, when cells are treated with DFP and allowed to recover in complete medium the rates of appearance of the dimeric and tetrameric forms is linear with respect to time and extrapolates back to zero (Rotundo, in preparation). Thus, assembly must have occurred at or shortly after the time of synthesis. Pulse-chase studies of catalytically active, or isotopically labeled AChE molecules indicate that once individual molecular forms are assembled they do not interconvert, although they may subsequently be degraded. A second line of evidence indicating that the globular forms of AChE are assembled in the RER comes from the analysis of the AChE oligosaccharides (16). In these studies we have used lectins that recognize specific sugar residues which are added to AChE molecules either in the RER or the cis or trans elements of the Golgi apparatus respectively. At the earliest times post-synthesis all dimeric and tetrameric AChE molecules can bind con-

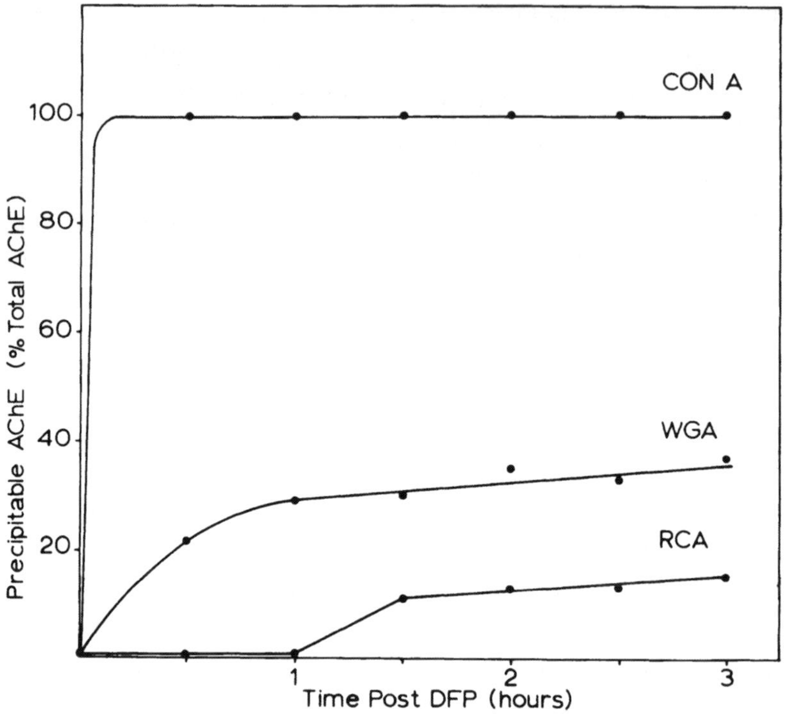

Figure 5. Time Course of AChE Oligosaccharide Processing in Tissue Cultured Quail Muscle Cells
Muscle cultures were treated with DFP and allowed to synthesize new AChE molecules in the presence of complete medium. At the designated time intervals, duplicate cultures were rinsed with HBSS and extracted in detergent containing buffer. Aliquots of each supernatant were incubated with immobilized concanavalin A (ConA), wheat germ agglutinin (WGA), or ricin I (RCA) which specifically bind to the sugars mannose, N-acetylglucosamine, and galactose, respectively. The AChE remaining in the supernatants was determined using the radiometric assay of Johnson and Russell (20) and the percent AChE bound (percent precipitable AChE) was calculated as the difference between samples incubated with lectins or an identical volume of underivatized sepharose 4B beads. Copyright PNAS, with permission.

canvalin A (ConA), which recognizes mannose residues added in the RER, whereas newly synthesized AChE does not bind either wheat germ agglutinin (WGA) or ricin (RCA) which recognize sugars added in the

Golgi apparatus (Figure 5). We conclude at this point that the globular forms of AChE are asembled in the RER and subsequently transferred to the cis elements of the Golgi where additional processing of the AChE molecules occurs. Details of these processing events will be discussed in a later section.

The assembly of collagen-tailed asymmetric AChE form occurs much later than the globular forms (16). In contrast to the dimeric and tetrameric forms which appear immediately after DFP treatment, the asymmetric form of AChE does not appear until about 90 minutes post treatment (see Figure 6). Based upon our current knowledge of the time course of processing events in muscle cells these results suggested that the collagen-tailed form of the enzyme was being assembled in the Golgi apparatus. Since we know that the addition of mannose, GlcNAc, and Gal occur sequentially in defined subcellular compartments (17) we could take advantage of that observation to ask the question, in which organelle does assembly occur? From our earlier studies we knew that the transport of AChE from the RER to the earliest Golgi compartment required about 15 minutes. This is based upon the time required for addition of GlcNAc which is believed to occur in the Golgi cisternae most proximal to the RER. The AChE molecules appear to reside in the Gogli for about two hours prior to export either to the cell surface or secretion into the extracellular milieu. This is based on the observation that it requires approximately 45-60 minutes post-synthesis for the first appearance of Endo-H resistant AChE polypeptides (Rotundo, submitted for publication), an event which requires processing in the Golgi apparatus, and that the addition of the terminal galactose residues only occurs about 90-120 minutes after synthesis of the AChE polypeptide chains (Figure 5). The addition of terminal sugars such as galactose, sialic acid, and fucose all appear to occur in the most distal, or trans, cisternae of the Gogli. When we analyze the oligosaccharides on the newly synthesized and assembled asymmetric AChE molecules we find that all

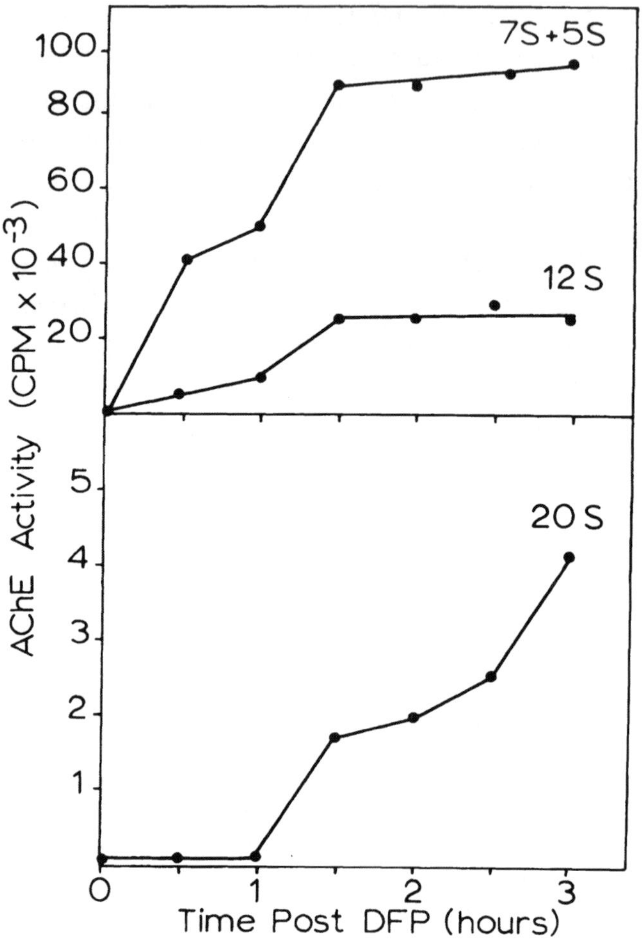

Figure 6. Recovery of AChE Molecular Forms in Quail Muscle Cultures after DFP Treatment
Muscle cultures were treated with DFP at 30 minute intervals and returned to the incubator in complete medium for the designated period of time. At the end of the time course AChE was extracted in detergent buffer and the molecular forms analyzed by velocity sedimentation. The total activity for individual AChE molecular forms was calculated by summing the areas under their respective peaks. The 7S dimers and 5S monomers are not well resolved on these gradients, hence their total activities were combined. However, the 5S AChE constitutes only a small fraction of the 7S + 5S activity. Copyright PNAS, with permission.

have GlcNAc residues indicating that they must have been assembled from subunits which have already acquired complex sugars and hence must have been residing in the Golgi. We conclude that the A12 AChE molecule is assembled in the distal elements of the Golgi apparatus.

Processing of AChE

Although the evidence for several processing events has already been described in preceeding sections, a brief summary, along with some additional material, will be presented here. We have already mentioned that the α and β polypeptides of AChE are synthesized independently and hence are distinct proteins. They differ in apparent molecular weight by about 5000 daltons. Based upon the shift in apparent mobility on SDS gels after endo-H treatment (Figure 4) as well as their apparent molecular weights when synthesized in the presence of tunicamycin they also appear to be glycosylated in a similar manner and contain about the same amount of carbohydrate per polypeptide chain. Pulse-chase studies indicate that the polypeptide portions of the AChE molecules do not undergo any obvious modifications during their transit through the cell, as revealed by SDS gel electrophoresis. When the secreted forms of AChE are treated in such a way as to remove the asparagine-linked oligosaccharides we find that the apparent mobilities of the α and β chains are unchanged compared to the cell associated enzyme. However small covalent modifications of the AChE polypeptides such as phosphorylation or fatty acid acylation would not be detected by these techniques.

The major modifications of the AChE molecules which we can detect are those which involve processing of oligosaccharides. Although the structures of the AChE oligosaccharides have not been elucidated, from our lectin studies we do know that they contain mannose,

GlcNAc, and Gal. We have not detected any appreciable amounts of sialic acid using limulus lectin.

Based upon the time and order of addition of the different marker sugars we postulate that the same types of processing events occur on the AChE oligosaccharides as have been shown to occur for other asparagine-linked oligosacchararides in other cell types.

Degradation of AChE

During our initial studies on the assembly of the AChE molecules in tissue cultured muscle using isotopically labeled AChE and pulse-chase paradigms we noticed that the vast majority of the newly synthesized AChE polypeptides were lost very rapidly by a process which appeared to exhibit first order decay kinetics with a half-life of just under one hour. This apparent loss of AChE molecules does not appear to be simple loss of antigenicity because both our monoclonal and polyclonal antibodies recognize denatured enzyme as well as proteolytic fragments of the AChE molecules down to about 20,000 daltons molecular weight. Because of this we feel that a fraction of the AChE population is being degraded intracellularly. Approximately 80% of the newly synthesized AChE molecules are lost in this manner. Most interesting, however, is the observation that the rapidly degraded AChE molecules do not appear to be catalytically active, and for the most part consist of the monomeric forms of the enzyme. A portion of the G2 enzyme is also degraded, however once assembled the G4 AChE molecules appear to be stable. This peculiar aspect of AChE metabolism is currently being investigated.

Transport of AChE

The transport time for AChE as we define it is the time required for the newly synthesized molecules to reach the plasma membrane, either to be inserted as the membrane bound form or to be secreted into the medium or extracellular milieu. Following treatment of muscle cells with DFP we can show that it requires approximately two to three hours for the newly synthesized enzyme molecules to reach the plasma membrane (18,19). After that time they either accumulate on the plasma membrane or accumulate in the culture medium. Identical results are obtained when cells are incubated in the presence of isotopically labeled amino acids and the time of first appearance of labeled AChE molecules into the medium measured by immunoprecipitation and SDS gel electrophoresis followed by fluorography. This transport time, then, is the total time required for the AChE molecules to transit through all the cellular organelles involved in their processing and translocation. Based upon our current understanding of the intracellular trafficking of glycoproteins, the intracellular transport of the AChE molecules is presumably mediated via coated vesicles.

Summary and Conclusions

Like all exportable glycoproteins studied to date, AChE is synthesized on the RER with the addition of approximately four asparagine-linked oligosaccharides occurring cotranslationally. The AChE molecules are synthesized as two separate polypeptide chains of about 100,000 and 105,000 daltons each. The polypeptide chains are assembled shortely after synthesis into the dimeric and tetrameric forms of the enzyme. Based upon analyses of the oligosaccharides on newly synthesized AChE molecules we conclude that the assembly of the globular AChE forms must be occurring in the RER. Following their assembly, the molecules are then transported to the most proximal elements of the Golgi apparatus (cis Golgi) where processing of the high mannose type of oligosaccharides to complex sugars begins. The time for transport from RER to the cis Golgi appears to take about fifteen minutes on the average. Entry into the cis Gogli is marked by the addition of GlcNAc, hence acquisition of WGA binding. Two other events which are also known to occur in the Golgi are the acquisition of endo-H resistance, which for AChE occurs about 45-60 minutes post-synthesis, and the addition of terminal sugars such as galactose in the most distal or trans elements of the Golgi. This latter event, for AChE, occurs at about 90 minutes post-synthesis. Only late in this scheme is the asymmetric form of the enzyme assembled; based upon the types of sugars associated with the AChE polypeptides at the time of assembly we conclude that the asymmetric forms must be assembled from subunits, presumably tetramers, which have already entered the Gogli. These findings suggest that the regulation of AChE synthesis, activation, and assembly to multimeric forms may involve several post-translational events. In the case of the asymmetric AChE molecule, our studies suggest the interesting possibility that assembly might be regulated at the level of the Golgi apparatus.

This research was supported by grants from the National Science Foundation (BNS80-15778), the Muscular Dystrophy Association, and a Sloan Foundation Fellowship to RLR. The technical assistance of Ms. Abbie Mays and Ms. Susan Satchell's preparation of the manuscript are gratefully acknowledged.

References

1. Massoulié, J., Rieger, F.: Eur. J. Biochem. 11, 441-455 (1969).
2. Massoulié, J., Bon, S.: Ann. Rev. Neurosci. 5, 57-106 (1982).
3. Rosenberry, T.L., Richardson, J.M.: Biochem. 16, 3550-3558 (1977).
4. Anglister, L., Silman, I.: J. Mol. Biol. 125, 293-311 (1978).
5. Lwebuga-Mukasa, J.S., Lappi, S., Taylor, P.: Biochem. 15,

1425-1434 (1976).

6. Lee, S., Taylor, P.: J. Biol. Chem. 257, 12292-12301 (1982).
7. Vigny, M., Koenig, J., Rieger, F.: J. Neurochem. 27, 1347-1353 (1976).
8. Koenig, J., Vigny, M.: Nature 271, 75-77 (1978).
9. Rubin, L.L., Schuetze, S.M., Weill, C.L., Fischbach, G.D.: Nature 283, 264-267 (1980).
10. Lømo, T., Slater, C.R.: J. Physiol. 303, 191-202 (1980).
11. Rieger, F., Koenig, J., Vigny, M.: Devel. Biol. 76, 358-365 (1980).
12. Weinberg, C.B., Hall, Z.W.: Devel. Biol. 68, 631-635 (1979).
13. Weinberg, C.B., Sanes, J.R., Hall, Z.W.: Devel. Biol. 84, 255-266 (1981).
14. Rotundo, R.L., Fambrough, D.M.: J. Biol. Chem. 254, 4790-4799 (1979).
15. Bulger, J.E., Randall, W.R., Nieberg, P.S., Patterson, G.T., McNamee, M.G., Wilson, B.W.: Develop. Neurosci. 5, 474-483 (1982).
16. Rotundo, R.L.: Proc. Natl. Acad. Sci. (1983) in press.
17. Lennarz, W.J. (ed.): The Biochemistry of Glycoproteins and Proteoglycans, Plenum Press, New York (1980).
18. Rotundo, R.L., Fambrough, D.M.: Cell 22, 583-594 (1980).
19. Rotundo, R.L., Fambrough, D.M.: Cell 22, 595-602 (1980).
20. Johnson, C.D., Russell, R.L.: Anal. Biochem. 64, 229-238 (1975).

ONTOGENIC AND AGRANULATION-INDUCED ALTERATIONS IN CHOLINESTERASES AND IN CHOLINESTERASE mRNA IN THE RODENT CEREBELLUM

Ruti Parvari, Israel Silman and Hermona Soreq

Department of Neurobiology,
Weizmann Institute of Science,
Rehovot 76100, Israel.

Introduction

Ontogenic variations in the level, localization and properties of cholinesterases (ChEs) have been extensively studied in the brain by both biochemical and histochemical techniques (for reviews see 1, 2). In the rodent cerebellum both approaches were used to study the ontogenic pattern of ChEs. Transient ChE activity was histochemically localized in the Purkinje cell layer in slices of cerebellum obtained during the 2nd postnatal week (3), and was implicated in the direct connection of Purkinje cells to mossy fibers at this stage (4). Most of the nerve cells in the mature cerebellar cortex (Purkinje, granule, basket and stellate) were found to be noncholinergic, with the exception of Golgi type II neurons. Climbing fibers, parallel fibers and basket terminals were also found to be non-cholinergic, whereas in the granular layer most of the acousticovestibular mossy fibers and their glomeruli terminals were positively stained (4), as were nerve cells in deep cerebellar nuclei (5).

The developmental changes in location of cerebellar ChE are accompanied by biochemical variations in the enzyme, which was reported to be composed principally of 4S and 10S forms, the 4S form being predominant at birth and decreasing with cerebellar maturation (6). In the mouse cerebellum, the specific activity of AChE was found to increase progressively throughout the first 2 postnatal weeks, during the period in which Golgi type II cells mature and synapses with granule cells are established by both mossy fibers and Golgi terminals (5). However, histochemical and biochemical analyses were inadequate to reveal which fraction of the enzyme is synthesized within intrinsic cerebellar cell bodies and which part of it is contributed by incoming fibers. An analysis of mRNA levels offers an approach to answering this question, since mRNA is found exclusively in cell bodies and is absent from processes (7). Thus, increases in ChE levels which were not accompanied by a corresponding increase in ChEmRNA would indicate, at a first approximation, that this enzyme was being contributed by incoming fibers.

In order to reveal whether the ontogenic changes in the level and properties of cerebellar ChE depend on the presence of specific cell types and the formation of correct circuitry, we investigated the alterations in specific activity, substrate specificity and molecular forms of ChE during development of normal and X-irradiated rat cerebellum (8-10), and in the agranular cerebellum of adult staggerer mice (11, 12). So as to define whether these changes are regulated at the level of mRNA, we translated cerebellar mRNA from all of these sources into catalytically active ChE in microinjected Xenopus oocytes (13). Our results indicate that in the mature cerebellum most of the ChE activity is contributed by incoming fibers and is not regulated at the level of cerebellar mRNA. Minor cell populations contribute a small fraction of the enzyme both in the normal and the agranular cerebellum, and biosynthesis of ChE is most intense in the neonatal cerebellum, decreasing progressively with maturation.

Results and Discussion

As can be seen in Fig. 1, specific activity of ChE increases during cerebellar development from birth up to 4 weeks of age, and the total content of ChE increases likewise. A similar age-dependence is noted in the X-irradiated cerebellum, which is depleted of most of its granule neurons (8-12) and which displays higher specific activity of ChE than the corresponding controls throughout this period (Fig. 1, left) in agreement with Valcana et al.(14). However, Fig. 1 (right) clearly

Figure 1. **Increased specific activity and unchanged content of ChE throughout ontogenesis of irradiation-agranulated rat cerebellum, as compared to control cerebellum.**

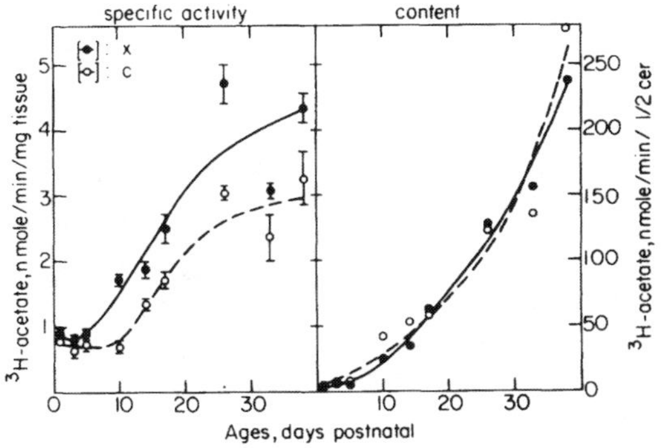

Sprague-Dawley rats were raised and irradiated as described (10). ChE activity was determined radiometrically (16) in triplicate in tissue homogenates (13). Data are presented as ^{3}H-ACh degraded per mg tissue (left) and as ^{3}H-ACh degraded per cerebellar hemisphere (right). Standard deviations are indicated by bars.

shows that the total content of ChE per cerebellar hemisphere, in control and X-irradiated cerebella, is identical during this period. It is interesting to note that parallel observations were made for the ontogenesis of density and content of muscarinic binding sites in the irradiated cerebellum (15).

Fig. 2 (left) shows the change during development in the percentage of total ChE activity which is resistant to the AChE-specific inhibitor BW 284C51 (17). In both normal and irradiated cerebellum, this figure decreases from over 30% at birth to ca. 15% at day 30, indicating that a substantial fraction of the ChE activity in neonatal cerebellum corresponds to pseudo-ChE. A similar observation was made for ChEs in neuronal perikarya from developing rat cerebral cortices by Ochoa and coworkers (18). When molecular forms of ChE were analysed by sucrose

Figure 2. BW 284C51-resistant ChE activity in irradiation-agranulated and control rat cerebellum: ontogenic decrease and sedimentation pattern.

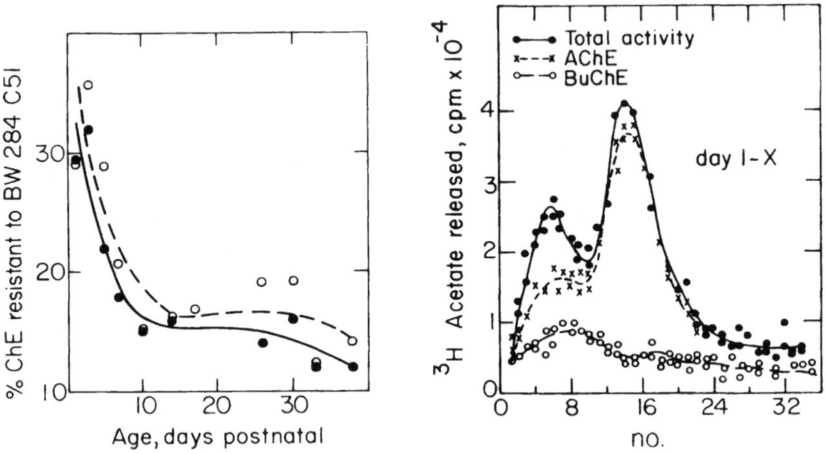

Left: ChE activity was determined in cerebellar homogenates from control (-o-) and irradiated (-●-) rats, in the presence or absence of BW 284C51. The percentage activity resistant to inhibitor, representing pseudo-ChE, was calculated for each sample. Right: Homogenates of pools of 5 irradiated cerebellar hemispheres from 1 day old rats were centrifuged on linear sucrose gradients and ChE activity determined radiometrically (19). (-●-): no inhibitors added (total ChE). (-x-): samples were preincubated 30 min with 10^{-4} M iso-OMPA and activity measured in the presence of inhibitor (AChE). (-o-): assay carried out in the presence of 10^{-4} M BW 284C51 (pseudo-ChE). Bovine catalase (11.4S) peaked in fraction 18.

gradient centrifugation of extracts of fresh tissue, a major peak of 10S and a smaller peak of 4S were observed in both irradiated and normal cerebellum. Fig. 2 (right) shows, by use of BW 284C51 and the corresponding pseudo-ChE-specific inhibitor iso-OMPA (17), the relative contributions of AChE and pseudo-ChE to these two peaks in day 1 irradiated cerebellum. It can be seen that the 10S peak is almost all accounted for by AChE, whereas a substantial part of the 4S peak is contributed by pseudo-ChE. Day 1 control cerebellum yields a similar pattern (not shown).

Figure 3. Ontogenic and malformation-induced alterations in the migration pattern of ChE molecular forms.

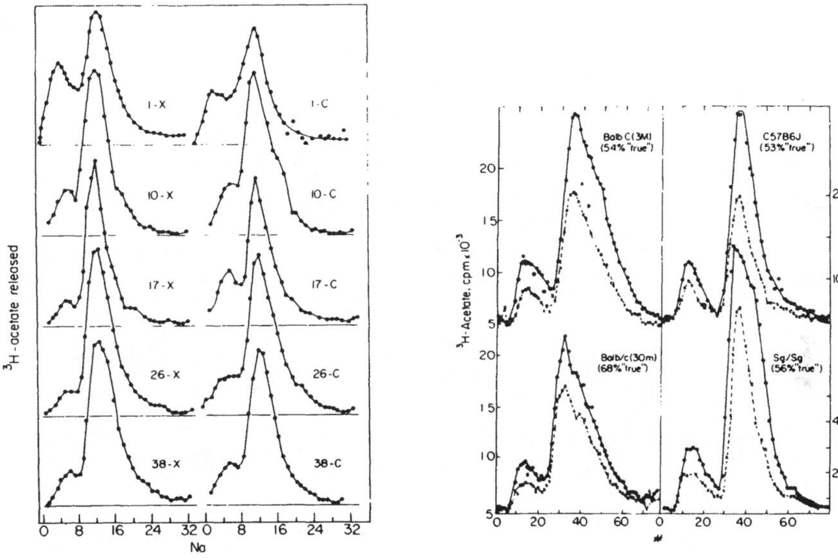

Extracts of the appropriate samples were centrifuged on sucrose gradients and ChE activity assayed radiometrically in the fractionated gradients. Left: Sucrose gradients of extracts of cerebellar hemispheres from control (C) and irradiated (X) rats, at the denoted ages (days). Right: Sucrose gradients of cerebellar extracts from BalbC mice (3 and 30 months old) and from 5 month old C57B6J mice and homozygous staggerer mutants. ChE activity was determined in the absence (-●-) or presence (-x-) of 10^{-4} M BW 284C51.

In the neonatal cerebellum, the 4S peak accounts for ca. 30% of the total ChE activity in both normal and irradiated hemispheres, and its contribution decreases with age in the two cases (Fig. 3, left). These results are at variance with those of Timiras and Wade (6) who found the 4S peak to be predominant at birth, to decrease transiently at day 10, and finally to decrease again in the adult.

Figure 4. Ontogenic and malformation-induced alterations in the level of translatable ChEmRNA in rodent cerebellum.

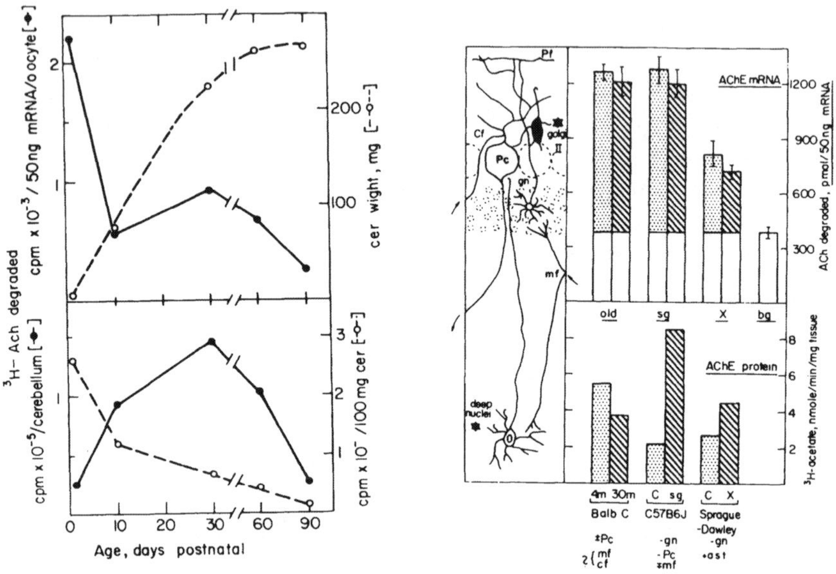

Polyadenylated RNA was extracted from cerebellar tissue as described (20). 50 ng of 1mg/ml cerebellar mRNA were microinjected into groups of 10 oocytes each. Oocytes were incubated for 20 hr at 21°C and ChE activity determined radiometrically (16) in triplicate (13).

LEFT: Developmental modifications in the level and content of rat cerebellar ChEmRNA. Upper: The data presented show total cumulative mRNA-induced ChE activities (oocyte homogenate + incubation medium) per single oocyte. The dotted line represents cerebellar weight. Endogenous ChE activity in control oocytes (700 pmoles ACh degraded per hr per oocyte) was subtracted. Lower: The relative content of ChEmRNA, expressed as cpm x 10^{-5} of ^{3}H-ACh degraded per cerebellum (-●-) was derived from ChEmRNA concentration per 50 ng of mRNA, and the total content of mRNA per cerebellum at the different developmental stages. The concentration of ChEmRNA, in cpm x 10^{-5} of ^{3}H-Ach degraded per 100 mg cerebellar tissue (-o-), was derived from the ChEmRNA concentration and the level of total cerebellar mRNA.

RIGHT: Expression of ChE and of ChEmRNA in the cerebellum of old and staggerer mice and of irradiated rats, as compared to the appropriate controls. Upper: ChEmRNA levels. mRNA was extracted from cerebella of 4 and 30 month BalbC mice, of normal and sg/sg C57B6J mice and control and irradiated hemispheres of cerebella of Sprague-Dawley rats (12). Up to 50 ng of mRNA were injected into groups of 10 oocytes, and ChE activity determined in triplicate after 20 hr incubation at 21°C in both oocyte incubation medium and oocyte homogenates. Values presented are the sums of both activities, the bars representing standard deviations. Control oocytes (bg), injected with 50 nl of Barth medium, displayed ChE activity degrading 390 pmole ACh/hr/oocyte. Lower: ChE specific activity. Pooled cerebella from several mice or rats were used to prepare homogenates for each determination. Assays were carried out in triplicate. Inset: The major cellular elements in the cerebellar cortex are schematically described. Cell types which are putative ChE producers are noted by stars (The elements defective in each of the malformations examined are noted below).

In the cerebellum of both staggerer mice and the corresponding C57B6J controls, and in old (30 months) BalbC mice and the corresponding 3 month adults, the 10S peak of ChE activity predominates, and the 4S peak is a minor component (Fig. 3, right). In all of the mature mouse cerebella, in contrast with the neonatal cerebellum, a large part of the 10S peak is also susceptible to inhibition by iso-OMPA. Altogether, the results presented in Figs. 1-3 indicate that, although ChE activity in the mature cerebellum resides primarily in the granular layer, agranulation does not alter the content, substrate specificity or sedimentation characteristics of ChE, nor does it affect ontogenic changes in these parameters.

The biosynthesis of cerebellar ChE is directed by poly(A)$^+$ mRNA, capable of inducing the production and secretion of active ChE in microinjected *Xenopus* oocytes (13). The amount of ChE produced in oocytes increased linearly with the quantity of unfractionated cerebellar mRNA injected, up to 100 ng/oocyte (13). Within this range, the amount of ChE synthesized in the oocytes reflects, therefore, the abundance of ChEmRNA in the injected mRNA population, and the biosynthetic potential of cerebellar cell bodies to produce ChE.

The *in ovo* bioassay for expression of ChEmRNA was employed in order to detect and quantify levels of ChEmRNA in the developing rat cerebellum. Poly(A)$^+$ mRNA was extracted from rat cerebellum at different developmental stages (20), injected into groups of 10 oocytes and ChE activity assayed radiometrically (13, 16). Cerebellar mRNA from all stages examined reproducibly induced the synthesis of significant activities of ChE, well above the endogenous activity of control oocytes injected with Barth medium. The capacity of equal amounts of mRNA to produce ChE in microinjected oocytes was found to change with development. A representative microinjection experiment, utilizing 50 ng of mRNA extracted from the cerebellum of rats at different ages, is displayed in Fig. 4 (left). The fraction of ChEmRNA out of total mRNA was found to be maximal in the neonatal cerebellum and to decrease thereafter (Fig. 4, upper left). This pattern clearly differs from that exhibited for the mRNA of the granular neuron enzyme plasminogen activator, which in a corresponding experiment peaks during interneuron proliferation (21).

The concentration of total mRNA, expressed as µg/gr tissue, changes with cerebellar development (20). The concentration of ChEmRNA per gr cerebellar tissue, at each of the stages examined, depends, therefore, both on the fraction of ChEmRNA out of total mRNA and on the concentration of total mRNA per gram cerebellum at that stage. Similarly, the total content of ChEmRNA in the cerebellum can be derived, at each stage, from the fraction of ChEmRNA and the total amount of mRNA in the cerebellum. It is evident from Fig. 4 (lower left) that the amount of ChEmRNA per cerebellum increases by about 5-fold from day 1 to day 30 after birth, when it reaches a maximal value and then falls sharply. However, the concentration of ChEmRNA decreases continuously throughout cerebellar development. Both of these biosynthetic patterns clearly differ from the ontogenic changes in the specific activity and content of cerebellar ChE (Fig. 1). This suggests that the major part of the cerebellar ChE is not regulated at the level of cerebellar mRNA.

The specific activity of ChE increases considerably in the agranular cerebellum of irradiated rats and of staggerer mutant mice, as compared to corresponding controls. In contradistinction, it decreases in cerebellum of "old" (30 months) mice, where afferent fibers appear to be defective (22), compared to control young adults (Fig. 4, lower right). Both observations corroborate the conclusion that most of the cerebellar ChE is contributed by incoming fibers. Unfractionated mRNA from cerebellum of old mice, from the agranular cerebellum of staggerer mutants and from the irradiated rat cerebellum all induced, in microinjected Xenopus oocytes, the production of rather similar levels of ChE to those induced in oocytes injected with mRNA from the appropriate control tissues (Fig. 4, upper right). This further supports the view that granular neurons do not produce ChE, and indicates that neither agranulation nor aging do substantially affect the minor production of ChE which takes place in the mature cerebellum.

Concluding Remarks

An approach combining biochemical assays with mRNA expression was used in our experiments to yield insight into contributions of exogenous and endogenous neuronal populations to maturation of cholinergic interconnections in the developing and agranular rodent cerebellum (for review see 23). We found ontogenic alterations in the level and biochemical properties of cerebellar ChE. However, our data indicate that most of the activity is contributed by incoming fibers. This conclusion is in agreement with an earlier report by Kasa et al. (24) who observed a pronounced decrease in cerebellar ChE activity following deafferentation. Our findings further suggest that the developmental changes in ChE do not depend on the presence of granular neurons, and do not appear to be regulated at the level of cerebellar mRNA.

Are different genes responsible for the production of the various ChE forms in different cerebellar cell types? If so, are these genes related to each other in their evolutionary origin, nucleotide sequence, orientation and regulation of expression? To answer these and related questions, we are now performing molecular cloning experiments, using the ChEmRNA bioassay to screen for ChEcDNA sequences so as to obtain DNA probes for cholinesterase gene(s).

Acknowledgements

We thank Mr. Daniel Eliyahu, Mrs. Rivka Zisling and Mrs. Esther Roth for their assistance throughout these experiments. This research was partially supported by grants from the Israel Centre for Psychobiology, Charles E. Smith foundation (Grant 34/81, to H.S.) and from the

Muscular Dystrophy Association (to I.S.). A preliminary report appeared in the abstracts of the 12th Annual Meeting of the Society for Neuroscience, 1982 (p.416).

References

1. Silver, A.: The biology of cholinesterases. North Holland publishing company,. Amsterdam, Oxford (1974).
2. Massoulié, J., Bon, S.: Ann. Rev. Neurosci. 5, 57-106 (1982).
3. Silver, A.: Intern. Rev. Neurobiol. 10, 57-109 (1967).
4. Altman, J., Das, G.D.: Exp. Neurol 28, 11-34 (1970).
5. Olschowka, J.A., Vijayan, V.K.: J. Comp. Neurol. 191, 77-101 (1980).
6. Wade, P.D., Timiras, P.S.: Dev. Neurosci. 3, 101-108 (1980).
7. Mahler, H.R.: Basic Neurochemistry, Siegal, G.J., Albers, R.W., Agranoff, B.W. and Katzman, R. (eds.), Little and Brown, Boston, pp. 391-400 (1982).
8. Altman, J., Anderson, W.J.: J. Compar. Neurol. 146, 55-405 (1972)
9. Soreq, H., Miskin, R.: Brain. Res. 216, 361-374 (1981).
10. Eliyahu, D., Soreq, H.,: J.Neurochem. 38, 313-321 (1982)
11. Sotelo, C.: Trends Neurosci. 3, 33-36 (1980).
12. Soreq, H., Safran, A., Eliyahu, D.,: Dev. Brain. Res. in press (1983)
13. Soreq, H., Parvari, R., Silman, I.: Proc. Natl. Acad. Sci. USA 79, 830-835 (1982).
14. Valcana, T., Liao, C., Timiras, P.S.: Env. Physiol. Biochem. 4, 58-63 (1974).
15. Soreq, H., Gurwitz, D., Eliyahu, D., Sokolovsky, M.: J. Neurochem. 39, 756-768 (1982).
16. Johnson, C.D., Russell, R.L.: Anal. Biochem. 64, 229-238 (1975).
17. Austin, L., Berry, W.K.: Biochem. J. 54, 695-700 (1953).
18. Ochoa, E.L.M., Brusco, A., Idoyaga-Vargas, V.P., Carminatti, H.: J. Neurochem. 38, 1236-1240 (1982).
19. Razon, N., Soreq, H., Bartal, A., Roth, E., Silman, I., submitted for publication.
20. Soreq, H., Safran, A., Zisling, R.: Dev. Brain Res. 3, 65-79 (1982).
21. Soreq, H., Miskin, R.: Dev. Brain Res., in press.
22. Peng, M.T., Lee, L.R.: Gerontology 25, 205-211 (1979).
23. Soreq, H. In: The Role of Cell Interactions in Early Neurogenesis, NATO advanced study institutes, in press (1983).
24. Kasa, P., Scillik, B., Joo, F., Knyihar, E.: J. Neurochem. 13, 173 (1966).

FUNCTIONAL ROLE OF CHOLINESTERASE IN DIFFERENT TYPES OF NEURO-MUSCULAR JUNCTION

L.G.Magazanik, V.V.Fedorov, R.A.Giniatullin, E.E.Nikolsky, V.A.Snetkov
Sechenov Institute of Evolutionary Physiology and Biochemistry, Academy of Sci. of the USSR, K-223 Leningrad, USSR

Introduction

There are several approaches to studying the functional role of AChE in cholinergic synapses: investigation of the type of AChE, quantitative estimation of AChE activity distribution within the synapse and correlation of AChE with ChRs (1, 2, 3). But data of this kind can not answer directly very important question: do AChE preclude the possibility of repetitive binding of ACh molecules with ChRs. Examination of the time course and amplitude of end-plate currents under various experimental conditions seems to be more informative in this respect. It is generally accepted that the rate of decay of postsynaptic currents induced by ACh quanta normally (when AChE is fully active) reflects the rate at which receptors undergo a conformational change (4, 5, 6). The coincidence of the decay time constant of miniature end-plate currents (τ_{mepc}) and the mean life-time of open synaptic channels (τ_n) may be considered as a sign of rapid hydrolysis of ACh by AChE: ACh molecules have only one chance to bind with ChRs before removal by AChE. On the contrary, the difference between τ_{mepc} and τ_n ($\tau_{mepc} > \tau_n$) may be considered as a measure of the functional insufficiency of AChE (7, 8, 9). This relative insufficiency retards the process of ACh removal. As a consequence a repetitive binding of a small part of the ACh molecules with ChRs prolongs mepc decay (10, 11).

We expected that AChE insufficiency would be more pronounced in junctions of slow muscle fibres, since there are biochemical and cytochemical data that show a lower quantity and density of AChE active sites in slow junctions (12, 13, 14, 15). Some AChE insufficiency also may be revealed during postsynaptic potentiation, when adjacent ACh quanta act upon the partially overlapping postsynaptic areas (16).

Methods

The experimental procedure consisted in recording (a) mepcs under voltage clamp or extracellular conditions and (b) current fluctuations induced by focal ACh application (7, 8). These records were made in intact preparations before and after treatment by anticholinesterase inhibitors. We used either the reversible inhibitor prostigmine (3×10^{-6}M), or the irreversible organophosphorous inhibitor, armin (preincubation in 1×10^{-6}M armin during 0.5 hour). Several hunderd mepcs were captured and analysed in each experiment, and mepc amplitude, rise time and half-decay time were estimated. The distribution of these values were diagrammed. Semilogarithmic plots of averaged mepc decay obtained by automatic digital averaging also were examined. The life time of ionic channels was computed from the autocorrelation function of ACh-induced noise.

Results

1. Comparison of the time course of mepcs in fast and slow muscle fibres of chicken. Isolated preparations of fast (m. posterior latissimus dorsi, PLD) and slow (m. anterior latissimus dorsi, ALD) muscles of the chicken (6-8 week old) were used. When AChE was fully active τ_{mepc} in slow muscle fibres (ALD) was 2.5 times higher than in fast ones (PLD). The results obtained with the voltage clamp method and by extracellular

<u>Fig. 1</u> Mepcs recorded extracellulary in chicken muscles at 37°C (17).

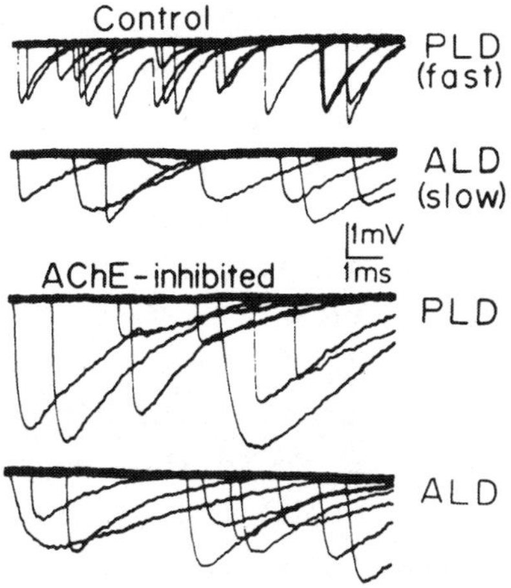

recording were in good agreement. Inhibition of AChE induced a more pronounced prolongation of τ_{mepc} in fast fibres (3.5 times) than in slow ones (1.5 times). As a result the difference between the mepc time courses in fast and slow fibres completely disappeared (Fig. 1). After inhibition of AChE the patterns of τ_{mepc} distribution became quite simillar (Fig. 2). There was no difference between the mean life time of open channels (τ_n) in PLD and ALD (17). Fig. 2 demonstrates that in both fibres the mean life time of channels coincided with the main peak of τ_{mepc} distribution of fast fibres.

<u>Fig. 2</u>
Distribution of τ_{mepc} recorded extracellulary in chicken muscle fibres at at 23°C (17). Arrows (⇩ -fast ↓ - slow) show the values of τ_n (18).

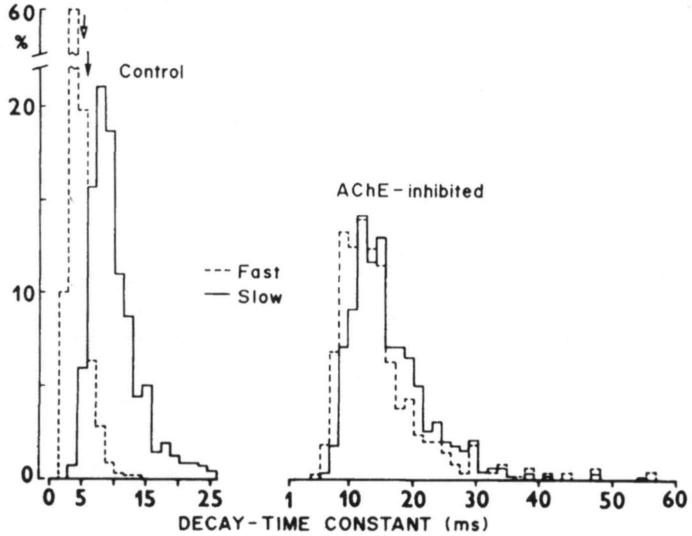

This indicates that the slowness of mepc decay in ALD is due to favorable conditions for repetitive binding of ACh molecules with ChRs. The properties of these ChRs in both kinds of fibres seems to be identical. It is known that the level of AChE activity is lower in ALD than in PLD muscles (2, 15, 19). Evidently AChE in ALD can not prevent the repetitive binding of ACh molecules.

2. Mepcs in fast and slow rat muscle fibres. A similar situation was found when mepcs recorded in fast (m. extensor digitorum longus) and (m. soleus) muscles of the rat were compared. When AChE was active, decay of mepcs was 1.4 times longer in slow fibres than in fast ones. But this difference practically disappeared after AChE inhibition (20, 21). The life time of open channels in both muscles appeared to be to be identical (22, 23). Thus, the relative slowness of mepc decay in rat soleus muscle also may be explained by insufficiency of AChE.

3. Postsynaptic currents in fast and slow frog muscle fibres. Mepcs in frog slow muscle fibres appeared to be more complicated. The decay of mepcs in slow muscle fibres was 4 times longer than in fast ones (7, 8, 20). The difference between the time courses of fast and slow fibres also became less after AChE inhibition (Fig. 3, 4). But unlike chicken and rat slow muscles the life time of ionic cgannels activated by ACh in frog slow muscle fibres was 2.8 times longer than in

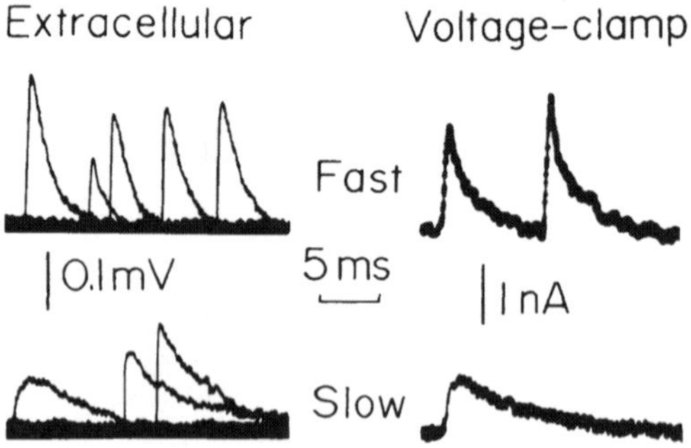

Fig. 3.
Mepcs recorded extracelulary and in voltage-clamped muscle fibres of m. cruralis of the frog (8).

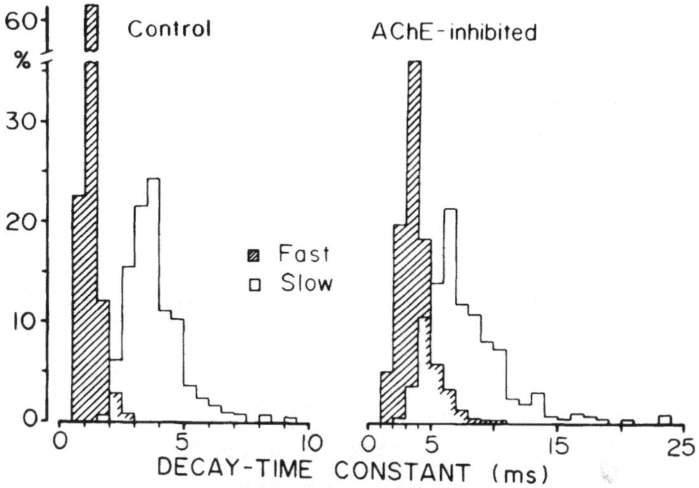

Fig. 4
Histograms showing τ mepcs recorded in the fibres of m. cruralis of the frog (8).

fast ones (Fig. 5) (7, 8). Miledi and Uchitel (24) considered that the main factor governing the integral time course of mepcs in slow frog muscle is the channel open time. We compared fluctuations induced by ACh and mepcs sampled in the

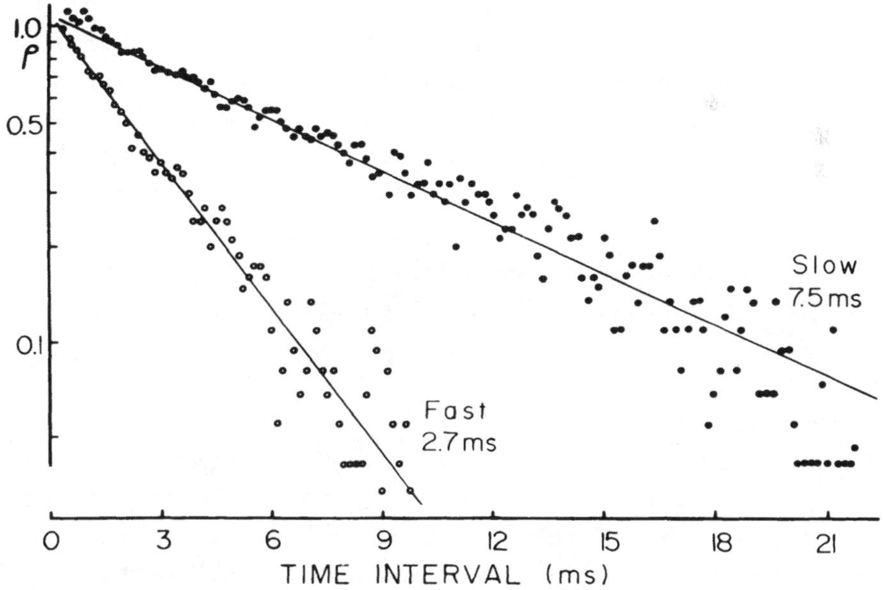

Fig. 5. Autocorrelation function of ACh-induced noise recorded in fibres of m. ileofibularis of the frog, $t^o = 8^oC$, MP = -80 mV (7).

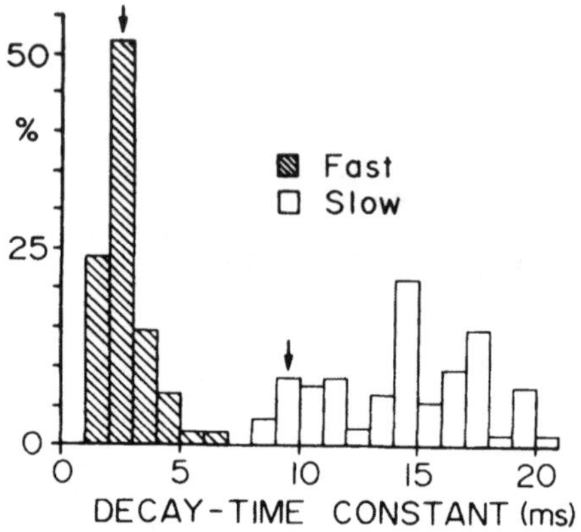

Fig. 6. Histograms of τ_{mepc} recorded in the fibres of m. ileofibularis of the frog. AChE is active. Arrows show the values of τ_n recorded in the same fibres, $t^o = 10^oC$, MP= -80 mV (7).

same junctions of m. ileofibularis. The mean time constant of mepc decay (τ_{mepc}) surpassed the mean life time of ionic channels (τ_n) in both types of fibres studied. In fast fibres this excess was rather small (only 17%), but in slow fibres τ_{mepc} was 1.7 - 2.4 times larger than the channel-life time. Figure 6 demonstrates that in the fast fibres the mean life time of channels coincides with the mean peak of distribution of individual mepc decay time constants. In contrast, in slow fibres the mean life time of ionic channels corresponded only with the decay time constant of the fastest mepcs. Thus the relative insufficiency of AChEs is not uniform in all compartments of slow junctions. In some compartments the removal of ACh seems to be so fast that its repetitive binding is impossible. In this case τ_{mepc} coincides with τ_n. But ACh appeared to be retarded in the great majority of compartments in slow slow junctions, leading to repetitive binding of ACh and prolongation of mepc time course.

4. The time course of mepcs and life time of open channels in lamprey muscle. Lamprey belongs to Cyclostomata, a relatively primitive branch of Vertebrata. One of the most interesting peculiarities of these muscles is the practicular regular sensitivity to ACh action along the whole surface of the muscle fibre (25). In this respect the lamprey muscle fibre resembles a chronically denervated muscle fibre of frog

or rat (26, 27). We compared current fluctuations induced by ACh in junctional and extrajunctional areas of the fibres from m. longitudinalis lingue of the lamprey Lampetra fluviatilis. τ_n in both areas was completely identical, 3.8 ms, MP=-80 mV, $t^o = 10^oC$ (Fig. 7). This means that junctional and extrajunctional ionic channels have the same kinetics of activation by ACh unlike the denervated muscle of frog (28, 29) or rat (30, 31), where the life time of open extrajunctional channels is longer than junctional ones. The decay time constant of mepcs recorded in lamprey muscle fibre was (5.3 ms, MP=-80 mV, $t^o = 10^oC$) larger than τ_n (3.8 ms). The life time of open channels here corresponded with the decay of the fastest mepcs just the same as in frog slow muscle fibres (Fig.6). Inhibition of AChE induced the prolongation of mepcs, and the distribution of τ_{mepc} became more skewed (Fig. 7). Evidently there is some deficiency of AChE in fast muscle fibres of lamprey (9). As a result, the repetitive binding of ACh in these junctions appears more probable than in fast fibres of frog, rat or chicken.

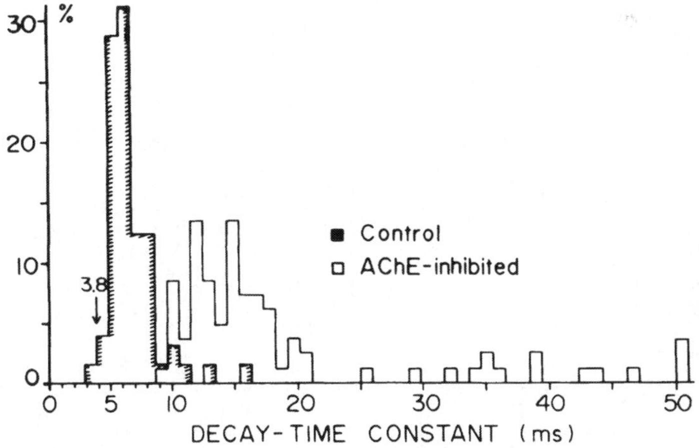

Fig. 7. Histograms of τ_{mepcs} recorded in lamprey muscle fibres. Arrow shows the value of τ_n recorded in the same fibre, $t^o = 10^oC$, MP= -80mV (9).

5. Shortening effect of α -bungarotoxin (α -BuTX) and d-tubocurarine (d-TC) on the mepc decay. An effective way of decreasing the probability of repetitive binding of ACh molecules to ChRs is to decrease the density of the free ChRs in the zone of ACh quantum action. It has been shown that α -BuTX and d-TC shorten synaptic current decay in frog fast muscle fibres but only after pretreatment by anticholinesterase drugs. No marked shortening effect of α -BuTX was found when AChE was fully active (10, 11). This may be explained by a very low probability of repetitive binding in normal fast frog junction. We expect that in any cases of prominent differences between τ_{mepc} and τ_n, a decrease of AChR density would induce the shortening of mepc decay despite the presence of intact AChE. Actually, in accordance with our data (similar results were also published earlier (10, 32, 33, 34) τ_{mepc} is only slightly longer ($\sim$ 10-17%) than τ_n in frog fast muscle fibres. But in the experiments on the frog slow muscle fibres, where this difference accounts for 66% (7, 8),

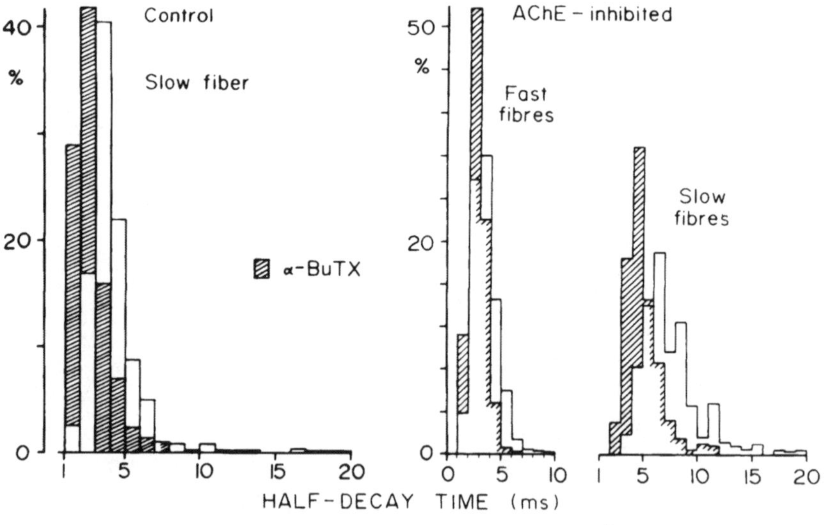

Fig. 8. Histograms showing the effect of α-BuTX on the **half - decay time** (ms) of mepc recorded in fibres of m. ileofibularis of the frog before (control) and after AChE-inhibition.

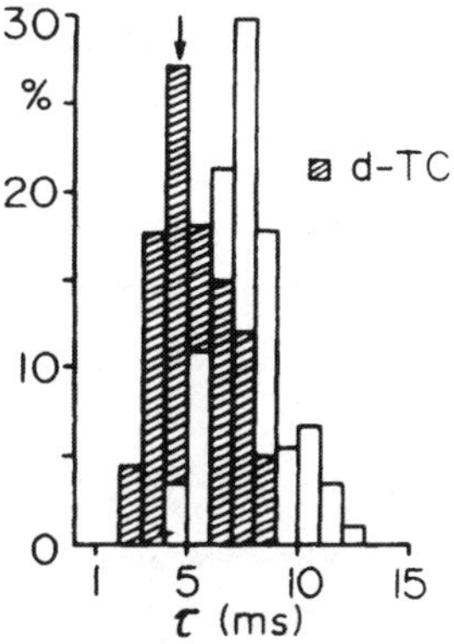

Fig. 9. Histograms showing the effect of dTC on the τ_{mepc} recorded in voltage-clamped muscle fibres of the lamprey (AChE is active). Arrow shows the value of τ_n. (9).

α-BuTX effectively shortened mepc decay when AChE was active (Fig. 8, Control). After AChE inhibition, the reduction of ChRs by α-BuTX is accompained by distinct changes of distribution of individual mepc decay rate (Fig. 8): all extremely slow mepcs disappeared after α-BuTX treatment. This seems to be in good agreement with our proposal of nonuniform AChE activity in different compartments of a slow junction. There are some compartments with low AChE activity and, as a result, have a high probability of repetitive binding of ACh molecules to ChRs. The shortening effect of α-BuTX appears well defined in this case.

Similar facts were found in the experiments on the fast muscle fibres of lamprey. dTC induced a distinct shortening effect on mepc decay when AChE was active (Fig. 9). In the presence of dTC, the main peak of distribution of individual mepc decay coincided with τ_n, the life time of open channels. This means that dTC greatly reduced the probability of repetitive binding which took place in lamprey neuromuscular junctions despite the presence of intact AChE.

6. Peculiarities of multiquantal end-plate currents evoked by single and repetitive nerve stimulation. Favourable conditions for the retardation of ACh molecules in the synaptic cleft and a resulting prolongation of current decay may appear during postsynaptic potentiation. It has been shown (16)

that adjacent quanta of ACh may interact on the postsynaptic membrane. This interaction could lead to repetitive binding of ACh to ChRs and to prolongation of current decay. But this phenomenon could be demonstrated on a snake nerve-muscle preparation only after AChE inhibition. It was proposed that fully active AChE can prevent postsynaptic potentiation during the generation of a multiquantal response. It is clear that the probability of the interaction of adjacent ACh quanta increases if the quantal content rises. We compared the time course of mepcs and multiquantal end-plate currents (epc) evoked by nerve stimulation recorded under voltage clamp conditions in the same end-plate of frog sartorius muscle (35, 36). Contractions of muscle fibre were abolished by glycerol pretreatment or by transverse cutting of muscle. When AChE was intact there was a small but significant excess of τ_{epc} over τ_{mepc} (~ 10%), if the quantal content of epc was more than 100- 150.

Repetitive stimulation may also favor the retardation of ACh in the synaptic cleft, if the quantal content of epcs is high enough and the interstimulus interval is short. But prolongation of the epc time course during repetitive stimulation was shown only after pretreatment by anticholinesterase drugs

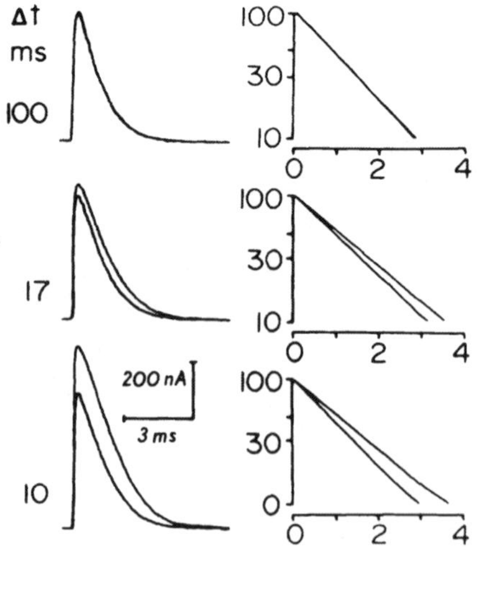

Fig. 10. Left: dependence of the time course of paired epc on the duration of interstimulus interval (Δ t). Cut muscle preparation. AChE is fully active. t° = 20°C, MP = -29 mV. Right: decay of these normalized currents plotted semilogarithmically as a function of time. The decay of the 2nd epc is slower than the decay of the 1st (36).

Fig. 11. Dependence of τ_{epc} on the amplitude of paired epcs with AChE fully active. Cut muscle preparation, MP= -31 mV. The $[Mg]_o$ in the bathing solution was slowly increased during the experiment. Mean amplitude of epc in (a) - 177 nA, in (b) - 93 nA (36).

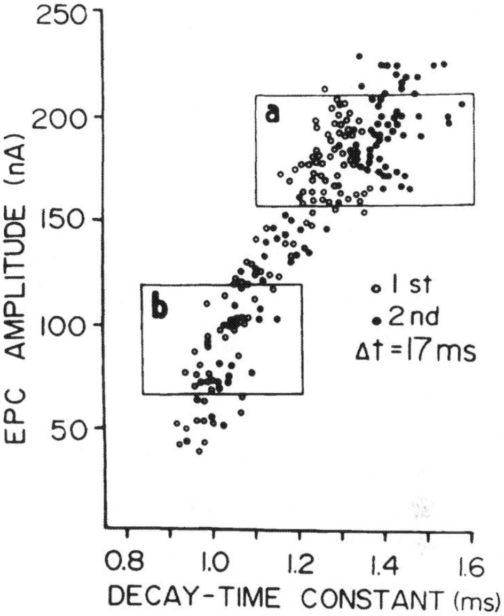

(4, 5, 16). We compared the time constants of decay of the 1st (τ_1) and the 2nd (τ_2) epcs delivered by paired stimuli. When AChE was intact, a statistically significant difference between τ_2 and τ_1 was seen only if the interstimulus interval (Δt) was less than 20 ms (Fig. 10). In a series of similar experiments, we followed the amplitude and decay time constant of a large number of epcs evoked by paired stimuli separated by 17 ms. During each experiment the concentration of Mg^{2+} ions in the bathing fluid was slowly rised from 0 to 7 - 8 mM. Decrease of the epc quantal content induced by Mg^{2+} led to a progressive reduction of the difference between τ_2 and τ_1 (Fig. 11). Treatment of AChE by inhibitors induced the augmentation of postsynaptic potentiation. The ratio of τ_{epc} to τ mepc increased from 1.2 (when AChE was active) to 2.8 after AChE inhibition, more than 2.3 times (the mean quantal content was equal to 135 $\pm$ 12 in this series of experiments, n= 21). The dependence of the decay rate of the 2nd epc upon the duration of interstimulus interval also became much more prominent. Thus τ_2 exceeded τ_1 even when Δ t was as long as 30 sec. We followed the dependence of the difference

Fig. 12. Dependence of the prolongation of 2nd epc ($\Delta\tau$) on the Δt. Means $\pm$s.d. from 8-16 experiments in the presence of anticholinesterase drugs (35).

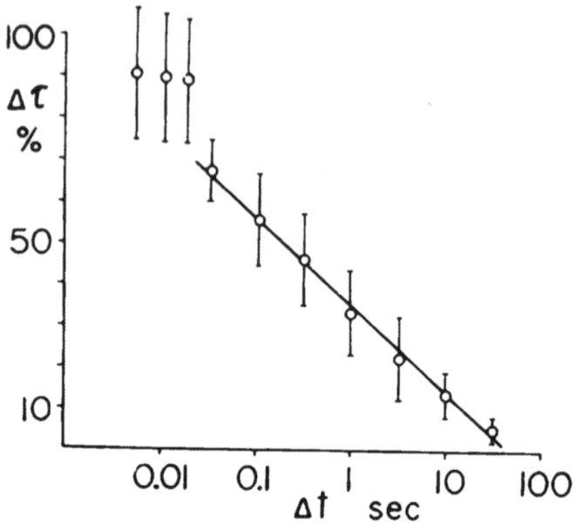

between τ_2 and τ_1 in a wide range of interstimulus intervals. The value of $\Delta\tau$ changed in inverse proportion to log Δt for the duration of the interstimulus interval (Fig. 12). The decrease of quantal content induced by Mg^{2+} ions led also to a reduction of the difference between τ_2 and τ_1.

Evidently there are favorable conditions for postsynaptic potentiation when AChE activity is relatively insufficient and especially after the treatment by anticholinesterase drugs. This may be revealed only if the quantal content is high enough.

Conclusions

Our data indicate that a previous conclusion about a high safety margin of AChE activity in neuro-muscular junctions is not correct. There is no surplus of AChE in a great number of neuromuscular junctions. The level of AChE activity in the junctions of fast muscles only guarantee the rather low probability of repetitive binding of ACh molecules to ChRs (37, 38). In some other cholinergic synapses, namely in junctions of slow muscles, the physiological requirement for such guarantee is not obligatory and a certain degree of repetitive binding does not hinder normal synaptic transmission. A relatively low level of AChE activity is in accordance with the functional properties of these muscles.

References

1. Silver, A.: The Biology of Cholinesterases. North-Holland Research Monographs "Frontiers of Biology", 36 (1974).
2. Barnard E.A., Chiu,T.H., Jedrzejczk, Porter,C.W., Wieckowski,J. In: Rang,H.P. (ed.) Drug Receptors. MacMilan, London, 225-24o (1973).
3. Peper,K., Dreyer,F., Sandri,C., Akert,K., Moor,H.,: Cell Tiss. Res.: 149, 437-455 (1974).
4. Kordaš, M.: J.Physiol.(Lond.), 224, 317-332 (1972).
5. Magleby, K.L., Stevens, C.F.: J.Physiol (Lond.), 223, 151-171 (1972).
6. Anderson, C.R., Stevens, C.F.: J.Physiol.(Lond.), 235, 655-691, (1973).
7. Fedorov, V.V., Snetkov, V.A., Magazanik, L.G.: Doklady Acad.Nauk USSR, 261, 1502-1506 (1981).
8. Fedorov,V.V., Magazanik,L.G., Snetkov,V.A., Zefirov,A.L.: Pflügers Arch., 324, 202-210 (1982).
9. Fedorov,V.V., Snetkov,V.A., Magazanik, L.G.: Neurofiziologia, 15, 428-431 (1983).
10. Katz, B., Miledi, R.: J.Physiol.(Lond.),231, 549-574 (1973).
11. Magleby,K.L., Terrar, D.A.: J.Physiol. (Lond.), 224, 467-495 (1975).
12. Barnard E.A., Lyles, J.M., Pizzey, J.A., J.Physiol.(Lond.) 331, 333-354 (1982).
13. Csillik, B., Schneider, J., Kaiman, G.: Acta Neuroveg. (Wien), 22, 212-224 (1961).
14. Heaton, J., Buckley, J.A., Evans, R.H.: Experientia, 22, 503-504 (1972).
15. Buckley, G.A., Heaton. J.: Nature New Biol., 231, 154--155 (1971).
16. Hartzell, H.C., Kuffler, S.W., Yoshikami, D.: J.Physiol. (Lond.), 251, 427-463 (1975).
17. Fedorov V.V.: Neurofiziologia, 13, 390-397 (1981)
18. Harvey, A.L., van Helden, D.F.: J.Physiol.(Lond.), 317, 397-411 (1981).
19. Scheuetze, S.M., J.Physiol. (Lond.), 303, 111-124 (1980).
20. Magazanik, L.G., Fedorov V.V., Snetkov,V.A.: Progr. Brain Res., 49, 225-240 (1979).

21. Fedorov, V.V.: Neurofiziologia, 12, 627-636 (1980).

22. Sakmann, B., Brenner, H.R.; Nature, 276, 401-402 (1978).

23. Sterz, R., Pagale, M., Peper, K.: Pflügers Arch., 398, 48-54 (1983).

24. Miledi, R., Uchitel, O.D.: Nature, 291, 162-165 (1981).

25. Itina, N.A., Skorobovichuk, N.F.: Zurn. Evol.Bioch.Fiziol., 3, 352- 358 (1967).

26. Axelsson, J., Thesleff, S.: J.Physiol.(Lond.), 147, 178--193, (1959).

27. Miledi, R.: J. Physiol. (Lond.), 151, 1-23 (1960).

28. Katz,B., Miledi, R.: J.Physiol.(Lond.), 224, 665-699 (1972).

29. Neher, E., Sakmann, B.: J.Physiol. (Lond.), 258, 705-729 (1976).

30. Dreyer,F., Müller, K.-D., Peper, K., Sterz, R.: Pflügers Arch., 367, 115-122 (1976).

31. Sakmann, B.,: Fed. Proc., 37, 2654-2659 (1978).

32. Colquhoun, D., Large, W.A., Rang, H.P.: J. Physiol. (Lond.), 266, 361-395 (1977).

33. Feltz, A., Large, W.A., Trautmann, A.: J.Physiol. (Lond.) 269, 109-130 (1977).

34. Gage, P.W., Van Helden, D.F.: J.Physiol.(Lond.), 288, 509-528,(1979).

35. Magazanik, L.G., Nikolsky, E.E., Giniatullin, R.A.: Doklady Acad.Nauk USSR, 272, 489-492 (1983).

36. Magazanik, L.G., Nikolsky, E.E., Giniatullin, R.A.: Pflügers Arch. in press,(1984).

37. Rosenberry, T.L.: Biophysical J., 26, 263-289, (1979)

38. Wathey,J.C., Nass, M.M., Lester, H.A.: Biophysical J., 27, 145-164 (1979).

III. SUB-CELLULAR LOCALIZATION, TRANSPORT AND SECRETION OF CHOLINESTERASES

INTRODUCTION TO SESSION III

Miro Brzin

Institute of Pathophysiology, Faculty of Medicine, University E. Kardelj, Zaloška 4, 61105 Ljubljana, Yugoslavia

The contributions to session 3 deal with the distribution of AChE and BuChE in tissues including their subcellular localization, sites of synthesis, cellular transport in regulation mechanisms in normal and experimentally designed conditions.

The first article (by Brimijoin and Mintz), describes the new powerful tool which has already shown its potency in neuroscience research. The authors report about the development of monoclonal antibodies to AChE and BuChE, starting with the purified enzymes isolated from human red blood cells and plasma. The monoclonal antibodies rised against human ChE did not freely cross-react with enzymes in other species. Furthermore, some of the selected clones produce highly species specific antibodies. Extension of this line of research, including the monoclonal antibodies to ChE of suitable laboratory animals, should in the near future bring new information about the metabolic and regulatory pathways of ChEs in health and disease.

The next contribution (by Brzin et al.) is a comparative survey focused on properties of AChE, its synthesis and regulatory influences in two typical cholinergic structures: the striated muscle and the superior cervical ganglion (SCG). AChE activity at the synaptic region in muscle originates predominantly from muscle cell and is about ten times higher than in a neuronal ganglionic cell. The differences between the two structures exist also in regard to the influence of innervation on AChE activity, distribution and the pattern of molecular forms of AChE in the postsynaptic cell. Furthermore, the regulatory effect of presynaptic neurons strongly depends on the maturity stage of the tissue. Thus, the junctional localization and the level of activity of the asymmetric molecular forms of AChE are strictly dependent on unimpaired innervation, whereas the establishment of synaptic contacts in a developing and not yet innervated SCG induces a decrease of these molecular forms. The innitially high level of the asymmetric form of AChE in the developing ganglion can be maintained till adulthood just by preventing the innervation. It is difficult to explain these differences at present but they probably reflect specific functional requirements at the two types of cholinergic synapses.

The third contribution to this session (by Kreutzberg et al.) describes the changes of AChE and BuChE localization and activity in motor neurons after the lesions of axons and during their regeneration. The two enzyme behave as most of transmitter-associated enzymes do in such situations: Their activity decreases during the intensive regenerative phase of the perikaryon and the normalization of activity is correlated with the normalization of axonal function. Interesting are certain species differences of intracellular and extracellular localization of AChE in response to axonal lesions. After axonal lesion BuChE activity in vagal neurons reapears later than AChE activity suggesting different regulation and confirming the previous evidence that BuChE and AChE are coded by different genes.

Numerous attempts have been made to find some functional role for AChE at sites where its presence is evidently not necessary for cholinergic neurotransmission. In this respect, the last contribution to the session 3 (by S. Greenfield) is particularly interesting: substantia nigra neurons which contain dopamine and AChE secrete the neurotransmitter and AChE under the same conditions, apparently unrelated to cholinergic mechanisms. Furthermore, soluble AChE when infused into substantia nigra unilaterally produced specific behavioral pattern, and this effect was not due to its hydrolytic activity but might be related to amplification of dopamine action on receptors. Tentative suggestions about various possible mechanisms of AChE action in substantia nigra are tempting and, if confirmed, would extend our understanding of the functional role of ACh beyond the classical cholinergic system.

IMMUNOCHEMICAL APPROACHES TO THE STUDY OF MAMMALIAN CHOLINESTERASES

S. Brimijoin, K.P. Mintz

Department of Pharmacology, Mayo Clinic, Rochester, MN 55905 USA

Among the more interesting aspects of the cholinesterases are their regulation, distribution and fate. These dynamic properties are currently less well understood than catalytic function and structure. Our recent investigations have focused on the axonal transport, subcellular localization, cellular release and turnover of AChE in mammalian nerve and muscles. Like others, we find that tetrameric globular AChE (G_4) and high molecular weight asymmetric AChE (A_{12}) are both subject to rapid bidirectional transport along axons (1, 2). Some of the transported G_4 enzyme is inserted locally into the axolemma or other external sites, where it becomes fixed in place (3). Much of the enzyme is destined for the terminal or paraterminal regions of the neuron, where it may be released upon electrical stimulation (4). Although released AChE is predominantly of the G_4 form, studies of enzyme turnover in muscle suggest that the released enzyme may actually arise from a labile pool of the G_1, monomeric form (5).

Cholinesterases, © Walter de Gruyter & Co., Berlin - New York, 1984

Further advances in understanding the regulation and interconversion of the molecular forms of the cholinesterases will be facilitated by the use of highly specific molecular probes. A promising class of probes are monoclonal antibodies (McAb's). For eventual use in studies of enzyme regulation, our research program has now turned towards producing and characterizing panels of McAb's to the cholinesterases of man and lower mammals.

The first steps were to isolate AChE and BuChE from human material. Plasma and red blood cells were chosen as rich sources of BuChE and AChE, respectively. The purification of BuChE involved affinity chromatography on N-methylacridinium-Sepharose 4B as described by Brimijoin et al. (6). Each liter of plasma yielded approximately 0.34 mg of protein with about 15% of the total starting BuChE activity. As assayed by the method of Ellman et al. (7), the specific activity of the product was 643 units/mg protein (1 unit = 1 micromole BuThCh hydrolyzed per min), representing a purification of 46,000-fold. The product was free of AChE activity, and its estimated purity was greater than 90%.

The purification of AChE began with the isolation of red cell ghosts by the procedure of Pazmino and Weinshilboum (8). AChE was extracted from the ghosts by homogenization in Tris buffer, pH 8, containing 1% Triton X-100. The purification scheme involved successive stages of affinity chromatography on N-methylacridinium-Sepharose and phenyl-trimethylammonium-Sepharose, followed by gel filtration on BioGel A-1.5 m resin. The final specific activity was 820 units/mg (1 unit = 1 micromole AThCh hydrolyzed per min), representing a purification of about 600-fold over the initial extract. The product, obtained in 60% yield, was free of BuChE activity and had a purity of about 25%.

The purified BuChE and partially purified AChE were used to immunize Balb/c mice, according to a standard protocol. A screening assay was developed to monitor the appearance and titer of specific antibodies in sera and culture media (6). Samples were mixed with a predetermined quantity of the antigen, in the presence of protein-A bearing staphylococcus cells (Pansorbin) precoated with rabbit antimouse IgG. The mixture was then centrifuged, and the precipitated ChE activity was measured by the method of Ellman et al. (7).

Most mice showed evidence of circulating anti-ChE antibodies within 1 month of immunization. Those with the highest titers were selected for hybridization of the spleen cells with mouse myeloma cells of the FO line. Cell-fusion was performed by a modification (6) of the procedure of Köhler and Milstein (9). Each fusion generated a few primary cultures containing anti-ChE secreting hybridomas. Positive cultures were defined as those whose conditioned media secreted specific antibody in quantities sufficient to bind all of the antigen added in the screening assay. Positive primary cultures were cloned by subculture at limiting dilution (average of 1/3 cell per culture well).

Most of the subcultures failed to secrete any detectable antibody to BuChE or AChE, but a few were positive (incidence ranging from 1% to 20% in different experiments). Daughter cultures derived from these positive subcultures via a second limiting dilution all secreted large amounts of specific antibody. These patterns of immunoreactivity are consistent with the selection of individual clones from mixed cultures. From a stochastic model, the probability of monoclonality was estimated at 98% for each cell line (6).

A few of the many antibody-secreting clones were selected for analysis in detail. Immunoglobulins from eight clones were subjected to isotype analysis; all were found to be IgG_1 or IgG_{2b}, with kappa light chains. Two-dimensional gel electrophoresis of these immunoglobulins showed that each consisted of a few charge isomers of single-sized heavy and light chains. Competition experiments showed that each of the antibodies was directed against a different ChE epitope. Guided by these immunochemical characteristics, we expanded as ascites tumors three clones secreting antibodies to AChE and two secreting antibodies to BuChE.

The monoclonal nature of the antibodies, suggested by the electrophoretic properties of the IgG fractions, was further tested by sucrose density gradient ultracentrifugation. In each case, preincubation with antibody caused an increase in the sedimentation velocity of AChE or BuChE, but the profile of enzyme activity on the gradient was not broadened or distorted (Figure 1). Studies with monomeric AChE (purified enzyme subjected to reduction and alkylation) indicated that only one type of complex was formed no matter how much antibody was used. On the other hand, when dimeric enzyme was added, two complexes formed: a fast sedimenting one predominated at high antibody concentrations; an intermediate-sedimenting complex predominated at low antibody

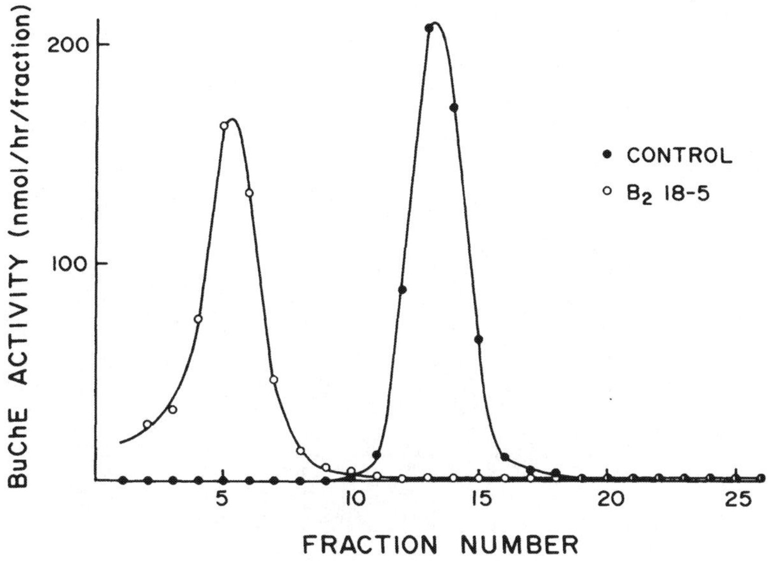

Figure 1. Effect of anti-BuChE McAb on sedimentation of BuChE. Approximately 5 micrograms of IgG were incubated for 1 hr at 37° with 14 milliunits of partially purified human plasma BuChE. The reaction mixture was centrifuged for 16 hr at 120,000 g av on a linear sucrose density gradient (5-20%). The untreated enzyme behaved as an 11 S tetramer. The shift to 18 S, induced by McAb B_2 18-5 was a typical result of antibody-treatment.

concentrations. We interpret these results to mean that our AChE antibodies recognize one epitope per enzyme monomer. On a dimer, only one site may be occupied when antibody is scarce, but both will be occupied when antibody-concentration approaches or exceeds Kd.

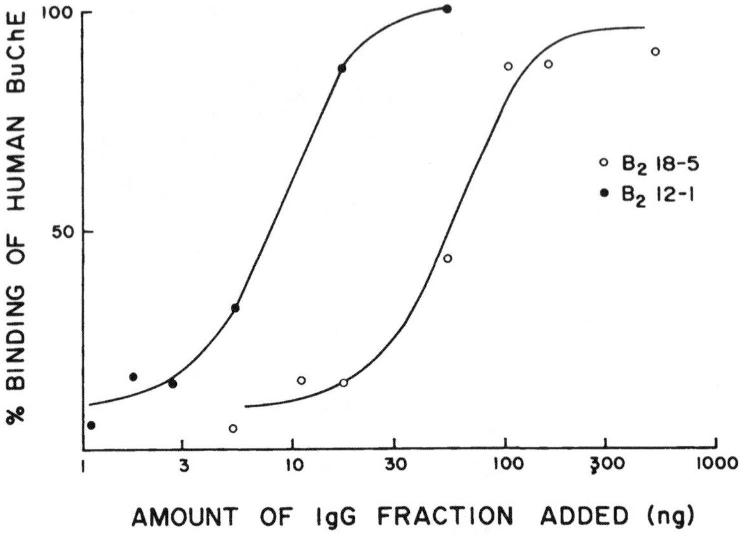

Figure 2. Dilution curves of anti-BuChE McAb's. All experiments were performed with 7 milliunits of BuChE from normal plasma. The standard screening assay was used (1 hr incubation at 37°). BuChE activity was measured in the bound phase and expressed as a percentage of the activity added.

McAb's isolated from the ascites fluids were tested in varying dilutions to determine their avidity for antigen (Figure 2). Assuming mass action behavior, with one epitope per enzyme monomer and two recognition sites per

IgG molecule, apparent Kd's were calculated from the equation:

$$Kd = \frac{2\ Ab}{\sqrt{1-B} - 1} - 2\ Ab$$

where "B" is the fraction of enzyme activity bound, and "Ab" is the molar concentration of IgG. Computer analysis of the dilution curves indicated that the Kd's of the anti-AChE McAb's ranged from 1.0 ± 0.1 nM to 2.9 ± 0.3 nM; those of the anti-BuChE antibodies were 2.2 ± 0.3 nM and 13 ± 2 nM (6).

Within experimental error, the same affinities were calculated when caudate nucleus was used instead of blood samples as the source of antigen. These findings imply that the ChE's of human brain and blood are immunologically equivalent with regard to the epitopes recognized by our monoclonal antibodies. Of course, the enzymes of different tissues might differ in primary structure at domains other than those recognized by the antibodies. For example, both of our anti-BuChE monoclonal antibodies had the same apparent affinity for normal human plasma BuChE (dibucaine number 80) and for homozygous atypical BuChE (dibucaine number 25). This result is expected since 1) normal and atypical BuChE probably differ at the active site only (10), and 2) our antibodies do not inhibit BuChE and therefore probably bind at some distance from the active site.

Clear differences in affinities became apparent when the antibodies were tested against antigens from different species. None of the antibodies had measurable affinity for AChE or BuChE from rat. The cross-reactivity of the

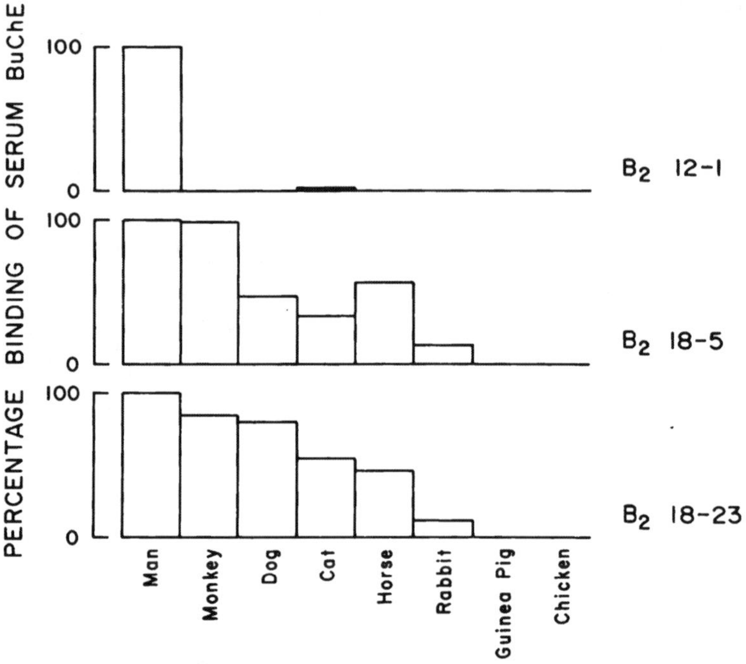

Figure 3. Reactivity of anti-BuChE McAb's with plasma BuChE from various animal species. Exactly 14 milliunits of BuChE from each species was present.

antibodies to enzyme of several other species is shown in Figs. 3 and 4. In general, binding was highly species-selective. At least 3 different patterns were seen: 1) binding only to human enzyme (samples from the great apes were omitted from the initial survey); 2) binding to human and monkey; 3) more widespread binding, including, antigen from species as remote as horse, guinea pig, and rabbit.

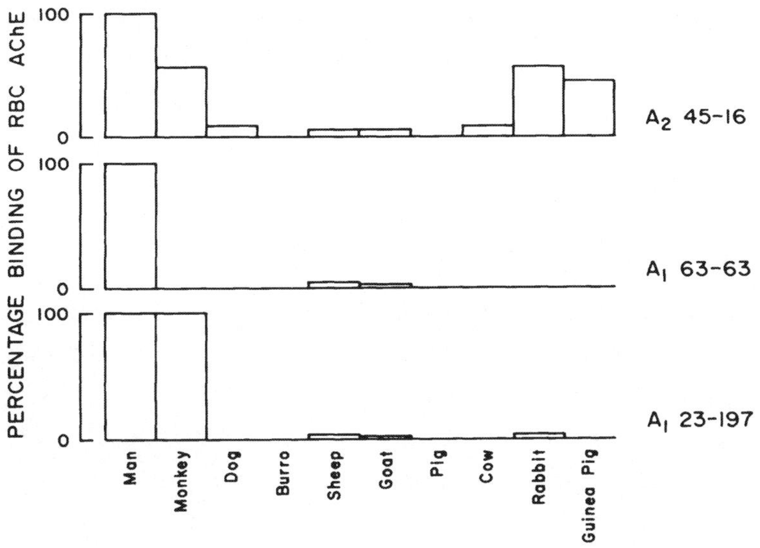

Figure 4. Reactivity of anti-AChE McAb's with erythrocyte AChE from various animal species. Erythrocyte extracts were prepared by homogenizing red cell ghosts in Tris buffer, pH 7.4, with 1% Triton X-100. Exactly 7 milliunits of AChE from each species was added. Rabbit AChE was from a Tris-Triton extract of brain (red cells had only trace activity).

The more selective anti-BuChE McAb (B_2 12-1) was tested further for clues to the changes in BuChE during evolution of the primates. This antibody, which lacked affinity for BuChE of squirrel monkey, was also unable to bind the enzyme from gibbon. On the other hand, in a typical screening assay, B_2 12-1 did bind 20% of the orangutan BuChE, 60-70% of the chimpanzee and pigmy chimpanzee BuChE, and all of the gorilla BuChE. This sequence of apparent affinities is consistent with current views on the genetic interrelationships within the primate order (11).

Given the selectivity of our McAb's with regard to corresponding antigens from closely related species, it is not surprising that the anti-AChE antibodies did not cross-react with BuChE and vice versa. In this sense the specificity was absolute, a property that will facilitate future experiments on regulation and disposition of the ChE's. It is now thought that AChE and BuChE are distinct proteins encoded by distinct genes (see 12, 13 for discussion). However, similarities in structural organization and mechanism of action argue for a common evolutionary origin (14). One would therefore expect the amino acid sequences to show some homology. If sufficient numbers of McAb's were examined, a few might well show cross-reactivity.

Because our initial panels of antibodies had at best moderate affinity for nonprimate ChE's, they are of limited use in studies of enzyme regulation in the more convenient experimental animals. Our next step was therefore to purify AChE from rabbit brain, to use in raising a new generation of monoclonal antibodies with the necessary specificities and affinities. To begin this purification, McAb A_2 45-16 was coupled to CNBr-activated Sepharose 4B as an immunoaffinity reagent.

An affinity column of this material bound over 90% of the AChE extracted from rabbit brain membranes by homogenization in Tris buffer, pH 7.4, with 1% Triton X-100. After extensive rinsing, half the bound AChE was recovered when the column was eluted with glycine buffer at pH 11. At this stage the enzyme had been purified 2000-fold and exhibited only one major band on silver-stained SDS electrophoresis gels. However, from its specific activity of 600 units/mg, we estimated a purity of only 20-25%. Therefore we subjected the preparation to an additional stage of purification, on a ligand-affinity column of phenyl trimethylammonium. The best fractions obtained by eluting the AChE with decamethonium-bromide (linear gradient, 0-100 mM) had a specific activity of 3000 units/mg. This material, representing 37% of the enzyme originally solubilized, was electrophoretically homogeneous.

Purified rabbit brain AChE has now been used to raise antibodies in Balb/c mice. Spleen cell fusions to form FO hybridomas have been carried out. It can be anticipated that the monoclonal cell lines to be derived will include several that secrete specific AChE-McAb's with desirable properties. Apart from their utility as histochemical and biochemical "labels" such antibodies could help in probing the mechanisms for regulation of the ChE's. For example, in studies of mRNA-directed in vitro synthesis (see the paper by Soreq et al, this volume) appropriate antibodies could be used to distinguish "endogenous" from "exogenous" enzyme. Polysomes highly enriched in specific RNA might be obtained by passing tissue extracts through a McAb immunoaffinity column. These sorts of preparations could aid in experiments designed to determine whether increases and decreases of tissue AChE activity, associated with various physiological and pathological states, are the consequences of changes in protein synthesis, degradation, or both. Applications such as gene cloning, presently more remote, may eventually become feasible as well.

References

1. Brimijoin, S., Wiermaa, M.J.: J. Physiol. 248, 129-143 (1978).
2. Brimijoin, S.: Mol. Pharmacol. 15, 641-648 (1979).
3. Brimijoin, S., Skau, K.A., Wiermaa, M.J.: J. Physiol. 284, 143-158 (1978).
4. Skau, K.A., Brimijoin, S.: Nature 275, 224-226 (1978).
5. Brimjoin, S., Carter, J.: J. Neurochem. 38, 588-590 (1982).
6. Brimijoin, S., Mintz, K.P., Alley, M.: Mol. Pharmacol. in press (1983).
7. Ellman, G.L., Courtney, K.D., Andres, V. Jr., Featherstone, R.M.: Biochem. Pharmacol. 7, 88-95 (1961).
8. Pazmino, P.A., Weinshilboum, R.M.: Clin. Chim. Acta 89, 317-329 (1978).
9. Köhler, G., Milstein, C.: Nature 256, 495-497 (1975).
10. Lockridge, O., LaDu, B.N.: J. Biol. Chem. 253, 361-366 (1978).
11. Dunnette, J.H., Weinshilboum, R.M.: Comp. Biochem. Physiol. 75, 85-91 (1983).
12. Massoulie, J., Bon, S.: Ann. Rev. Neurosci. 5, 57-106 (1982).
13. Brimijoin, S.: Prog. Neurobiol. in press (1984).
14. Augustinsson, K.-B.: In: Homologous Enzymes and Biochemical Evolution (N. van Thoai and J. Roche, eds.) Gordon and Breach, New York, pp. 299-311 (1968).

CHOLINESTERASES IN SKELETAL MUSCLE AND SYMPATHETIC GANGLIA

Miro Brzin, Biba Klinar, Janez Sketelj, Tomaž Kiauta, Zoran Grubić and Dušan Sket

Institute of Pathophysiology, Faculty of Medicine, University E. Kardelj, Zaloška 4, 61105 Ljubljana, Yugoslavia

Introduction

Muscle fiber and the sympathetic ganglionic cell represent two distinct types of cholinoceptive noncholinergic cells innervated by a presynaptic cholinergic neuron. Therefore, a brief comparison of differences and similarities between these two structures in regard to the localization of cholinesterases (ChEs), their origin, activity, molecular forms and regulation might be relevant for understanding their role in synaptic transmission or other functions.

Acetylcholinesterase (AChE) activity in skeletal muscles of adult vertebrates is distributed between the neuromuscular junction and extrajunctional regions of muscle cells (cf. 1). The junctional AChE is localized in the clefts between the nerve ending and muscle fibre and in Schwann cell - nerve ending interspace (Fig. 1) and is largely attached to the basal lamina (2,3). It constitutes, together with AChE in the T-tubules of muscle cell, the extracellular fraction of muscle AChE which is accesible from the intercellular space. The predominant part of intracellular AChE is located in the sarcoplasmic reticulum (SR), whereas AChE bound to intracellular membranes of the Schwann cells normally seems to contribute only a minute fraction to the total intracellular pool of adult muscle AChE. Although the junctional AChE makes only about 25 percent of the total muscle AChE activity, the direct measurements of AChE in isolated single endplates have revealed an activity of the order of 200 - 400 pmol/hr/e.pl. (4,5). Condensed in a synaptic space of about 300 μm^3, this activity corresponds to an enor-

Cholinesterases, © Walter de Gruyter & Co., Berlin - New York, 1984

mous enzyme concentration of about 100 or more EU/mg of the cleft substance and that puts the neuromuscular junction in an exceptional position when compared with other types of cholinergic synapses.

In the sympathetic ganglion the situation concerning AChE activity and localization differs from the one in muscle in quantitative and qualitative terms. The total AChE activity of a sympathetic ganglion is composed of preganglionic extracellular part which is mostly affiliated with the Schwann-cell-nerve ending interspace (Fig. 2b) and amounts to about 50 percent of the total activity (6), and an intracellular part located in the endoplasmic reticulum (ER) of neurons which accounts for the second half of ganglionic AChE (Fig. 2a)(6,7). No AChE activity can be readily demonstrated in the synaptic cleft as opposed to the neuromuscular junction. Furthermore, in a frog isolated ganglionic nerve cell which still has about one third of plasmalemma covered with nerve endings, AChE activity amounts to 5 - 30 pmol ACh split/hr/cell (7) which is about ten times less than found in an isolated motor endplate. The profound differences between the two holinoceptive cells in regard to the activity and localization of AChE probably reflect specific functional requirements based on differences in neurotransmission at the two types of cholinergic synapses.

Origin of AChE

AChE located at the neuromuscular junction may be supplied by the presynaptic neuron, muscle cell and Schwann cells affiliated with the motor endplate. Because the rate of synthesis of AChE in an adult muscle seems to be rather low, the developing muscle where the rate of protein synthesis is high, appears to be more suitable for the studies of possible contribution of different cells to the total AChE activity of muscle, and particularly to the enzyme at the motor endplate.

During the ontogenesis of rabbit muscle (cf. 8), AChE appears in myoblasts in early stages of their differentiation and attains a high specific activity before innervation. The first AChE activity which could be detected cytochemically is localized in the perinuclear membrane, SR and, shortly thereafter, at the myoblast plasmalemma (8). Later, when the nerve fibers penetrate into the muscle and the Schwann cells begin to appear, the latter also exhibit AChE activity at the nuclear membrane and in ER. During the formation and maturation of neuromuscular junction (9) AChE, synthesized throughout the muscle cell, seems to be transported from the sites of synthesis to the junction in tubulovesicular structures. The fusion of the AChE - containing structures with the postsynaptic membrane, and the contribution of AChE by the Schwann cell may represent the mechanism for the progressive accumulation of AChE activity at the junction (Fig. 3a,b). At that stage of development, the specific activity of the asymmetric molecular forms of the AChE in rat muscles is higher than in muscles of adult animals and these forms are still distributed in junctional and extrajunctional muscle regions (Fig. 5)(9,10,11). Once the maturation of the endplate has been completed AChE activity of SR and Schwann cell is greatly diminished. The 16 S form of AChE in extrajunctional regions nearly disappears and becomes restricted to junctional region.

Developmental studies therefore suggest that the muscle fibre and the Schwann cell may be the major sites of AChE synthesis in muscle. This view is strenghtened by the finding that in an adult muscle, the activity of AChE reapears at these locations during enhanced de novo synthesis after irreversible inhibition of AChE (12). Furthermore, the newly synthesized enzyme in adult muscle seems to be transported from the extrajunctional regions of muscle cell to the junctional membrane in tubulovesicular structures (Fig. 4), like in developing muscle.

The regeneration of total muscle AChE after inhibition is rather slow (12)(Fig. 6) whereas the initial recovery of junctional AChE is faster as directly shown by enzyme activity measurements in single isolated endplates as compared to homogenized endplates containing muscle region (Table 1). This fast accumulation of AChE activity at the endplate supports

Fig. 1 Motor endplate, rat diaphragm, 21 days pp. The reaction product indicates the sites of AChE activity on presynaptic and postsynaptic membranes (arrows), in the space between Schwann cell processes and nerve ending (crossed arrow) and in basal lamina in the synaptic cleft; MN: muscle cell nucleus, NE: nerve ending, thiocholine - KCNS method.
Bar: 0,1 µm.

Fig. 2 Rat SCG; a) Ganglion cell body; the reaction product in the endoplasmic reticulum. Bar: 0,5 µm b) Nerve ending in neuropile; reaction product in the Schwann cell- nerve ending interspace. Thiocholine - KCNS method. Bar: 0,2 µm.

Fig. 3 Developing neuromuscular junction. a) Diaphragm of 19 day rat fetus. The endings of ingrowing axons between muscle fibers. Reaction product caused by AChE activity in the intercellular space and inside of tubulovesicular structures of muscle cells. M: muscle cell; AX: axons. Bar: 0,5 µm. b) Motor endplate, diaphragm of three weeks old rat. Some regions of the junction appear not fully matured. AChE activity on pre- and postsynaptic membrane and in the synaptic clefts like in adult muscle, but at that stage of development, Schwann cell still exhibits distinct AChE activity (arrow) and tubulovesicular structures containing AChE activity are clearly visible in the sarcoplasm (crossed arrows). SN: Schwann cell nucleus; MN: muscle cell nucleus; NE: nerve ending. Bar: 1 µm.

Fig. 4 Motor endplate. Diaphragm of adult rat 24 hour after in vivo irreversible inhibition of AChE. After prolonged incubation the localization of de novo synthesized AChE appears almost normal, but tubulovesicular structures in subjunctional sarcoplasm with sequestered AChE, similar to those observed in developing muscle have repeared (arrows).
Bar: 0,5 µm.

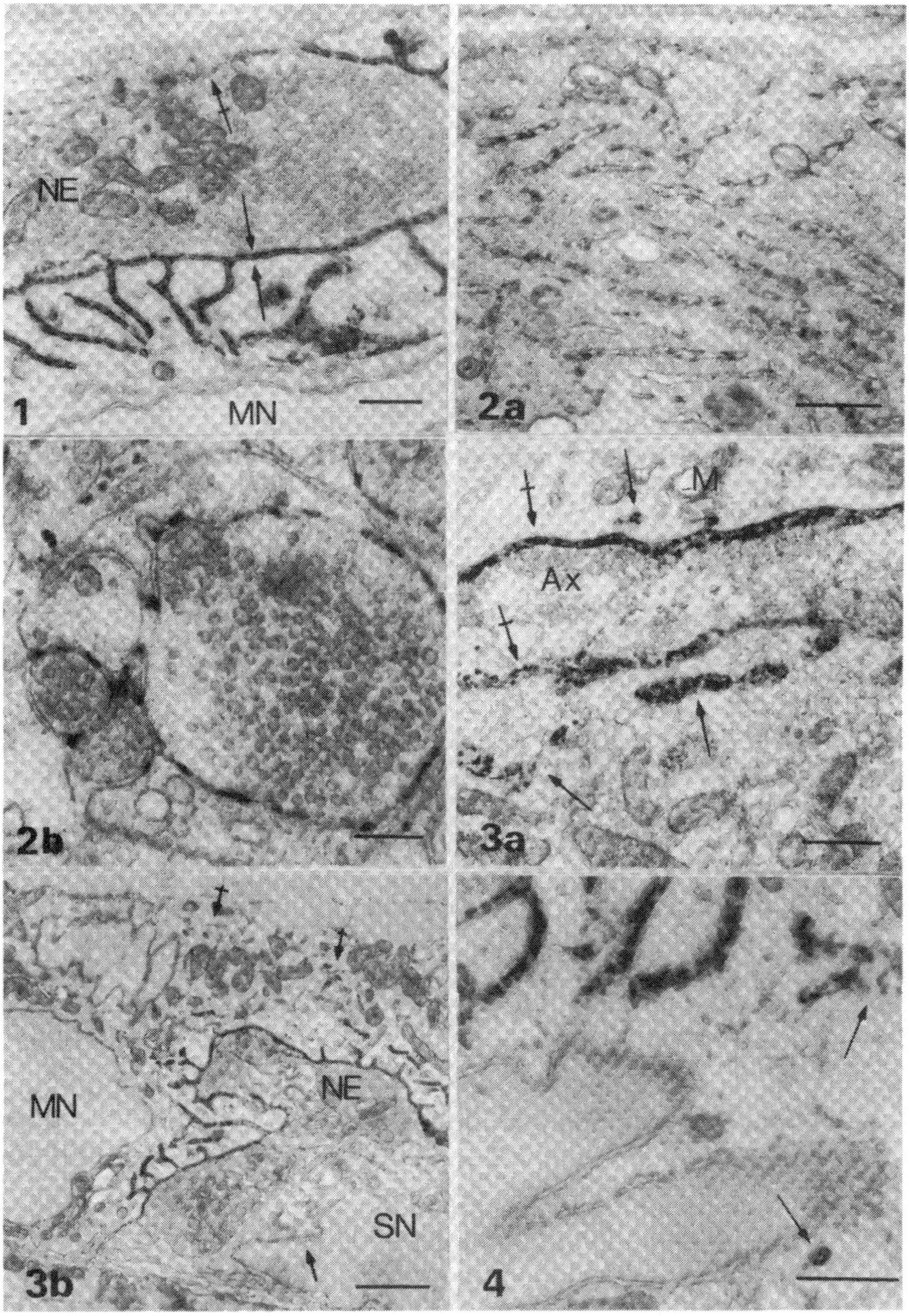
NE
MN
1
2a
2b
M
Ax
3a
MN
NE
SN
3b
4

the cytochemically indicated existence of a directed transport of the enzyme along the muscle fibre to the junction. The reapearing new AChE at the junction seems to be localized at both synaptic membranes and in the synaptic clefts, just like in the control muscle. This observation is relevant because the study of the reaperance of different molecular forms of AChE after irreversible inhibition has shown that the asymmetric forms are undetectable in muscle at the early stages of enzyme recovery (12), suggesting that the globular molecular form can be attached to the junctional structures and are responsible for the initial normalization of the neuromuscular transmission.

The above evidence strongly suggests that also in a normal adult muscle the muscle cell and the Schwann cell may be the main suppliers of junctional AChE but there the rate of synthesis and the amount of transported enzyme may be too low and, therefore, hard to demonstrate by existing methods.

The role of the presynaptic cholinergic neurons in maintaining the level of synaptic AChE is still poorly understood, but from above it seems obvious that the direct transfer of AChE synthesized in the neuron to the synaptic sites in muscle may not be functionally necessary. Synthesis of AChE in neurons (either cholinergic or cholinoreceptive) takes place in ER and AChE is then either extruded into the intercellular space or transported along the axon. The functional significance of the axonal transport of AChE is not clear at present. This is equally true both for the axons of cholinergic neurons where AChE, if transported into the nerve terminal, would interfere with the transmission (13) as well as for the axons of noncholinergic neurons where, according the present views, AChE at the synapse is not involved in synaptic transmission. Furthermore, the attempts to demonstrate AChE inside the nerve endings have not succeeded so far suggesting that the intraaxonal transport of AChE does not reach the nerve ending by a simple axoplasmic flow. The enzyme transported in the axoplasm may be connected with the maintenance of the stationary AChE of axons (14) located in the space between the axolemma and the myeline sheet and probably attached to axolemma (7,15).

The synthesis of AChE in cholinoceptive cells(cholinergic or noncholinergic) seems to represent a source of the enzyme performing its functional role in the extracellular space of the synaptic regions. Therefore, it seems justified to assume that different types of cholinoceptive cells, and to various degree the presynaptic cholinergic neurons, contribute most of AChE to the cholinergic synapse. Besides the postsynaptic cell, the Schwann cells can also synthesize a part of the enzyme located at the motor endplate during development. The contribution of AChE by Schwann cells to the synaptic regions of central and peripheral neurons is probable but has not yet been experimentally demonstrated. In the synaptic regions distributed in the neuropile arround the neurons of sympathetic ganglia the fraction of AChE activity originating from presynaptic neurons is obviously substantial as indicated by decentralization experiments.

The influence of innervation on ChE of cholinoceptive cells

The presynaptic axons have profound and manifold effects on the postsynaptic cells in regard to various properties of AChE such as the total activity, the pattern of molecular forms, subcellular localization and the intracellular transport. However, other mechanisms, humoral or intrinsic to the postsynaptic cell may be involved in the regulation of these properties, complementary to the innervation or in an independent manner.

The mechanisms of regulation of AChE in muscle cell either by the nerve trophic factors or by the muscle activity dependent upon innervation, have been intensively studied for a long period of time (cf. 16,17). Closer understanding for a particular regulation mechanism is obscured, however, by the quantitative differences in effects which the presence or absence of a regulatory factor may induce in muscles of different animal species or even in different types of muscles in the same animal. Thus, the denervation of muscles in adult animals causes a decrease of AChE activity in muscles of most vertebrates studied and this change affects both the junctional and extrajunctional muscle regions (1, 16). The exceptions of this rule which were studied to some details are the rabbit (18, 19, 20, 21) and the chicken (22, 23). In these animals the denervation of muscles induces a considerable increase of sarcoplasmic AChE activity which more than compensates for the decrease of junctional enzyme activity. Regarding the localization pattern and high activity of AChE, the denervated fibers in these animals resemble the immature muscles during embryonic development. However, it has been reported that sarcoplasmic AChE may increase also after denervation of developing rat muscles (24). The puzzling fact that denervation can produce either a decrease or an increase of sarcoplasmic AChE, depending on the animal species, makes any generalization premature but, in a long run, the comparative studies of such profoundly different responses in different species caused by the same experimental intervention might eventually help to reveal the basic molecular events in nerve-muscle interactions.

It seems to be a common property of muscles in all vertebrate species to exhibit a high sarcoplasmic activity of AChE during ontogenesis before and immediately after the contact between the nerve and muscle has been established. In developing muscles of most vertebrates the motor innervation induces a chain of gradual changes in localization, activity and molecular forms of AChE until the pattern, typical for the mature muscle is achieved exhibiting a high concentration of AChE at the junction and a low activity in extrajunctional regions.

The mechanism by which AChE activity concentrates at the endplate seems to be based to a large extent on the directed transport of AChE-containing tubulovesicular structures carrying and transfering the newly synthesized enzyme to the synaptic clefts (9).

Considering quite uniform intracellular distribution of AChE in muscle cells before they become innervated, it may be assumed that the first nerve contact initiates a directed transport of AChE in the developing fiber. Furthermore, once induced the transport mechanism seems to persist in the innervated and in the denervated adult muscles, as demonstrated by the rapid accumulation of AChE activity in motor endplates or former endplate sites of such muscles during resynthesis of irreversibly inhibited AChE (Fig. 4, Fig. 6, Table 1) (12, 25). In a denervated muscle some AChE activity remains concentrated on the postsynaptic membrane of the former endplate and in the secondary synaptic clefts for a long time. Since the asymmetric molecular forms of AChE are greatly diminished or partically disappear from denervated muscles in most animal species, it seems that the globular molecular forms can bind to the postsynaptic membrane and possibly basal lamina. Therefore, the collagen-like tail seems not to be absolutely essential for the attachment of AChE molecules in the neuromuscular synapse. The same suggestion was already discussed in connection with the reappearance of globular forms of AChE in the synaptic clefts after previous irreversible inhibition of the enzyme. It is the fact that the heavy asymmetric forms of AChE are located predominantly at the endplate region of mature muscles in most vertebrates (26) but the evidence also exists that considerable concentration of these molecular forms is present in extrajunctional regions of muscle fibers of adult chicken (27) and man (26, 28) and in immature developing rat muscle in vivo (9, 11, 29).

Besides the earlier described differences between muscle and sympathetic ganglia in activity of AChE and its extracellular and intracellular distribution, these two cholinergic structures differ also in regard to the influence the innervation exerts upon them. After decentralization or after a mild proteolytic treatment of intact ganglia (6), the extracellular enzyme activity is being abolished almost totally, whereas the intracellular neuronal activity remains. The activity of AChE left in ganglion cells after solubilization of extracellular enzyme and the activity remaining after decentralization of the adult ganglion are practically equal. Therefore, it appears that the presynaptic nerve exerts little if any regulatory effect on the total intracellular AChE of ganglion cells in an adult animal. That is just the opposite than in muscles where the direct contribution of neuronal AChE to the total muscle

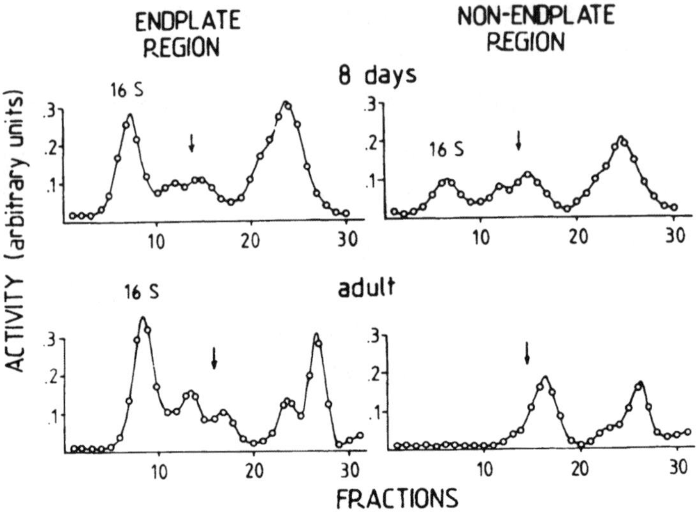

Fig. 5 Molecular forms of AChE in the endplate region and in the endplate free (= non-edplate) region of the diaphragm in 8 days old rats and in adult animals. The top of the gradient is on the right hand side. An arrow shows the position of catalase (11.4 S) in the gradient. AChE activity is expressed per unit of wet weight of a sample.

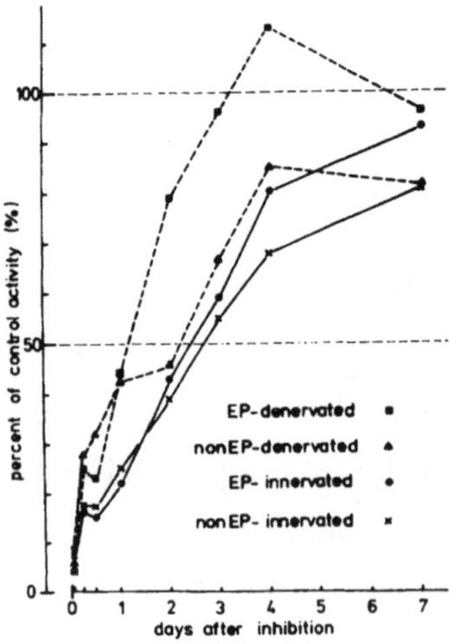

Fig. 6 Recovery of AChE activity in innervated and denervated rat diaphragm, after irreversible inhibition with phospholine in vivo.

Table 1 Recovery of AChE activity[+] in rat diaphragm 24 hours after *in vivo* inhibition by soman

	noninhibited controls	after soman 1hr	after soman 24 hrs	% recovery $\frac{c-b}{a} \times 100$
	a	b	c	
Isolated endplates pmol ACh/hr/epl.	180 ± 22 (n=9)	4,5 ± 1,3 (n=7)	34,3 ± 16,3 (n=11)	16,6
Endplate region homogenate nmol ACh/hr/mg	144 ± 23 (n=28)	5,4 ± 1,8 (n=9)	12,0 ± 3,4 (n=12)	4,6

[+]means ± SD

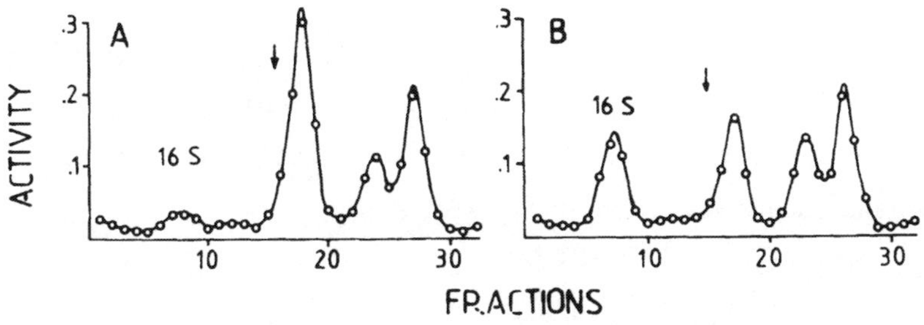

Fig. 7 Molecular forms of AChE in the superior cervical ganglion of 21 days old rat. A: normal ganglion; B: contralateral ganglion, denervated shortly after birth. The top of the gradients is on the right hand side. An arrow shows the position of catalase (11.4 S) in the gradient. AChE activity is expressed per unit of wet weight of the ganglion.

activity is small, but on the other hand the extracellular and intracellular activity of AChE of muscle origin is under distinct and substantial influence of innervation.

The asymmetric molecular forms of AChE are present also in sympathetic ganglia of the rat but their dependence on innervation seems to be quite different from that in muscles. In adult rats the percentage of the asymmetric forms is very low (4-5 %) but at birth it amounts to about 30 % of the total AChE activity (30, 31). This finding is particularly relevant considering that at birth only about 10 percent of ganglion cells have been contacted by the nerve and that a functional ganglionic transmission has not yet been established (32). Moreover, in pups where the preganglionic nerve was cut at birth, the high ratio of asymmetric AChE forms relative to total activity (20 %) persists during postnatal development and maturity and does not decrease like in contralateral control ganglion (Fig. 7), where the synaptogenesis has progressed to completion and a normal ganglionic transmission was established (33). This finding suggests that, contrary to muscle, the activity of the 16 S molecular form of AChE in the rat SCG is being depressed by the neural contacts and maturation of synapses. The above findings suggest that the asymmetric forms of AChE are succeptible to neural influence in a complex manneraffecting both relative activity and the distribution in the cells. This influence is expressed differently in different cholinoceptive tissues and depend on the developmental stage.

Conclusions

Muscle and sympathetic ganglion cells, two typical cholinergically innervated structures, differ considerably in regard to various aspects of AChE.

1. Very high concentration of AChE in muscle is present in the junctional region proper, whereas, in a sympathetic ganglion, the presynaptic AChE is distributed more diffusely in the neuropile and is located predominantly in the axolemma-Schwann cell interspace and not in the junctional regions.

2. Developmental studies and the studies of recovery of AChE activity after inhibition indicate that AChE at the endplate originates in the muscle

cell and is concentrated in the junction by a direct intracellular transport. When the rate of protein synthesis is enhanced, Schwann cells at the synapse synthesize AChE and it is possible that these cells may supply the enzyme also under normal adult conditions. The contribution of AChE to the endplate by the motoneuron via axonal transport seems to be only minor.

In the sympathetic ganglion the direct contribution of the preganglionic neurons is considerable and amounts up to 50 percent of the total ganglionic AChE activity.

3. AChE activity is already high and is distributed mostly intracellularly along the muscle cell when motoneuron first contacts the muscle fibre. After this the concentration of AChE at the neuromuscular junction increases whereas sarcoplasmatic AChE decreases.

The innervation of SCG is quite late, and the total ganglionic AChE is rather low at that time but increases extra- and intracellularly during the following stages of postnatal development.

4. In muscle, the neural contact has a profound effect on the activity of AChE of muscular origin. The denervation of muscle causes always a decrease of endplate AChE activity but can cause either a decrease or an increase of sarcoplasmatic activity of AChE.

Decentralization of the SCG in an adult animal results in loss of only the preganglionic extracellular AChE. AChE activity of ganglion cells decentralized at birth increases until the normal intracellular activity is reached at maturation. It seems that, in contrast to the muscle, the intracellular AChE activity in SCG is not regulated by the nerve.

5. The appearance and maintenance of the asymmetric molecular forms of AChE in muscles depend upon innervation. These molecular forms are induced in developing muscle by the nerve contact and they are drastically decreased after denervation.

The asymmetric AChE molecular forms in adult rat SCG are rather low but they do not decrease after preganglionic denervation as in muscles. These forms are present in an immature, only partly innervated SCG at birth. Preganglionic nerves probably restrain their activity during further development since much higher activity of the asymmetric forms was found in ganglia, decentralised at birth than in control, normaly innervated ganglia. The mechanisms regulating the activity of these forms in both cholinoceptive tissues are evidently very different.

1. Brzin, M., Sketelj, J., Klinar, B.: Handbook of Neurochemistry, Volume 4 (Lajtha, A., Ed.) Plenum Press, New York and London, pp. 251-292 (1983).

2. McMahan, U.J., Sanes, J.R., Marshall, L.M.: Nature 271, 172-174 (1978).

3. Sketelj, J., Brzin, M.: Histochemistry 61, 239-248 (1979).

4. Brzin, M., Zajiček, J.: Nature 181, 626 (1958).

5. Barnard, E.A.: The Peripheral Nervous System (Hubbard, J.J., Ed.) Plenum Press, New York and London, pp. 201-224 (1975).

6. Klinar, B., Brzin, M.: Cell. molec. Biol. 26, 459-467 (1980).

7. Brzin, M., Tennyson, V., Duffy, P.: J. Cell Biol. 31, 215-242 (166).

8. Tennyson, V., Brzin, M., Slotwiner, P.: J. Cell Biol. 51, 703-721 (1971).

9. Brzin, M., Sketelj, J., Tennyson, V.M., Kiauta, T., Budininkas-Schoenebeck, M.: Muscle and Nerve 4, 505-513 (1981).

10. Vigny, M., Koenig, J., Rieger, F.: J. Neurochem. 27, 1347-1353 (1976).

11. Sketelj, J., Brzin, M.: Neurochem. Res. 5, 653-658 (1980).

12. Grubić, Z., Sketelj, J., Klinar, B., Brzin, M.: J. Neurochem. 37, 909-916 (1981).

13. Tauc, L., Hoffmann, A., Tsuji, S., Hinzen, D.H., Faille, L.: Nature 250, 496-498 (1974).

14. Lubińska, L., Niemierko,S.: Brain Res. 27, 329-342 (1971).

15. Brzin, M.: Proc. nat. Acad. Sci. 56, 1560-1563 (1966).

16. Guth, L.: Physiol. Rev. 48, 645-687 (1968).

17. Drachman, D.B.: Biology of Cholinergic Function (Goldberg, A.M., Hanin, I., Eds.) Raven Press, New York, pp. 161-186 (1976).

18. Ginetzinsky, A.G., Shamarina, N.M.: Uspekhi sovremenoi Biol. 15, 283-293 (1942).

19. Brzin, M., Majcen-Tkačev, Ž.: J. Cell Biol. 19, 349-358 (1963).

20. Tennyson, V.M., Kremzner, L.T., Brzin, M.: J. Neuropathol. exp. Neurol. 36, 245-275 (1977).

21. Bacou, F., Vigneron, P., Massoulié, J.: Nature 296, 661-664 (1982).

22. Linkhart, T.A., Wilson, B.W.: J. exp. Zool. 193, 191-200 (1975).

23. Sketelj, J., McNamee, M.G., Wilson, B.W.: Exp. Neurol. 60, 624-629 (1978).

24. Lubińska, L., Zelená, J.: Nature 210, 39-41 (1966).

25. Kiauta, T., Brzin, M., Dettbarn W-D.: Exp. Neurol. 56, 281-288 (1977).

26. Sketelj, J., Pavlin, M., Peršič, M., Rus, M., Brzin, M.: Abstracts of the 2nd Intern. Meeting on Cholinesterases, Bled, p. 55 (1983).

27. Koenig, J., Vigny, M.: C.R. Soc. Biol. 172, 1069-1074 (1978).

28. Carson, S., Bon, S., Vigny, M., Massoulié, J., Fadeau, M.: FEBS Lett. 97, 348-352 (1979).

29. Koenig, J., Rieger, F.: Dev. Neurosci. 4, 249-257 (1981).

30. Gisiger, V., Vigny, M., Gautron, J., Rieger, F.: J. Neurochem. 30, 501-516 (1978).

31. Verdière, M., Derer, M., Rieger, F.: Dev. Biol. 89, 509-515 (1982).

32. Smolen, A., Raisman, G.: Brain Res. 181, 315-323 (1980).

33. Klinar, B., Sketelj, J., Sket, D., Brzin, M.: J. Neurosci. Res. 9, 437-444 (1983).

CYTOCHEMICAL CHANGES OF CHOLINESTERASES IN MOTOR NEURONS DURING REGENERATION

Georg W. Kreutzberg, Wolfram Tetzlaff
Max-Planck-Institut für Psychiatrie
Abteilung für Neuromorphologie
D-8033 Martinsried b. München
BRD

Lajos Tóth
Department of Anatomy
University Medical School
Kossuth L. 40
H-6701 Szeged 1
Hungary

Introduction

The response of motor neurons to transection of their axons is described as chromatolysis or axon reaction and is believed to display the attempt of the neurons to regenerate the lesioned axon. A number of enzymes involved in glucose and RNA metabolisms increase during this process (for review see 8). Enzymes involved in transmitter metabolism show decreasing activity. AChE and BuChE in general are following this latter scheme, however, cytochemistry on the EM level shows interesting changes in the subcellular distribution of the enzymes. It thus appears that both AChE and BuChE are enzymes which respond dynamically to functional changes of neurons.

Material and methods

Changes in ChEs were studied in young adult guinea pigs and Sprague-Dawley or Long-Evans hooded rats, 6-8 weeks old. Transection of the right facial nerve was at the stylomastoid foramen. The vagus nerve was cut at the level of the nodose ganglion and the ciliary nerve was interrupted by removing one eye. The animals were sacrificed at times varying between 12 hrs and 6 months. Unfixed 20μ thick cryostat sections were cut and incubated for AChE and BChE in a medium according to Gomori's modification of the Koelle and Friedenwald technique (1). For cytochemical studies the animals were perfused with glutaraldehyde plus paraformaldehyde and postfixed with OsO_4. Thick sections cut on the tissue chopper were incubated for 3 hrs at $4^{o}C$ according to Lewis and Shute (7). Control incubations with substrate lacking media or with specific inhibitors such as ethopropazine, DFP, BW284C51 were carried out to ascertain specificity of the cytochemical reaction. The biochemical measurement of AChE was performed in homogenates of the facial nuclei by a radiochemical assay (12). Histochemical sections were also submitted to densitometric measurement based on a computerized texture analysis system, T.A.S. Leitz.

Results and Commentary

ChEs in the facial nucleus. Normal motor neurons demonstrate AChE activity in the perinuclear cisternae, in the granular and in smooth-ER cisternae of the perikaryon, the axon and the dendrites. Reaction product is also seen in subsurface cisternae approaching the dendritic membranes and on the outer surface of plasmalemma of dendrites irrespective of their functioning as postsynaptic side or of being covered by satellite glial cells. In the neuropil activity is often present in the extracellular spaces especially of bundles of small axons of the C-fiber type. Intraaxonal activity is rarely seen and seems restricted to motor axons. Glial cells and vascular cells show no intracellular activity. However, occasionally parts of the basal laminae are stained. BuChE is not seen in facial neurons, but is present in the granular ER cisternae of endothelial cells. The association of the ChEs to subcellular organelles and compartments as described here is in agreement with the early reports from the laboratories of G. Koelle and of P. Lewis, confirmed by many others as reviewed by Ann Silver (11). It reflects (i) the site of synthesis and probably of processing in the ER systems of the perikaryon, (ii) the transport within dendrites and axons, (iii) the presence in the dendritic membrane and the release from there to the extracellular space.

Changes in the facial nucleus following transection of the nerve. In the rat AChE activity drops rather (Fig.5-6) rapidly in both the neuronal perikarya and the neuropil. In histochemical sections this becomes visible after 24 h and reaches a plateau almost 7 d following the operation. Figure 9 shows that quantitative measurements reveal a decrease to approximately 60% of normal values for 3 weeks. Thereafter activity recovers.

In the guinea pig facial nucleus changes of AChE during motorneuronal axonal reaction are very different although the chromatolytic changes are very similar in both species (5). It has been reported that "light microscopic histochemistry shows an unchanged or even increased AChE activity in the cell bodies of the motoneurons. Yet, distribution of activity decreases dramatically in the neuropil. This is because there is less activity in the dendrites and especially in the dendritic membrane (Fig. 3). Rather than in these normally positive structures, the enzyme accumulates in the basement membrane of the capillaries (Fig.4)(4,6,). It appears that the dendritic membrane becomes leaky to AChE or that the enzyme can no longer be fixed on the outer surface of the membrane, and is therefore released into the extracellular spaces. From here, it reaches the basement membranes (basal lamina) of the capillaries, which are known to form a specialized part of the extracellular space. By some yet unknown mechanism, basement membrane material seems to be able to concentrate AChE. This has also been demonstrated after injection of exogeneous AChE into rat brain (3)."

Recovery of AChE in the motoneurons of the facial nucleus is slower in the rat compared to the guinea pig. Reappearance of the enzyme in the rat is also related to the type of trauma and may correlate to the degree of regeneration (Fig. 9). Following a nerve excision of 1 cm, AChE levels decrease to 60% of control (after one week) and little recovery occurs (72% after 70 days). In contrast AChE recovery is almost complete after nerve crush (96%) and less complete after transection with suture (88%, 70 days post OP). These unpublished observations suggest that the AChE recovery is related to regeneration, since functional restitution is delayed in the case of nerve transection plus excision.
A further response of AChE has been studied following a so-called "conditioning lesion". This paradigm at present is the basis for delayed sutures of lesioned nerves in peripheral neurosurgery. It has been observed that a second lesion of a nerve two or three weeks after the initial cut leads to an enhanced growth of axon sprouts from the proximal stump (9, 10). It is assumed that while the first lesion conditioned the neuron and triggered the "regeneration program", the second lesion could set an additional stimulus to booster the response of the motor neurons. We now found (Fig. 10) that AChE shows an additional drop in activity after the second lesion.However, recovery of enzyme activity is not enhanced. Thus it seems that the second lesion does not simply repeat what a single lesion is doing, it rather forces the cell to further reduce its synthesis of the transmitter related enzyme AChE. The significance of this for the regeneration process still remains unclear. So far the semi-quantitative observations of Tuncbay (13) indicate that, 90 days after secondary nerve suture, AChE is less active in the spinal cord than after a

primary suture of the sciatic nerve of the cat. This is an indication that the further decrease of AChE is not fully reversible which might reflect a certain impairment to regeneration.

BuChE is present in the brain mainly in glial cells and in capillaries. However, there are a number of brain stem and forebrain areas where BuChE is associated with neuronal structures. The most striking examples of this are the dorsal motor nucleus of the vagus nerve and the Edinger-Westphal nucleus (EWN) both serving parasympathetic function. As shon in fig. 8 neuronal BuChE activity is seen in the perinuclear cisterna and in the cisternae of the granular-ER which in these neurons show no Nissl body like arrangement. No activity is seen in the plasmalemma of the neurons and of the dendrites but faint activity is visible in the axolemma of weakly myelinated most probably vagal axons (Fig. 8). Activity is also present in the axoplasmic reticulum of peripheral vagal nerve fibers. After a lesion BuChE disappears rapidly from the neurons of both the dorsal motor nucleus of N.X and the EWN. As seen in fig. 7 only background staining (glial) is visible 4 d p. op. The recovery of BuChE is remarkably different from the reappearance of AChE. While vagal neurons show some activity of the latter enzyme already two weeks p. op., BuChE activity can be seen in the same neurons only three weeks after nerve lesion. This suggests that the synthesis of the two ChEs is coded by two different genes which are also regulated by different mechanisms. The functional significance of BuChE in the nervous systems is as unclear as its function in the liver or the serum. However, its highly selective appearance in some neuronal systems is impressive and its correlation to certain anatomical structures e.g. in the lateral geniculate nucleus of the macaque monkey (2) is tempting to speculate on its role in synaptic function. However, when attempting to correlate BuChE positive neuronal systems with one of the known neurotransmitters or neuromodulators including various peptides no such parallelism was detected in the rat. However, with respect to the decrease during chromatolysis BuChE behaves like a transmitter related enzyme.

References

1. Gomori, G.: Microscopic Histochemistry. University Press, Chicago (1952).

2. Graybiel, A.M., Ragsdale, D.W.: Nature 299, 439-442 (1982).

3. Kreutzberg, G.W., Kaiya, H.: Histochemistry 42, 233-237 (1974).

4. Kreutzberg, G.W., Tóth, L.: Naturwissenschaften 61, 37 (1974).

5. Kreutzberg, G.W., Tóth, L., Kaiya, H.: Advances in Neurology 12, 269-281 (1975).

6. Kreutzberg, G.W., Tóth, L., Weikert, M., Schubert,P.: Pathology of Cerebral Microcirculation, J.Cervós-Navarro (Ed.) pp. 282-288 (1974).

7. Lewis, P.R., Shute, L.C.: J. Microsc. 89, 329-342 (1969).

8. Lieberman, A.R.: Int. Rev. Neurobiol. 14, 49-124 (1971).

9. McQuarrie, I.G.: Brain Res. 167, 185-188 (1979).

10. McQuarrie, I.G., Grafstein, B.: Arch. Neurol. 29, 53-55 (1973).

11. Silver, A.: The Biology of Cholinesterases, North-Holland, Amsterdam (1974).

12. Sterri, S.H., Fonnum, F.: Europ. J. Biochem. 91, 125-222 (1978).

13. Tuncbay, T.O.: Neurology 14, 657-667 (1964).

Legends

Fig. 1. Cytochemical demonstration of intracellular AChE activity in a normal rat facial motorneuron. Electron dense reaction products indicate activity in the cisternae of the rough ER and in the perinuclear cisterna. x 18000

Fig. 2. AChE in the neuropil of normal rat facial nucleus. Activity is present in the smooth ER of dendrites (D) on the dendritic plasmamembranes and in the extracellular spaces of C-fiber bundles (arrows). No activity at the capillaries. x 5700

Fig. 3. AChE activity in a typical chromatolytic facial neuron of the guinea pig 21 days post axotomy. The dispersed cisternae of the ER are filled with reaction products. The neuronal plasmalemma is almost free of activity. x 5700

Fig. 4. AChE activity accumulates in the basal laminae and the abluminal interendothelial clefts where it stops at the tight junction. No intraendothelial activity except for cytoplasmic vesicles suggesting cytosis across the endothelial cell. Guinea pig 2 weeks (4a) and 3 weeks (4b) p.op., magnification a x 54000, b x 18000.

Fig. 5. Rat facial neurons respond to axotomy with decreased AChE activity. In the motorneuron shown 4 d p.op. only a few cisternae of the r-ER have weak reaction products. x 18000

Fig. 6. 8 d p.op. AChE activity is weak in the operated right facial nucleus (rat).

Fig. 7. BuChE is present in capillaries throughout the brain and also in neurons of selected areas, e.g. the dorsal motor nucleus of NX. 4 d after transection of the vagus nerve activity has disappeared almost completely from the right nucleus.

Fig. 8. Distribution of BuChE activity in rat vagus motoneuron. Perinuclear and ER cisternae are positive in the neuron, in a dendrite (D) and an axon (A). The axolemma also shows activity but otherwise plasmamembranes are negative. x 25000

Fig. 9a. Time course of AChE changes in the axotomised facial nucleus of the rat expressed as a percentage of the contralateral, nonoperated control side. Quantifications by biochemical assay (12) and by computerized densitometry of histochemical sections are in good accordance.
n=10 for each biochemical timepoint. n=6 animals x 10 sections each for each histochemical value; the vertical bars indicate standard deviation.

Fig. 9b. Recovery of AChE activity in the facial nucleus of the rat after different surgical procedures. Evaluation of histochemistry in 2 animals, 10 sections each for each timepoint; $\pm$ SD. The data suggest reappearance of AChE is related to the severity of the lesion.

Fig. 10. AChE activities in the rat facial nucleus after single (e-h) and after double (a-d) nerve section.
The left (a-d) side was sectioned in a 1st operation.

In a 2nd operation 14 days later both sides were transected. The left, double lesion side displays consistently less activity than the right, single lesion side. a and e 7d, b and f 12d, c and g 20d, d and h 28h post 2nd op. (Tetzlaff and Kreutzberg, in preparation).

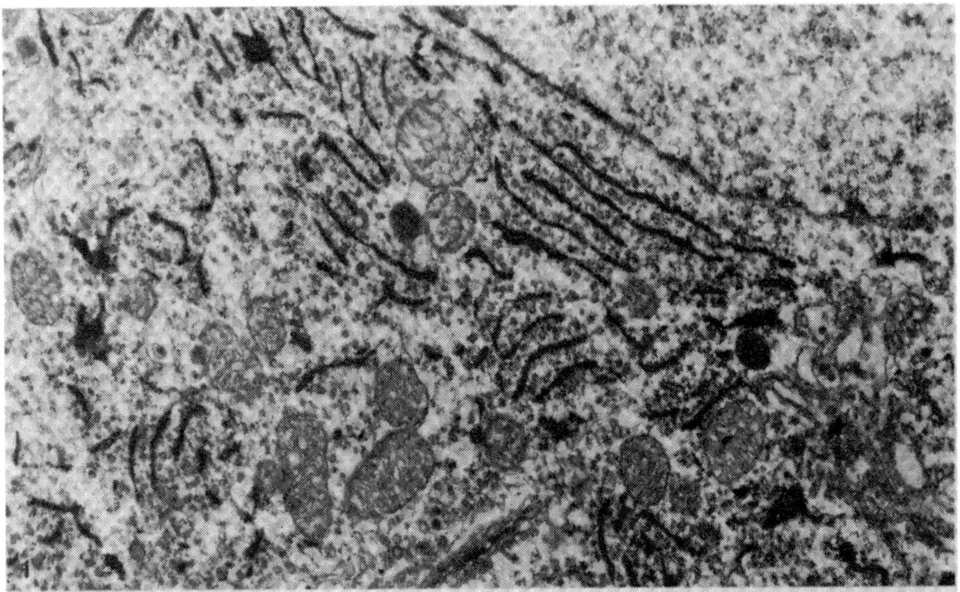

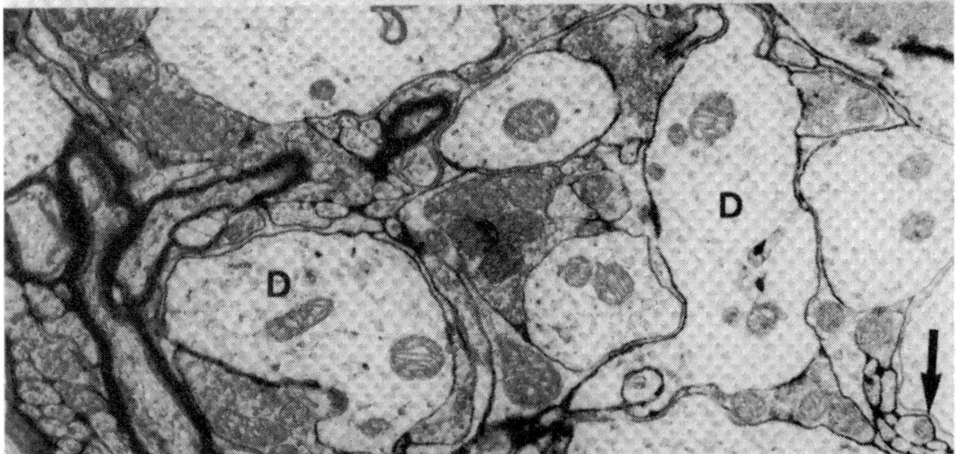
D
D
D
2

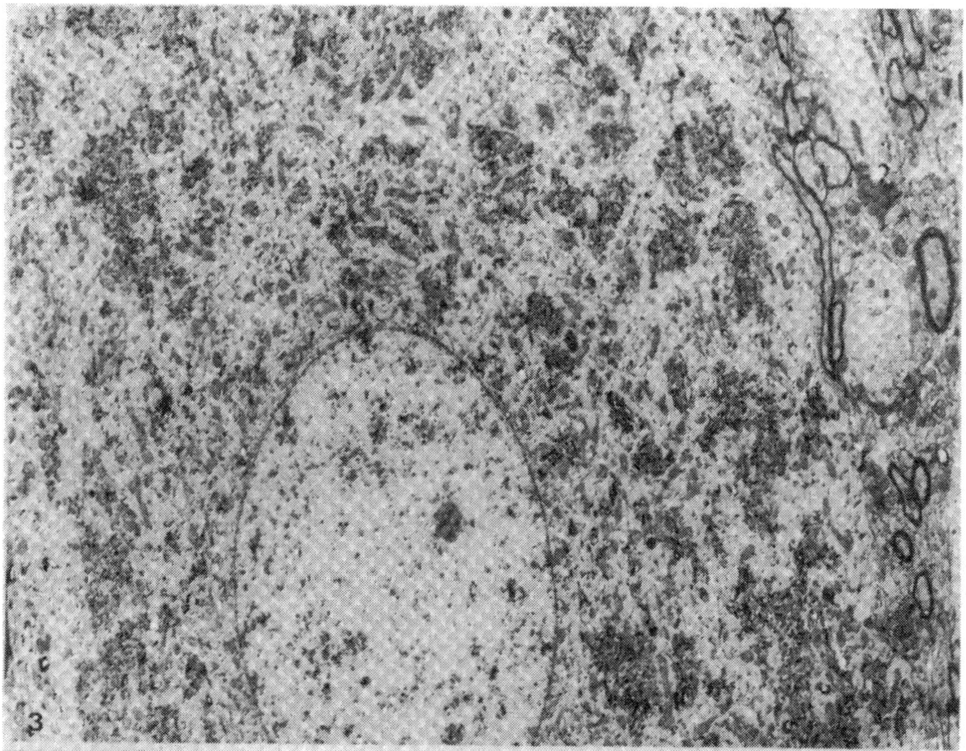
3

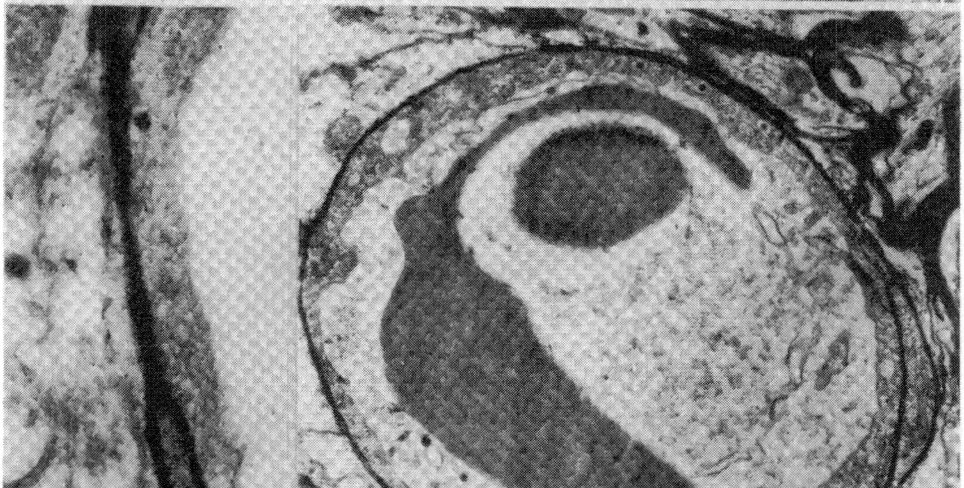
4a
4b

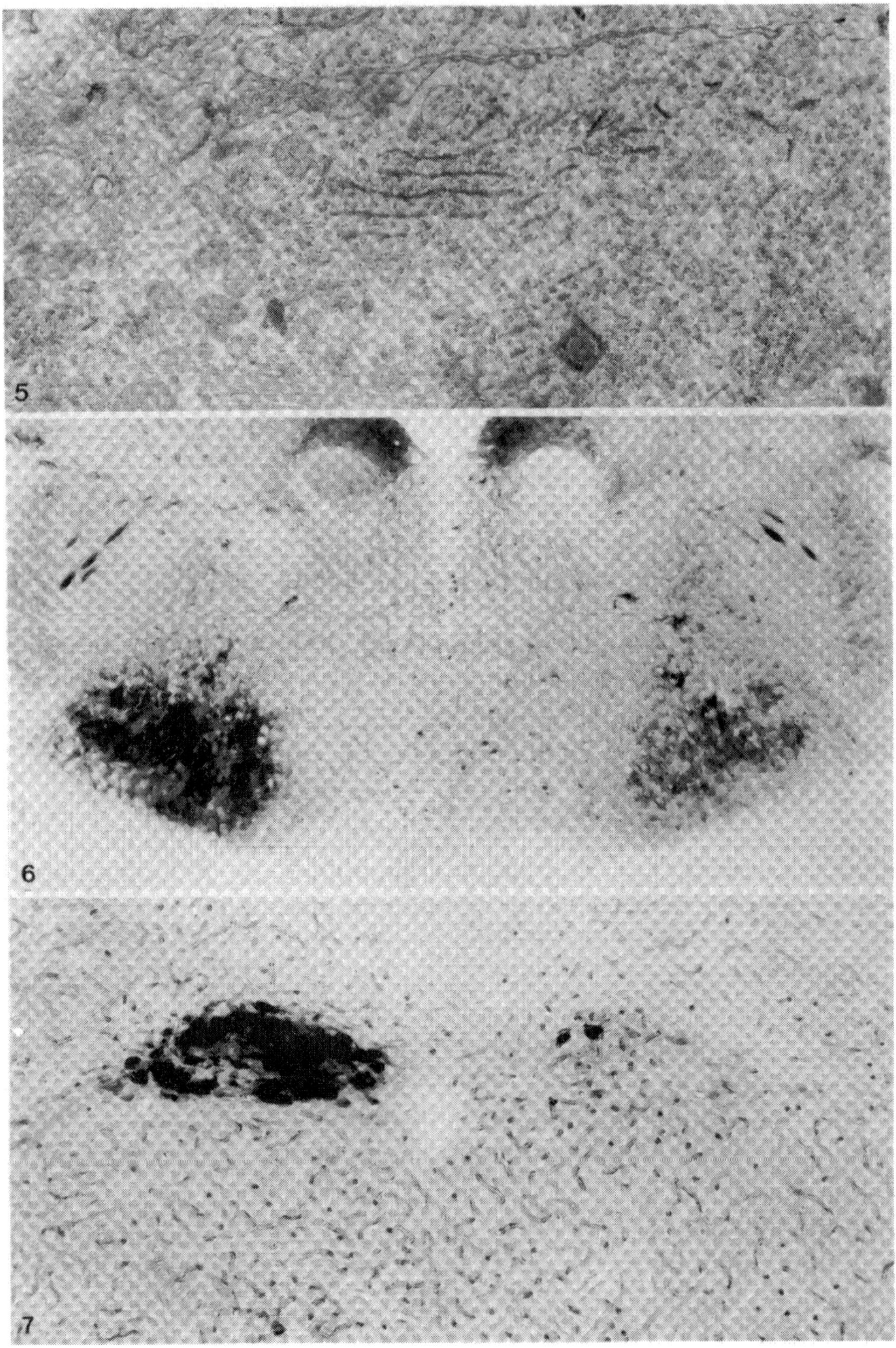
5
6
7

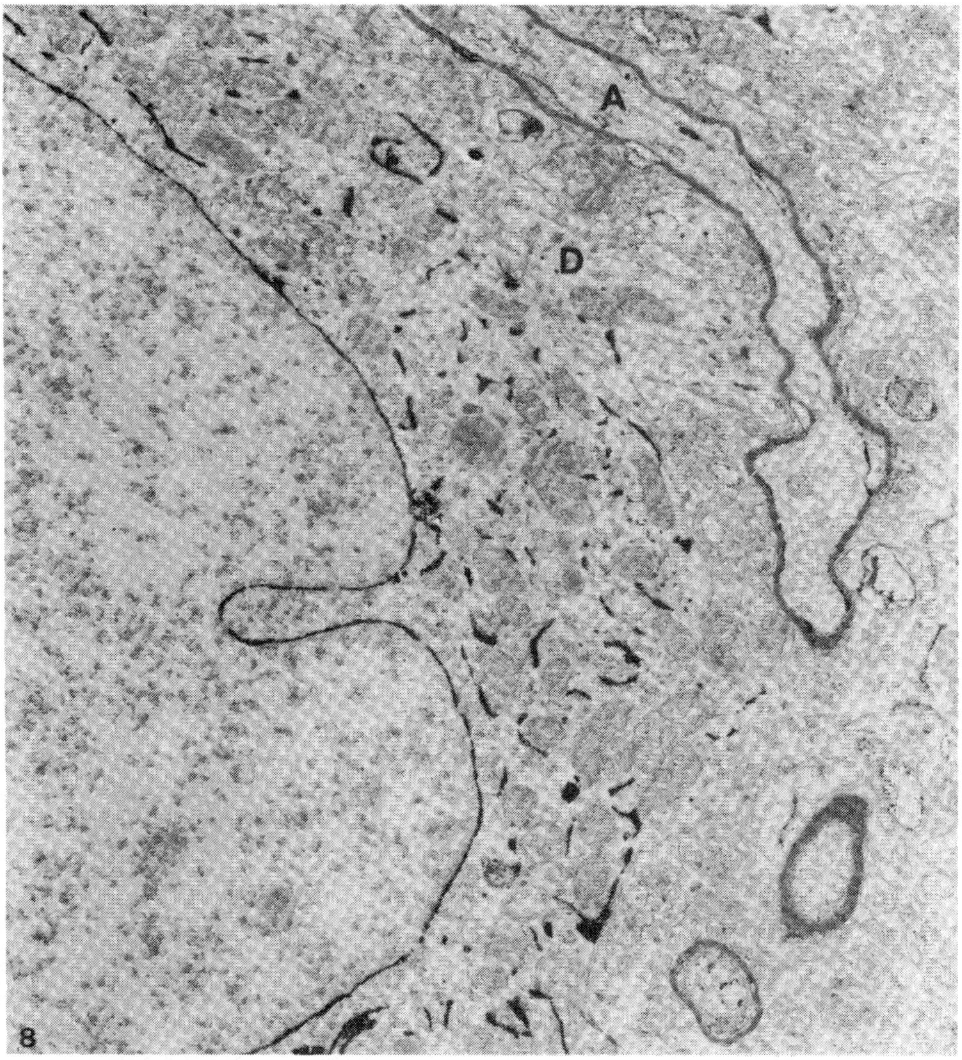
A
D
8

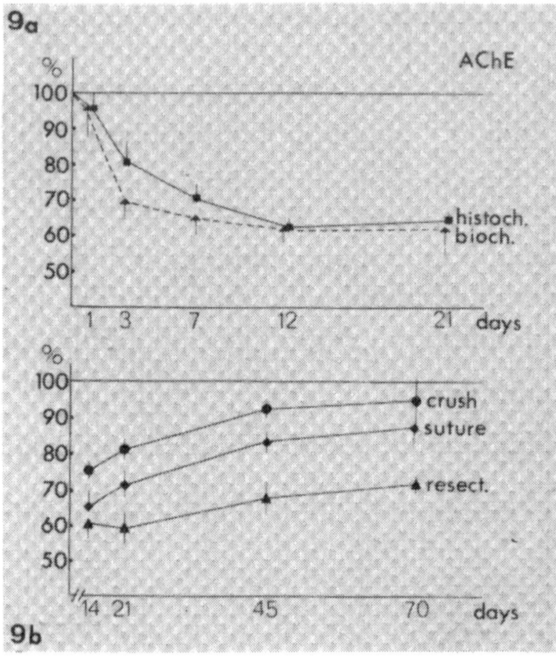
9a
%
AChE
100
90
80
70
60
50
histoch.
bioch.
1
3
7
12
21
days
%
100
90
80
70
60
50
crush
suture
resect.
14
21
45
70
days
9b

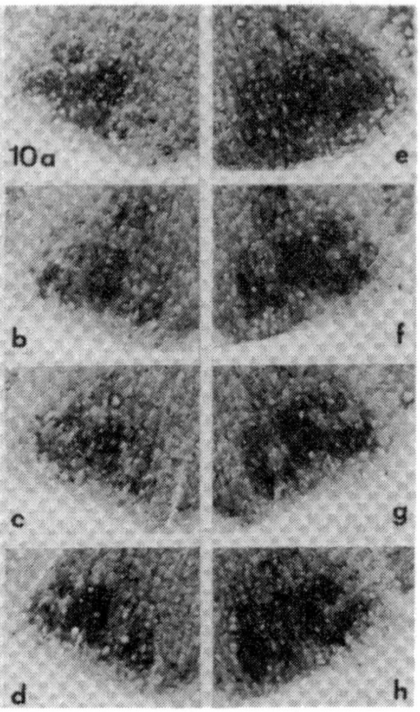
10a
e
b
f
c
g
d
h

A NOVEL FUNCTION FOR ACETYLCHOLINESTERASE IN NIGRO-STRIATAL NEURONS

Susan A. Greenfield,

University Laboratory of Physiology,
Parks Road,
Oxford,
OX1 3PT,
U.K.

(A) Introduction

It is not a new idea that AChE could have a function or functions independent of the hydrolysis of ACh. This theory was first advanced almost ten years ago by Silver (1), who based her conclusions on the not-infrequent occurrence of high levels of AChE accompanied by little or no CAT and ACh. Excessive amounts of AChE, superfluous to or even in the absence of, cholinergic transmission, occur in both the periphery (e.g. erythrocytes, platelets, placenta) and also in certain parts of the CNS (1). One such region in the brain is the substantia nigra. Not only are levels of nigral ACh and CAT very low compared to AChE (2, 3, 1, 4, 5) but furthermore, there is no convincing evidence for cholinergic synapses in this area (6, 7).

A clue to the puzzling presence of AChE in the substantia nigra arose initially out of a discovery made by Chubb and Smith working with peripheral tissue. In the isolated splanchnic nerve-adrenal medulla preparation, one of the five soluble isoenzymes of AChE is released; this release is evoked by K^+ and is Ca^{++}-dependent (8, 9). A similar phenomenon occurs in the CNS, in vivo. A soluble isoenzyme of AChE, of similar electrophoretic mobility to that released from the adrenal medulla, is present in cerebrospinal fluid (CSF) and increases following peripheral nerve stimulation

(10). We can be virtually certain that AChE in CSF is derived from a soluble fraction in neurons as opposed to plasma (11, 12, 13, 14, 10). However, release of AChE from central neurons into the ventricular system does not necessarily reflect release of ACh from the brain. Release of ACh into the ventricular system is depressed by anaesthesia (15). However, this was not the case for AChE, which was unaffected by anaesthesia, in rabbit cisternal CSF (Greenfield and Smith, unpublished observations). In addition, the concentration of released ACh is highest in the lateral ventricles, compared to the rest of the ventricular system (16, 17): yet AChE activity is greatest in CSF from the cisterna magna (18). It would seem then that although structures in the caudal part of the brain were releasing relatively little ACh, much AChE in CSF was derived from these regions. This idea was corroborated by experiments involving direct electrical stimulation. Following stimulation of the rabbit caudate nucleus, which borders on the lateral ventricle, there was a large increase in AChE in cisternal but not ventricular CSF (18). Thus the enzyme was probably actually released from a structure or structures caudal to the caudate nucleus following activation by it. The substantia nigra is situated in the ventral mesencephalon and has direct reciprocal connections with the caudate nucleus (19). Following a unilateral electrolytic lesion of the nigra, two striking effects occur. First, stimulation of the caudate nucleus no longer leads to an increase in the concentration of AChE in cisternal CSF and secondly, the resting level of the enzyme drops by approximately 50% (18). These findings suggest that stimulation of the caudate nucleus causes AChE to be released from the substantia nigra: furthermore, it would appear that a large proportion of the enzyme normally present in cisternal CSF, is derived from nigral neurons. If the substantia nigra is stimulated directly, there is a marked increase in the concentration of AChE in CSF: this stimulation-evoked release is not blocked by systemic pre-treatment with the cholinergic receptor antagonists atropine (18) or mecamylamine. In conclusion, there is thus indirect evidence that AChE is released from neurons in the substantia nigra. This release does not parallel that of ACh and is independent of blockade of the ACh receptor. Perhaps then, release of AChE is unrelated to cholinergic transmission, in the substantia nigra.

(B) Nigro-Striatal Neurons, Dopamine and AChE

The substantia nigra is divided into two main zones: the pars compacta and pars reticulata. Briefly, the pars compacta is rich in neuronal somata, approximately 90% (20) of which are dopamine-(DA) containing cells which send a monosynaptic input to the striatum. The pars reticulata contains far more neuropil, including afferent axon terminals and also very long dendrites extending from the DA-containing, nigro-striatal somata of the pars compacta. Nigro-striatal neurons appear to be cholinoceptive, but not to receive a cholinergic input (19, 7). They do, however, contain large amounts of AChE (21, 6, 22 and Fig. 1). In fact, AChE and DA develop in parallel in these cells during ontogeny (21). Furthermore, both AChE (23) and DA (24) are detectable in the smooth endoplasmic reticulum (SER) of the dendrites. An interesting property of nigro-striatal neurons is that DA is released from the dendrites. This release is K^+-evoked, Ca^{++}-dependent but unaffected by blockade of Na^+ channels with tetrodotoxin (TTX) (25). Since AChE was present in nigro-striatal neurons and there was already indirect evidence (Introduction) that the enzyme might be released from nigral cells, we attempted to obtain direct evidence that AChE was indeed released from the substantia nigra. Glowinski's group have modified with great success the technique of local perfusion via push-pull cannulae in the anaesthetized cat, in order to study release of DA directly from the substantia nigra (26). Using the same preparation we found that AChE was released from nigral neurons in a fashion that

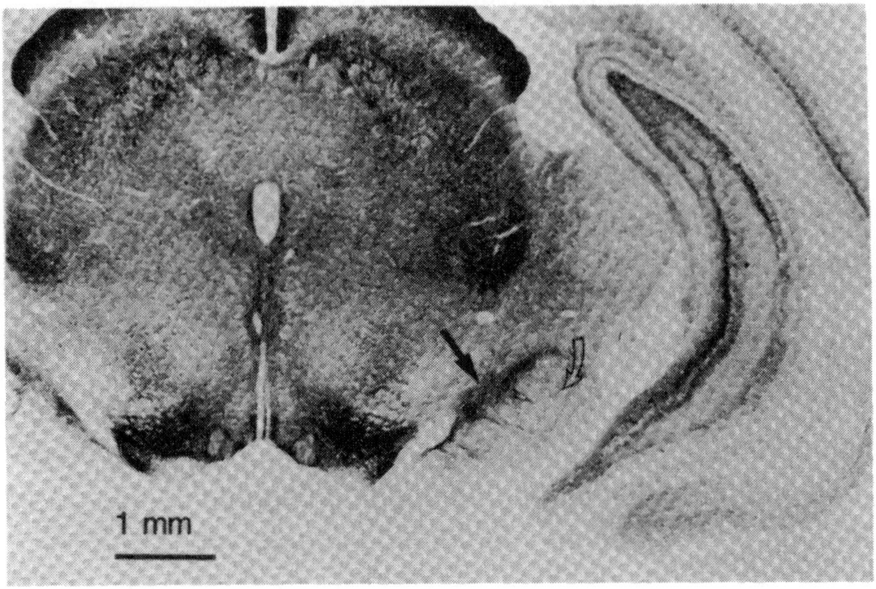

Fig. 1: Coronal section of rat brain stained for AChE. Black arrow indicates pars compacta; open arrow, pars reticulata.

was, like DA, K^+-evoked (27), Ca^{++}-dependent (28) and resistant to TTX (Greenfield and Chesselet, unpublished observations). However, we could not be sure that the AChE detectable in nigral perfusates did in fact come from DA-containing nigro-striatal neurons. Although histochemical observations suggest that nigral AChE is stored almost exclusively in these cells (21), biochemical studies indicate that only 40% of nigral AChE is present in the same cells as DA (6). In addition, Henderson (22) has identified a second, rarer type of AChE-containing nigral cell that is probably an interneuron and non-DA containing. It was therefore important to ascertain whether or not AChE released in the substantia nigra was actually derived from DA-containing nigro-striatal neurons. The rat nigro-striatal pathway was lesioned with the neurotoxin 6-hydroxydopamine such that striatal DA was depleted by about 90%. Following this procedure, release of AChE from the substantia nigra could no longer be evoked by K^+ and the resting level fell to about 15% of control values (29). It appears therefore that AChE is not only stored in DA-containing nigro-striatal neurons, but is released exclusively from their non-terminal processes, probably dendrites. This phenomenon prompts two basic questions. Firstly, how is AChE released from nigro-striatal neurons and secondly, does released AChE have a function? These issues will be discussed in the following two sections.

(C) Release of AChE in the Substantia Nigra

As we have seen, depolarizing concentrations of K^+ can enhance the release of AChE from nigro-striatal neurons. However, this effect tells us little about specific transmitter systems with which release of AChE would normally be associated. Working in vitro with isolated slices of rat substantia nigra, Cuello et al. (30) found that, as in vivo (previous section), release of AChE was K^+-evoked and Ca^{++}-dependent. However, neither carbachol nor ACh itself affected release of nigral AChE. This finding is consistent with earlier observations on the inefficacy of ACh receptor blockers in preventing release of AChE (c.f. Introduction). We can conclude therefore that release of AChE from nigro-striatal neurons is independent of synaptic activation by its familiar substrate, ACh.

Recently, a less familiar substrate for AChE has been described. It has been shown that, in vitro, purified AChE can hydrolyse the peptide substance P (31). Substance P, unlike ACh, is present in large amounts in the substantia nigra (32); furthermore, substance P-containing afferent axons have been shown to form synaptic contacts with the soma and dendrites of pars compacta neurons (33). It is therefore an attractive possibility that AChE is released to hydrolyse nigral substance P. Unfortunately, however, substance P, like ACh, does not modify the release of AChE from nigral neurons (30). Furthermore, we have shown that the endogenous isoenzyme of AChE released from nigro-striatal cells is not an aminopeptidase, at least not an aminopeptidase that will break down the substrate leucine-beta- naphthylamide (34). Release, therefore, of AChE appears not to be evoked by known potential substrates. Since both AChE and DA are released from the same neurons, it was possible that release of the enzyme was in some fashion associated with nigral DA transmission. Following (in vivo) local perfusion of the substantia nigra with the DA agonist amphetamine, there was a marked increase in the release of AChE (34). However, this finding was surprising. It had previously been assumed that AChE was released from central neurons in direct relation to their activity (18). Yet infusion of amphetamine into the substantia nigra depresses the firing rate of pars compacta cells (35). The finding that amphetamine evoked an increase in the release of AChE raises two, not necessarily mutually exclusive possibilities. First, AChE could be co-stored in the same SER as DA. Hence, amphetamine could displace AChE when it displaced DA, without this being the normal physiological mechanism for release of the enzyme. Secondly, release of AChE may not be directly related to the frequency of firing rate. This second possibility certainly seems to be the case for dendritic release of DA, which has no clear relationship to pars compacta cell activity. Serotonin and ACh both increase DA release (25): however, iontophoretic studies show that the former has a depressant affect on these cells (36) whereas the latter is excitatory (37). Substance P also increases pars compacta cell discharge (Walker et al., 1976), but unlike ACh, application of this peptide leads to a decrease in DA release (25). Finally, gamma-aminobutyric acid (GABA), iontophoresed onto identified nigro-striatal neurons, produces a rapid and marked inhibition of their firing (38): however, DA levels in nigral perfusates are unaffected by addition of this transmitter (25). In order to understand electrophysiological events underlying dendritic release of both DA and AChE, it is clearly necessary to identify the ion channels operative in nigro-striatal neurons. To this end Llinas, Jahnsen and I have recently recorded intracellularly from pars compacta cells in slices of guinea pig mesencephalon. We have identified two conductances that appear to function in the dendrites of these neurons. In both cases, current is carried by Ca^{++} ions and can occur in the presence of TTX or absence of Na^{+} ions. It is tempting to associate release of DA and AChE with these dendritic Ca^{++} potentials. Their ability to occur both in the presence and absence of repetitive firing of the fast Na^{+} spike, might explain the difficulty in correlating changes ir dendritic release with changes in firing frequency.

(D) Action of AChE in the Substantia Nigra

The release of AChE into the extracellular space might simply reflect the fate of a soluble form of the enzyme, but in addition it could actually have a physiological function. In an attempt to answer this question, we have infused exogenous AChE into the extracellular space of the substantia nigra and recorded the firing rate of identified pars compacta cells, in vivo (39). Following application of AChE, either by micro-injection or pressure ejection (40), there was a marked inhibition of pars compacta cell firing rate. Other cells in the vicinity of the substantia nigra, which did not display the characteristics of nigro-striatal neurons, were unaffected by infusion of the enzyme. When the caudate nucleus is stimulated, nigro-striatal cells respond with an early synaptic excitation, believed to be subserved by striatal substance P afferents, followed by a long-latency inhibition, probably mediated by GABA (19). AChE enhanced the stimulus-induced inhibition, but had no affect on the early synaptic excitation. Thus again, it seems unlikely that substance P serves as a substrate for AChE in vivo (c.f. previous section). Furthermore, it is improbable that the AChE-induced inhibition of neuronal firing is via the hydrolysis of ACh: BuChE, given at ten times the activity used for AChE, had no effect on either the spontaneous or stimulus-linked activity of pars compacta cells (39).

Comparisons can be drawn with the putative action of dendritically released DA on nigro-striatal cells. It has been shown that exogenous DA and DA agonists also inhibit the firing rate of these neurons (41). A commonly held theory to explain this finding, is that DA released from dendrites mediates a local negative feedback to the same cell via 'autoreceptors' (35). A similar function has also been postulated for AChE (39). However, the release, diffusion and action of either dendritic DA or AChE may not be completely analogous with that of inhibitory substances released in the synaptic cleft. First, the fact that both these compounds are stored in the SER (Section B) rather than vesicles of dendrites, suggests that release in this situation may be rather more continuous. Secondly, dendro-dendritic synapses in the substantia nigra are rare (42, 43) with the dendrites generally in a post-synaptic position to other neurons (44). These observations imply that the action of released DA and AChE would normally be slow in onset, non-specific and involve a large population of target sites, c.f. (45). Hence, these anatomical features would argue against the 'autoreceptor' theory and suggest that both DA and AChE are acting in a more modulatory capacity.

We have recently obtained behavioural evidence that AChE can, in fact, exert long-term changes in the activity of nigro-striatal neurons. Ungerstedt (46) showed that rats will turn in circles in a direction away from the side of the brain where there is a higher level of available striatal DA. When we infused exogenous AChE into one substantia nigra of the rat, animals circled in a direction away from the side of injection (Greenfield et al., unpublished observations). The direction of circling implied that AChE infusion had enhanced the activity of the nigro-striatal pathway (47). The degree of circling did not depend on the over-all activity of the AChE preparation used, but rather on the amount of the secretory form of the enzyme it contained. Furthermore, BuChE in very high concentrations, did not affect the rats' motor behaviour in any way. We concluded that AChE appeared to have a functional significance specific to the secretory form, independent of ACh hydrolysis, and serving to enhance the activity of the DA nigro-striatal pathway. More surprisingly, a single infusion of AChE led to a continuation of circling behaviour lasting for days after the treatment. It seemed possible that the single injection of AChE was exerting its long-term effect via a change in the sensitivity of striatal DA receptor, for the following reason. If AChE were acting directly or indirectly in the substantia nigra to produce a tonic increase in striatal DA release (as implied by the direction of chronic circling), then a down-regulation of the striatal post-synaptic DA receptor would be expected (46, 48). If a drug was then administered systemically, which activated DA receptors directly (e.g. apomorphine), the striatum on the non-AChE treated side would be preferentially stimulated and the animal would transiently circle towards, not away from, the injected side. We found that this was the case: rats continuing to circle for a long period of time following a nigral infusion of AChE, transiently reversed their direction of circling whilst apomorphine was present (Greenfield et al., unpublished observations).

(E) Conclusions

In nigro-striatal neurons AChE may have a function independent of cholinergic transmission (Table I). Rather, it seems that release of AChE is in some fashion associated with DA transmission in the substantia nigra (Table II).

Table I. Reasons for believing AChE has a novel role in the substantia nigra

(1) Levels of ACh and CAT are disproportionately low compared with high levels of AChE.

(2) Cholinergic synapses in the substantia nigra have not been demonstrated.

(3) Release of AChE into the ventricular system, which originates largely from the substantia nigra, does not parallel release of ACh.

(4) Release of AChE from nigral neurons is not prevented by cholinergic receptor blockers.

(5) Release of AChE from nigral neurons is not enhanced by cholinomimmetics.

(6) Exogenous AChE affects the firing of nigral neurons, BuChE does not.

(7) Unilateral application of AChE to the substantia nigra induces circling behaviour, BuChE does not.

(8) The potency of AChE in inducing circling is not related to its degree of activity towards ACh.

However, two critical questions remain unanswered that would further our understanding of the possible interaction between AChE and DA. First, whether or not the two compounds share the same subcellular compartment in nigro-striatal cell dendrites (c.f. Sections B and C). If AChE and DA are in fact co-stored, we could postulate that the enzyme might function to amplify or extend the DA 'signal'.

AChE would be admirably suited for this role, since its rate of diffusion is slow, 'one to two millimetres per hour' (49) and it would probably be broken down far less rapidly than DA. On the other hand, if AChE and DA are in different SER, it is conceivable that they are released following different types, intensities or durations of stimuli. Any further speculation as to what would be the function of AChE release, in this case is hampered by a lack of knowledge of the selectivity of different stimuli for AChE, compared to DA release.

The second problem with describing more precisely the degree of association between AChE and DA arises from not knowing how AChE acts on target neurons. There are several, probably not exhaustive, possibilities. First, released AChE could exert its effects indirectly through breakdown of a substrate that has as yet not been identified. Secondly, the enzyme could act on the ACh receptor itself: we already know that nigro-striatal neurons are cholinoceptive (Section B) and recent evidence suggests that AChE might interact with the ACh receptor, independent of the hydrolysis of ACh (50). Thirdly, the secreted form of AChE might be able to change the DA receptor, by influencing either its turnover or its affinity. Fourthly, AChE could act, not at the level of a receptor but directly on an ion channel that may or may not be the same as that influenced by activation of DA receptors by DA. Lastly, the

Table II. Possible interaction of AChE and DA in the substantia nigra

(1) Both AChE and DA are present in the nigro-striatal cells of the pars compacta.

(2) AChE and DA accumulate in parallel in nigro-striatal cells during development.

(3) Both AChE and DA are present in the SER of nigro-striatal cell dendrites.

(4) Both AChE and DA are released from nigro-striatal cells in a fashion that is K^+-evoked, Ca^{++}-dependent and TTX-resistant.

(5) The release of both AChE and DA from nigral neurons is evoked by amphetamine.

(6) Both AChE and DA depress pars compacta cell firing.

(7) Application of AChE to nigral neurons induces long-term changes in motor behaviour involving modifications to striatal DA receptors.

effects of the enzyme might not be receptor or ion-channel specific, but simply change the properties of the cell membrane.

All that can be said at the moment, therefore, is that the release and action of AChE in the substantia nigra has little to do with the hydrolysis of ACh: rather, it appears associated with DA transmission. The nature of this interaction will not be understood properly until it is known whether or not AChE and DA are co-stored in the same subcellular compartment and secondly, to what extent AChE and DA share a common mechanism of action on target neurons. In any event, a very basic issue is to explore the physiology of the apparent 'modulatory' role of substances released from dendrites.

References

1. Silver, A.: The Biology of the Cholinesterases, Elsevier, Amsterdam (1974).
2. Bull, B., Hebb, C., Ratkovic, D.J.: J. Neurochem. 17, 1505-1516 (1970).
3. McGeer, E.G., Fibiger, H.C., McGeer, P.L., Brooke, S.: Brain Res. 52, 289-300 (1973).
4. Fonnum, F., Grofova, I., Rinvik, E., Storm-Mathisen, J., Walberg, F.: Brain Res. 71, 77-92.
5. Levey, A.I., Wainer, B.H., Mufson, E.J., Mesulam, M.-M.: Neuroscience 9, 9-22 (1983).
6. Lehmann, J., Fibiger, H.C.: Neurochem. 30, 615-624 (1978).
7. Kimura, H., McGeer, P.L., Peng, J.H., McGeer, E.G.: J. Comp. Neurol. 200, 157-201 (1981).
8. Chubb, I.W., Smith, A.D.: Proc. R. Soc. B. 191, 245-261 (1975a).
9. Chubb, I.W., Smith, A.D.: Proc. R. Soc. B. 191, 263-269 (1975b).
10. Chubb, I.W., Goodman, S., Smith, A.D.: Neuroscience 1, 57-62 (1976).
11. Augustinsson, M.-B.: Acta Physiol. Scand. 15, 1-182 (1948).
12. Tower, D.B., McEachern, D.: Can. J. Res. E. 27, 105-119 (1949).

13. Kalsbeck, F., Cohen, J.A., Bovens, B.K.: Biochim. Biophys. Acta 5, 548-560 (1950).

14. Yaksh, T.L., Filbert, M.G., Harris, L.W., Yamamura, H.I.: J. Neurochem. 25, 853-860 (1975).

15. Beleslin, D., Carmichael, E.A., Feldberg, W.: J. Physiol. 173, 368-376 (1964).

16. Portig, P.J., Vogt, M.: J. Physiol. 204, 687-715 (1969).

17. Carmichael, E.A., Feldberg, W., Fleischauser, K.: J. Physiol. 173, 354-367 (1964).

18. Greenfield, S.A., Smith, A.D.: Brain Res. 177, 445-459 (1979).

19. Dray, A.: Neuroscience 4, 1407-1439 (1979).

20. Gulley, R.L., Wood, R.L.: Tissue and Cell 3, 675-690 (1971).

21. Butcher, L.L., Talbot, K.: In 'Cholinergic-Monoaminergic Interactions in the Brain' (Ed. Butcher, L.L.) Academic Press, London, pp. 25-95 (1978).

22. Henderson, Z.: J. Comp. Neurol. 197, 185-196 (1981).

23. Liesli, P., Panula, P., Rechardt, L.: Histochemistry 70, 7-18 (1980).

24. Mercer, L., Del Fiacco, M., Cuello, A.C.: Experientia 35, 101-103 (1979).

25. Glowinski, J., Cheramy, A.: In 'Chemical Neurotransmission: 75 Years' (eds. Stjarne, L., Hedquist, P., Lagercrantz, H., Wennmalm, A.) Academic Press, pp. 285-299 (1981).

26. Nieoullon, A., Cheramy, A., Glowinski, J.: Nature 266, 375-377 (1977).

27. Greenfield, S.A., Cheramy, A., Leviel, V., Glowinski, J.: Nature 284, 355-357 (1980).

28. Greenfield, S.A., Cheramy, A., Glowinski, J.: J. Neurochem. 40, 1048-1057 (1983a).

29. Greenfield, S.A., Grunewald, R.A., Foley, P., Shaw, S.G.: J. Comp. Neurol. 214, 87-92 (1983b).

30. Cuello, A.C., Romero, E., Smith, A.D.: J. Physiol. 312, 14P (1981).

31. Chubb, I.W., Hodgson, A.J., White, G.H.: Neuroscience 5, 2065-2072 (1980).

32. Emson, P.C.: Prog. Neurobiol. 13, 61-116 (1979).

33. Somogyi, P., Priestley, J.V., Cuello, A.C., Smith, A.D., Bolam, J.P.: Cell Tiss. Res. 223, 469-486 (1982).

34. Greenfield, S.A., Shaw, G.: Neuroscience 7, 2883-2893.

35. Groves, P.M., Wilson, C.J., Young, S.J., Rebec, G.V.: Science 190, 522-529 (1979).

36. Dray, A., Gonye, J.J., Oakley, N.R., Tanner, R.: Brain Res. 113, 45-57 (1976).

37. Walker, R.J., Kemp, J.A., Yajima, H., Kitagawa, K., Woodruff, G.N.: Experientia 32, 214-215 (1976).

38. Scarnati, E., Pacitti, C.: Exptl. Brain Res. 46, 377-382 (1982).

39. Greenfield, S.A., Stein, J.F., Hodgson, A.J., Chubb, I.W.: Neuroscience 6, 2287-2295 (1981).

40. Isenberg, G.: Pflugers Arch. Ges. Physiol. 371, 51-59 (1977).

41. Bunney, B.S., Aghajanian, G.K., Roth, R.H.: Nature 245, 123-125 (1973).

42. Cuello, A.C., Iversen, L.L.: In 'Interaction Between Putative Neurotransmitters in the Brain' (Eds. Garattini, S., Pujol, J.F., Samanin, R.) Raven Press, New York, pp. 127-149 (1978).

43. Wassef, M., Berod, A., Sotelo, C.: Neuroscience 6, 2125-2139 (1981).

44. Grofova, I., Rinvik, E.: Exp. Brain Res. 11, 249-262 (1970).

45. Hefti, F., Lichtensteiger, W.: J. Neurochem. 30, 1217-1230 (1978).

46. Ungerstedt, U.: Acta Physiol. Scand.: 367, 69-93 (1971).

47. Pycock, C.J.: Neuroscience 5, 461-514 (1980).

48. Weston, J., Greenfield, S.A.: Neuroscience 7 (Suppl.) S5227 (1982).

49. Kreutzberg, G.N., Kaija, H.: Histochimie 42, 233-237 (1974).

50. Fossier, P., Baux, G., Tauc, L.: Nature 301, 710-712 (1983).

Acknowledgements:

I would like to thank Dr. Z. Henderson for preparing the section shown in Fig. 1 and Professor D. Fisher and Dr. M. Fillenz for their helpful advice and comments. Part of the work described was funded by a Medical Research Council Grant (G.810/79/93N).

IV. BIOLOGICAL FUNCTIONS OF ACETYLCHOLINESTERASE AND BUTYRYLCHOLINESTERASE, AND CHANGES IN DISEASE STATES

INTRODUCTION TO SESSION IV

Miro Brzin

Institute of Pathophysiology, Faculty of Medicine, University E. Kardelj, Zaloška 4, 61105 Ljubljana, Yugoslavia

The subject about mechanisms regulating the activity and other properties of ChEs, which was dealt with in a general way in previous chapters is elaborated here in more detail. Origin and nature of humoral factors are described including mutual regulatory interactions of presynaptic neurons and postsynaptic cells. The possible link between the mechanisms regulating tissue ChEs and the changes of activity, molecular forms pattern and secretion rates of ChEs in various neural or muscular pathological states is critically discussed. The scope of the last contribution to this session extends beyond the limits of the classical cholinergic system in the search for new functions for AChE in CNS, which would clarify its puzzling distrib tion often uncorrelated with cholinergic structures.

The first article (by Koelle et al.) presents the evidence that the extracts prepared from brain, spinal cord and sciatic nerve of cat contain a trophic factor which can maintain AChE and BuChE levels in perfused denervated SCG _in vivo_. The substance(s) present in extracts differ from NGF and its suggested site of action may be connected with the conversion of G_1 molecular form of AChE into G_4 in the postsynaptic ganglionic cells.

The next article (by Festoff et al.) discusses trophic factors in extracts of different tissues and their influence on the development of cultured chicken muscle and on the pattern of molecular forms of AChE during myoblast differentiation and following steps of myogenesis. The isolated neurotrophic factor (NTF) seems to be transferrin and its presence in the motor nerve might result from its synthesis in motor neurons or its uptake from serum by the nerve endings. NTF regulates the activity of AChE, the pattern of molecular forms and the secretion of the enzyme from the muscle cells.

In humans, the level of AChE activity in different body fluids is changed in different pathological conditions. Particularly, the correlation between the level of AChE activity or changes in its molecular forms in CSF or serum and various pathological changes in nerve tissue and muscle opens a possibility to obtain new diagnostic tools in these diseases.

A comprehensive overview of ChEs in tissues in regard to genetic variations and the reflection of neural and muscular diseases on properties of human ChEs is presented in the article on human ChEs (by Toschi et al.). With the increasing availability of new powerful tools of immunology and immunochemistry, new possibilities for detailed studies of the metabolism and molecular properties of human ChEs are emerging and that, in the future, may bring more insight into etiology of some human neurological and muscular disorders.

There is rather strong evidence that ACh in CNS can act not only at the central cholinergic synapses but also on other structures in a modulatory, essentially nonsynaptic fashion. Therefore the apparently puzzling lack of correlation between AChE activity and the concentration of CAT and ACh in various regions of the brain might just reflect diversity in the spatial organization, distribution and density of cholinoceptive structures with distinctly different physiological functions. Different spatial organization of cholinergic components in domains where either cholinergic synaptic transmission or various modulatory functions predominate may explain the uncorrelated distribution of cholinergic components in different regions of CNS but this requires further investigation. However, whatever the outcome it would not per se exclude a possible function of AChE beyond the scope of the cholinergic system.

Thus the evidence and suggestions presented in the last article of the session (by I. Chubb), that AChE may have other catalytic properties, besides the esteratic one, is relevant and may be opening new directions in neurochemical research.

DEMONSTRATION OF A NEUROTROPHIC FACTOR FOR THE MAINTENANCE OF ACETYLCHOLINESTERASE AND BUTYRYLCHOLINESTERASE IN THE PREGANGLIONICALLY DENERVATED SUPERIOR CERVICAL GANGLION OF THE CAT

George B. Koelle, Gerard A. Ruch, Eiji Uchida

Department of Pharmacology, Medical School/G3,
University of Pennsylvania, Philadelphia, PA 19104, USA

Introduction

Sawyer and Hollinshead (1) showed in 1945 that preganglionic denervation of the cat superior cervical ganglion (SCG) results within 3 days in a loss of >80% of its AChE and >30% of its BuChE contents, and that no further changes occur over the course of several weeks. These results were confirmed quantitatively (2) and by light microscopic histochemistry with the copper thiocholine (CuThCh) method (3,4). In the latter studies it was found that AChE disappears completely from the neuropil in the denervated SCG, whereas the BuChE activity of the neuropil shows a moderate fall. For these and other reasons it was concluded that in the normal SCG, AChE is confined to the preganglionic fibers and their terminals, and BuChE is present exclusively in the capsular glial cells. The subsequent development of a reliable electron microscopic histochemical method for the localization of AChE and BuChE (5) forced us to revise these views. Direct visualization at the subcellular level showed that in the normal cat SCG, AChE is located at the plasma membranes of both the presynaptic terminals and the dendrites and perikarya of the ganglion cells; BuChE is present chiefly at the latter, postsynaptic sites (6). Following denervation, AChE disappears from pre- and postsynaptic sites, and BuChE shows a moderate fall (7), in confirmation of results obtained by light microscopy. This raised the question of why the integrity of the preganglionic fibers is necessary for the maintenance of postsynaptic AChE, and a portion of the postsynaptic BuChE. The most likely explanation appeared to be that the preganglionic fibers provide a neurotrophic factor for the maintenance of the postsynaptically located enzymes. This hypothesis was tested in the present study (8).

Methods

Cats were anesthetized with sodium pentobarbital, 35 mg/kg, i.p. A 1-cm segment was excised from each cervical sympathetic trunk, and the operative wound was sutured. The following day they were reanesthetized and atropinized; the saphenous vein was catheterized for the infusion of a standard glucose-NaCl solution; the trachea was intubated for artificial respiration by a Palmer pump; the external carotid (EC) and lingual (L) arteries were exposed and ligated bilaterally following the i.v. injection of heparin, 50 units/kg. The right common carotid artery was exposed, and a 27 hypodermic needle was inserted. The needle was attached via tygon tubing to a reservoir containing an extract of cat brain, spinal cord, and sciatic nerves in an ice-water bath. The extract was delivered by a Harvard Peristaltic Pump at approximately 0.1 ml/min for 24 hr, with a mercury manometer interposed to monitor approximate arterial and infusion pressures. Additional pentobarbital, atropine, and mephentermine were given as required. At exactly 48 hr post-denervation the SCG were excised, frozen, and homogenized. Acetylcholinesterase and BuChE were assayed by a modification of the method of Ellman et al. (9); protein was determined according to Lowry et al. (10).

The extract was prepared by homogenizing the brain, spinal cord, and sciatic nerves (approximately 35g) of a cat with approximately 7 volumes of water in a Waring Blender in the cold room. Following the addition of NaCl solution to bring the final concentration to 0.9%, the preparation was rehomogenized. It was then adjusted to pH 4.5, homogenized again, and centrifuged at 1,000 g for 30 min. The supernatent was recovered, adjusted to pH 7.0, and centrifugation was repeated. The supernatent, approximately 150 ml, was stored in the refrigerator overnight prior to infusion. In the initial series of experiments, aprotinin (Trasylol) was included to prevent autolysis of proteins. However, this was found to be unnecessary; results reported here are all on extracts prepared without aprotinin.

Results and Discussion

The most important results are summarized in Table 1.

Table 1. Effects of intraarterial infusion of an extract of cat brain, spinal cord, and sciatic nerves on the AChE and BuChE contents of preganglionically denervated cat SCG

Procedure	nmol substrate hydrolyzed/mg protein/min	
	AChE	BuChE
1. Normal cat SCG (8)	449 ± 42	590 ± 61
2. Preganglionically denervated SCG; EC and L arteries ligated at 24 hr; ganglia excised at 48 hr post-denervation (8)	167 ± 10	412 ± 29
3. Preganglionically denervated SCG; EC and L arteries ligated, and extract infused 24-48 hr post-denervation (6)	354 ± 35*	602 ± 65+

Numbers of SCG in parentheses

* More than preganglionically denervated, arterially ligated controls, $P < 0.001$.

\+ More than preganglionically denervated, arterially ligated controls, $P < 0.05$

Infusion of the extract to a great extent prevented the fall in AChE and BuChE contents of the SCG that otherwise occurs 48 hours following preganglionic denervation. There was no significant difference between the AChE or BuChE contents of the right and left SCG in the infused cats, indicating that extensive anastomoses exist between the paired internal carotid arteries. It is unlikely that AChE or BuChE was taken up by the SCG from the infused extract. In an earlier study conducted in this laboratory, the common carotid artery of similarly arterially ligated cats was perfused with normal cat plasma (which contains over ten times the AChE and BuChE contents of the extract) for periods up to ten hours, following inactivation of BuChE by iso-OMPA. There was no evidence of ganglionic uptake of AChE or BuChE (unpublished observations).

These results suggest that the preganglionic fibers release a neurotrophic factor, also present in the central nervous system, that normally maintains the postsynaptic AChE and BuChE contents of the cat SCG. Whether the extract acts by preventing degeneration of the presynaptic terminals (11), or by maintaining the postsynaptic enzymes in spite of such is now under investigation by electron microscopic histochemistry.

The other major question is of course the identity of the neurotrophic factor in the extract. Preliminary findings suggest that it is a protein. We are now attempting to isolate and characterize the active material.

Two authentic compounds have been tested by the same procedure. Two cats were infused for 24 hours with acetylcholine bromide (total, 2.8 and 15.8 mMol, respectively). The mean enzyme-contents of their SCG, removed 48 hours post denervation, were AChE, 185 ± 11, and BuChE, 267 ± 9 nMol substrate hydrolyzed/mg protein/min. These values do not differ appreciably from the controls (Table 1).

Nerve growth factor (NGF) was infused for 24 hours in three cats (0.1 mg 7S-NGF in one, 0.5 mg 2.5S-NGF in each of two). Mean values for AChE and BuChE, respectively, were 257 ± 21 and 291 ± 12. While the value for AChE is above that of the controls, it is considerably below that for cats infused with extract (Table 1). In view of the limited concentrations of NGF found in mammalian brain (12-14), it is unlikely that NGF could have played more than a minor contributory role in the effects of the extract.

In subsequent experiments it has been found that continual anesthesia with sodium pentobarbital during the time from denervation to excision of the ganglia at 48 hours also retards significantly the fall in ganglionic AChE and BuChE, although to a considerably less extent than infusion of extract. This effect is to a great extent prevented by ligation of the EC and L arteries at 24 hours post-denervation (15). No explanation for these findings can be offered.

If the neurotrophic factor is found to act at postsynaptic sites, the following working hypothesis is proposed for its mechanism. Massoulie and Bon (16) and others have shown that AChE exists as at least six molecular aggregates: the globular forms, G_1, G_2, and G_4, consisting of monomers, dimers, and tetramers of the basic enzymatic unit, and the asymmetric or collagen-tailed forms, A_4, A_8, and A_{12}. In the SCG of the rat and steer, all six forms are present, but G_1, G_4, and A_{12} are the predominant types (17,18,19). G_1 is believed to occur in the cytoplasm, G_4 at the plasma membranes, and A_{12} at synaptic sites. Following preganglionic denervation, we have shown that AChE disappears from the neuropil but remains unchanged in the perikarya of the ganglion cells. Thus, the putative neurotrophic factor may regulate the conversion of G_1 to G_4, and subsequently to A_{12}. This proposal is now under investigation.

Acknowledgement

This study was supported by research grant NS 00282-30,31 from the National Institute of Neurological and Communicative Disorders and Stroke, National Institutes of Health, U.S.A. We thank Dr. Ruth Hogue Angeletti for a generous gift of 2.5S-NGF.

References

1. Sawyer, C.H., Hollinshead, W.H.: J. Neurophysiol. 8, 137-153 (1945).
2. Koelle, G.B., Davis, R., Koelle, W.A.: J. Histochem. Cytochem. 22, 244-251 (1974).
3. Koelle, G.B.: J. Pharmacol. Exp. Ther. 103, 153-171 (1951).
4. Koelle, W.A., Koelle, G.B.: J. Pharmacol. Exp. Ther. 126, 1-8 (1959).
5. Koelle, G.B., Davis, R., Smyrl, E.G., Fine, A.V.: J. Histochem. Cytochem. 22, 252-259 (1974).
6. Davis, R., Koelle, G.B.: J. Cell Biol. 78, 785-809 (1978).
7. Davis, R., Koelle, G.B.: J. Cell Biol. 88, 581-590 (1981).
8. Koelle, G.B., Ruch, G.A.: Proc. Natl. Acad. Sci. USA 80, 3106-3110 (1983).
9. Ellman, G.L., Courtney, K.D., Andres, V., Jr., Featherstone, R.M.: Biochem. Pharmacol. 7, 88-95 (1961).
10. Lowry, O.H., Rosebrough, N.J., Farr, A.L., Randall, R.J.: J. Biol. Chem. 193, 265-275 (1951).
11. Lubinska, L.: Brain Res. 223, 227-240 (1982).
12. Shine, H.D., Perez-Polo, J.R.: J. Neurochem. 27, 1315-1318 (1976).
13. Barde, Y.A., Edgar, D., Thoenen, H.: Proc. Natl. Acad. Sci. USA 77, 1199-1203 (1980).
14. Schwartz, M.J., Ghetti, B., Truex, L., Schmidt, M.J.: J. Neurosci. Res. 8, 205-211 (1982).
15. Koelle, G.B., Ruch, G.A., Uchida, E.: Proc. Natl. Acad. Sci. USA 80, 6122-6125 (1983).
16. Massoulie, J., Bon, S.: Ann. Rev. Neurosci. 5, 57-106 (1982).

17. Gisiger, V., Vigny, M., Gautron, J., Rieger, F.: J. Neurochem. 30, 501-516 (1978).

18. Verdiere, M., Derer, M., Rieger, F.: Developmental Biol. 89, 509-515 (1982).

19. Bon, S., Vigny, M., Massoulie, J.: Proc. Natl. Acad. Sci. USA 76, 2546-2550 (1979).

Key-words for Index

Acetylcholinesterase

Butyrylcholinesterase

Nerve growth factor

Neurotrophic factor

Superior cervical ganglion

Trophic factor

NEUROCRINE REGULATION OF ACETYLCHOLINESTERASE IN HEALTH AND DISEASE

BARRY W. FESTOFF, HEINZ POPIELA, ROBERT L. BEACH

Neurobiology Research Laboratory, Veterans Administration Medical Center, Kansas City, Missouri and Department of Neurology, University of Kansas Medical Center, Kansas City, Kansas, USA

Introduction

In skeletal muscle, AChE (EC 3.1.1.7) is the enzyme that hydrolyzes AChE at the neuromuscular junction to terminate its action there. The regulation of AChE activity and its localization at the synaptic area has been the subject of intense research efforts over the past several years (1-5) and a controversy as to the relative influence of activity or soluble, humoral-like "factors" contained within and released by nerves for action on or in the muscle continues. Increasing evidence has accumulated demonstrating that regulation of this enzyme occurs by both activity-dependent and independent processes. More recently, evaluation of the activity of AChE in plasma of patients with neuromuscular disease as well as the levels of this cholinergic enzyme in other fluids such as CSF suggests its utility in diagnosis and prognosis.

This paper reviews data pertaining to the neurotrophic regulation of asymmetric 16S AChE at rat neuromuscular junctions, the discovery of a nerve-derived factor essential for myoblast cell division and subsequent myogenesis, relationship of this factor--found to be homologous or identical to transferrin and called NTF--to the appearance of asymmetric 19.5S AChE in cultured chick muscle and release of AChE from muscle and nerve into the circulation in patients with various neuromuscular disorders.

Results

Rodent end-plate AChE molecular forms and neurotrophic regulation

As reported by a number of workers in other muscles (4-7) we found 2 major forms of AChE in extra-junctional regions of rat gracilis muscle corresponding to 10S and 4S AChE (8,9). More recent work has shown that as with Torpedo electric organ (10) non-end-plate regions of vertebrate skeletal muscle contain other globular and asymmetric forms (11). However, the absence of the "heaviest" form of AChE, 16S in the rat, in non-end-plate regions and its concentration in the junctional area has withstood subsequent experimentation. Figure 1 shows the major forms of AChE found in extra-junctional regions (Fig.1a) and in end-plate areas of rat gracilis (Fig.1b).

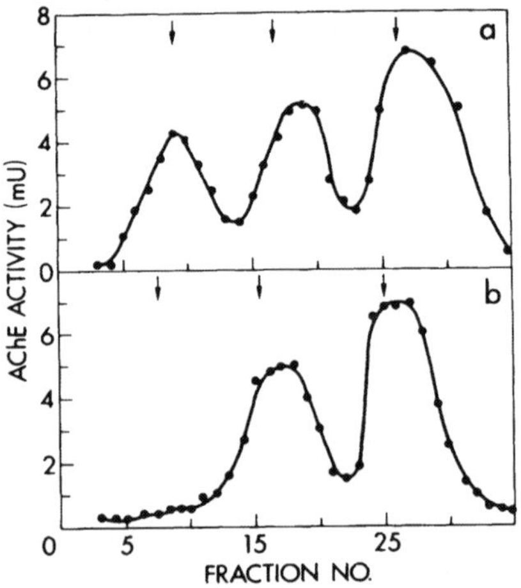

Fig. 1 Sucrose gradient profiles of AChE molecular forms in non-end plate (a) and end-plate regions (b) of rat anterior gracilis (9).

To determine the possible neurotrophic regulation of 16S enzyme we employed the long-short nerve-stump paradigm: simply stated, impulse transmission and, hence, nerve-evoked muscle activity ceases immediately whether the nerve is severed close to the muscle or close to the spinal cord (12). However, if differences are detected in a particular muscle function which are time-dependent in experiments of this type then the length of nerve, and, the material contained within the axons, are considered to underly such differences. Using such a model we axotomized rat obturator nerves either close to or far from their innervation site at the gracilis muscle, excised the end-plate regions under direct visualization, separated the AChE forms by velocity sedimentation on sucrose gradients and estimated the enzyme activity (9). Figure 2 shows that a striking rapid decrease in the amount of A_{12} (16S) AChE was found in the short-stump preparations while a 4-5 day delay in the $t1/2$ for decrease of A_{12} was found with long-stump muscles. We interpreted these results as indicating the presence of an activity-independent factor that was contained within the axoplasm of the obturator nerves (9).

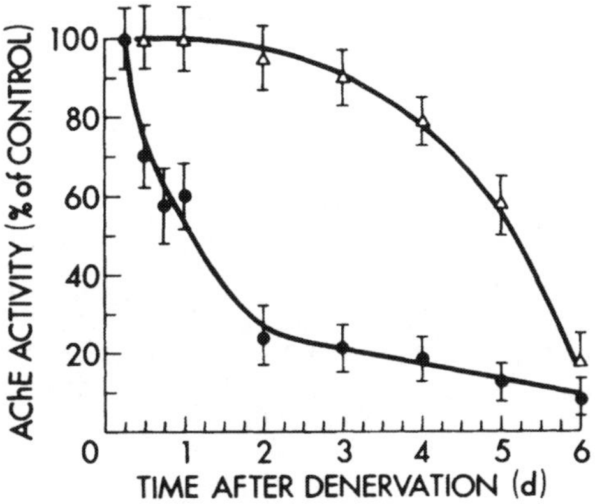

Fig. 2 Effect of axotomy on 16S AChE content in gracilis end-plates (O-O, long-stump; ●-●, short stump; 9).

One possible explanation for these results was that short-stump section more rapidly eliminated the source of 16S AChE, namely, the obturator axoplasm. It had previously been shown that a small fraction of AChE is transported within nerves in the fast compartment (13-15). We found that almost all of the AChE transported in sciatic nerves migrated at 400 mm/day, consistent with and confirming previous studies (13-15) and, furthermore, this was all 16S AChE (16). We estimated that the amount of 16S AChE in the axoplasmic compartment together with the rapid rate was only 1/10th to 1/100th the amount present in the end-plate regions of the gracilis muscle (9). Therefore, we concluded that although 16S AChE is present within motor nerves (8,16) and transported at a rapid rate (16) some other factor was largely responsible for regulating its location at the end-plate surface of skeletal muscle in the adult animal. Further information relating to such "maintenance" neurotrophic effects came from using an organ culture model of the rat gracilis. It was found that an extract of either sciatic or obturator nerves prepared essentially as described previously (17) could prevent the drop in end-plate 16S AChE that occurred during the 48 hrs in organ culture (18) and that if denervation was performed prior to removal of the nerve-muscle preparation into the culture containing the extract the AChE activity approximated the control preparations (18).

AChE molecular forms in nerve-extract-treated chick muscle culture

Trophic factors may operate during maintenance of the adult, innervated condition, during regeneration of the adult situation or during development (19). It is likely that a single factor is not responsible for such various and diverse neurotrophic influences at such widely disparate ages of the organism although no a priori reason exists for this statement. We were interested in determining whether adult axoplasmic material exerted trophic influence on embryonic chick muscle cells undergoing differentiation in vitro. We had previously found that an extract of rat sciatic nerve increased myotube formation, numbers of acetylcholine receptors (AChRs) and their maintenance, and levels of AChE in chick muscle culture (20). The extract had been used to immunize sheep and an antisera was obtained (17) that could inhibit the trophic effects of the extract (termed SNP) in culture. We had found that the sheep suffered a transmission-block type paralysis in response to booster doses of the axoplasmic antigens (17) among which was the enzyme CAT. This syndrome was reproduced by others in guinea pigs using a purified preparation of CAT from caudate nucleus (21). The major protein band on sodium dodecyl sulfate-polyacrylamide gel electrophoresis (SDS-PAGE) migrated at Mr 65,000 ± 5,000 daltons (65K). One of the minor bands had a Mr of 80,000 ± 2,000 daltons (80K). The 65K protein was further resolved into a doublet, the more intensely staining higher molecular weight band (about 68K) was subsequently identified as rat serum albumin (RSA; Festoff, et al., in preparation; 22).

Since we had shown a cross-species increase in AChE content in SNP-treated chick muscle culture (20) we studied the effects of an adult chicken extract obtained from ischiatic-peroneal nerves. This extract, NE, was shown to replace embryo extract (EE) as essential for chick myogenesis in vitro (23, 24) and was the source of relatively purified "neurotrophic factor" (NTF; 23). In the absence of EE or NE (or in some experiments, NTF) no myotubes and, little AChE could be detected. However, in the absence of EE but in the presence of 0.3mg/ml NE 3 forms of AChE could be resolved from sucrose gradient centrifugation of muscle culture extracts by day 8 in culture (Figure 3).

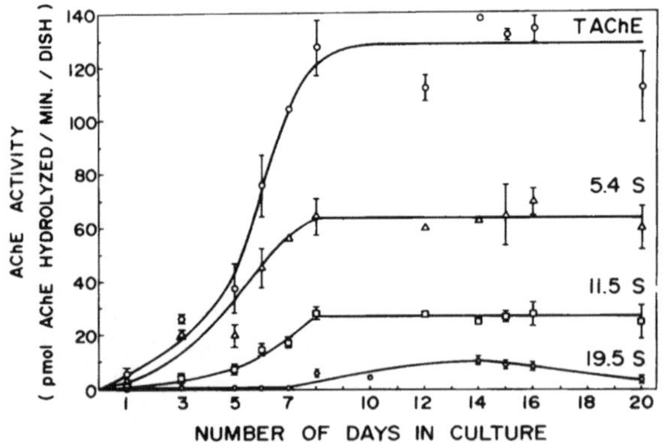

Fig. 3 Appearance of AChE molecular forms with time in culture. Sums of activities of molecular forms as well as total activity (T AChE) are shown with time in culture.

From day 1, the earliest sampling time, until day 7 only 2 forms, co-sedimenting at 5.4S and 11.5S respectively, could be identified. In fact, in cultures not exposed to either EE or NE but assayed at day 3 in culture small amounts of these 2 molecular forms of AChE could be detected (data not shown). By day 8 in culture, asymmetric, 19.5S AChE could be readily detected using our assay system (25,26). Representative gradient profiles are shown in Figure 4. In non-supplemented cultures assayed at early times (i.e., day 3) patterns similiar to the 2nd panel in this figure were found. Note that as with total AChE in the cultures the globular (G_2 and G_4) forms, 5.4S and 11.5S, increase until day 8 or 9 and then appear to plateau (Fig.3) while A_{12}, 19.5S AChE, slowly increases until day 14 and then declines. At day 3, 5.4S represents 80% of the total AChE in the culture but after plateau accounts for 50% of the enzyme activity. The 11.5S AChE is about 20% of the total activity from day 8 to day 20. A_{12} AChE, not detected before day 6, reaches a peak of 10% of total at day 14 and then drops to about 1% by day 20. This is shown more dramatically in Figure 5 where the calculated amount of 19.5S AChE (area under the curve generated by a computer program) is shown as a function of culture time. Thus, the A_{12} form, considered to be that form of AChE most under neural regulation (5) is the only form in our cultures that appears to depend on the presence of some factor(s) present in nerve axoplasm for appearance and regulation. Of interest is the temporal course of 19.5S in these studies: delayed appearance and then a 10-fold reduction in amount despite the fact that the cultures at day 20 were highly differentiated and healthy-appearing. The maintenance of 19.5S in culture by NE was not accomplished in contradistinction to the organ culture studies with rat muscle (18) mentioned above.

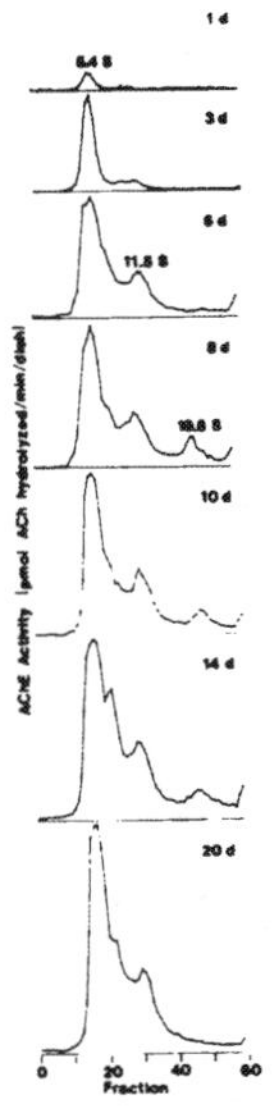

Fig. 4 Appearance of AChE molecular forms during chick muscle culture development in culture. Muscle cells were cultured in the presence of 300 ug/ml of nerve extract for the indicated times and then activities of AChE molecular forms were determined.

Neurocrine secretion in the neuromuscular system

Extensive studies of ortho- and retrograde interactions between motor neurons and target skeletal muscle fibers have been reported (19,23-33). Diagrammatic representation is shown in Fig. 6. Trophic, or activity-independent influences are more difficult to study in the intact neuromuscular system due to the pervasive presence of activity. With the exception of the long/short axotomy model, cold block and colchicine block of axonal transport have been used in vivo. Tissue culture has also been used to explore neurotrophic influences of nerve extracts or, more recently, extracts of basal lamina (37) on properties of cultured skeletal muscle cells. Thus, in the neuromuscular system one can identify 4 major categories of putative trophic factors based on their source and site of action:

1. Neuron-elaborated, muscle-supporting agents. Presumably these agents are synthesized in the motor neuronal cell soma, transported orthograde (and, perhaps retrograde as well, in order to provide some sort of feed-back signal to cell soma synthetic apparatus), and released from the nerve terminals in spontaneous and/or nerve-evoked fashion to then interact with specific cell surface or intracellular receptors in the skeletal muscle cell. We would consider these agents neurocrine factors. In addition to factors synthesized in neurons for release it is also possible that neurons at their pre-synaptic terminals at the NMJ have specific high affinity uptake mechanisms for concentrating certain substances from the blood. In this regard, the presence of albumin (Festoff, et al., in preparation; (22) and a protein homologous with or identical to transferrin has been found in peripheral nerves and motor neurons (29-33).

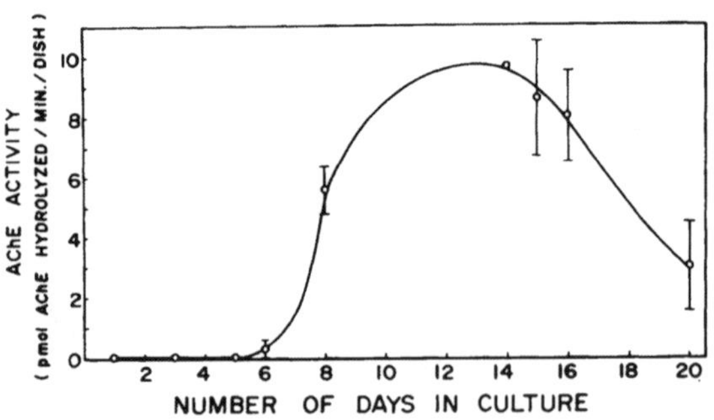

Fig. 5 The appearance of A_{12} AChE with time in culture. The 19.5 S AChE activity is not detected prior to 6 days in cultured, but then increases and maximizes between 12-14 days. Following this maximum 19.5 S AChE declines.

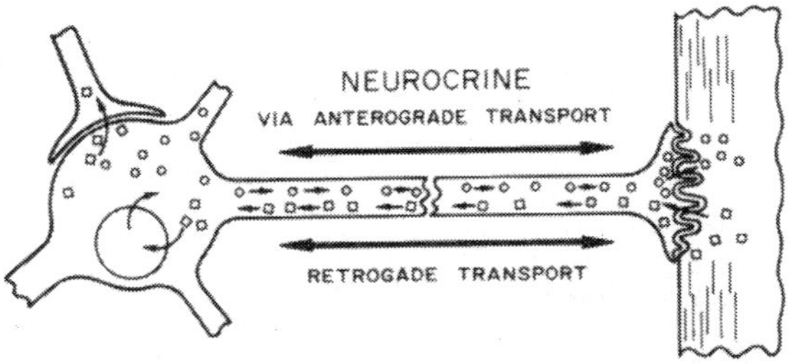

Fig. 6 Model of neurocrine (and retroneurocrine) secretion in neuromuscular systems (19).

Our interest in such factors, including SNP and NTF, intensified with the studies on AChE as described above. We were interested in the identity of the factor in NE that myoblasts depended on for successful completion of myogenesis in culture. With the finding of an identical factor in chicken serum (29) and the finding that sciatin, a protein very similiar to NTF, had amino acid composition similiar to transferrin (30, 31) we compared one-dimensional peptide maps according to the methods of Cleveland et al (34) with biologic potency of NTF and several transferrin preparations. We were encouraged in these studies not only by the works of others but by our own showing that various extracts having muscle-supporting activity all had a protein band migating at about 80K (Figure 7). Peptide maps of the avian proteins could not distinguish NTF from either ovotransferrin (OTF), chicken serum transferrin (TF) or embryo extract TF (EETF). When a measure of biologic potency, that had been used to follow the purification of NTF (23), was used to compare the various avian proteins, no difference in activity was found (32). This is shown in Table 1. Since our culture media routinely contained human transferrin and species specificity of TF requirement had recently been shown for chick reticulocytes (35) we compared a number of mammalian TFs with the avian proteins on chick muscle ^{3}H-thymidine incorporation and found that the mammalian TFs had very little effect on stimulating incorporation (Table 1). We next compared peptide maps of the avian and mammalian proteins as shown in Figure 8. Although the avian TFs appear identical, major differences that probably account for the markedly reduced biologic effect, were detected for the mammalian proteins. This was found despite the fact that a great many properties of the TFs are shared by mammalian as well as the avian proteins: about 80K subunit molecular weight, salmon-colored in concentrated solution, acidic glycoproteins, bind iron at 2 different binding sites, etc.

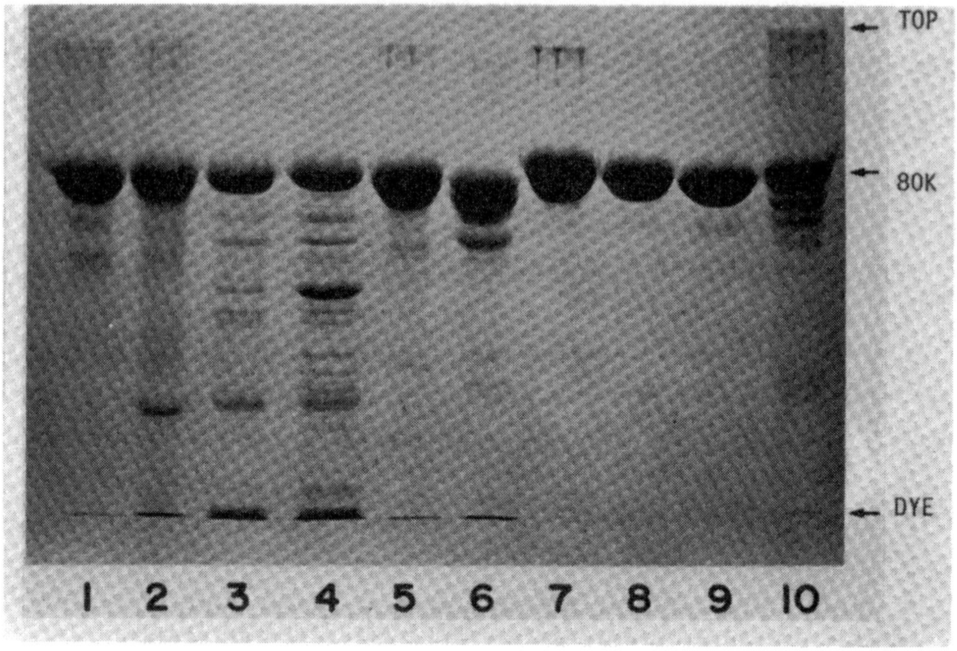

Fig. 7 SDS-PAGE of muscle-supporting proteins: Lanes 1,OTF; 2, TF(chicken); 3, EETF; 4, NTF; 5, TF(human); 6, TF(bovine); 7, TF(rabbit); 8, TF(rat); a, TF(mouse); 10, TF(horse) all 50 mg load.

TABLE 1*

Protein Added	% Control
None	100
Ovotransferrin	438
Neurotrophic Factor (Chicken)	428
Embryo Extract Transferrin	401
Chicken Transferrin	414
Rabbit Transferrin	86.7
Rat Transferrin	106
Mouse Transferrin	105
Human Transferrin	109
Bovine Transferrin	81.5
Horse Transferrin	102

*^{3}H-thymidine incorporation into chick myoblasts under influence of various proteins added (33).

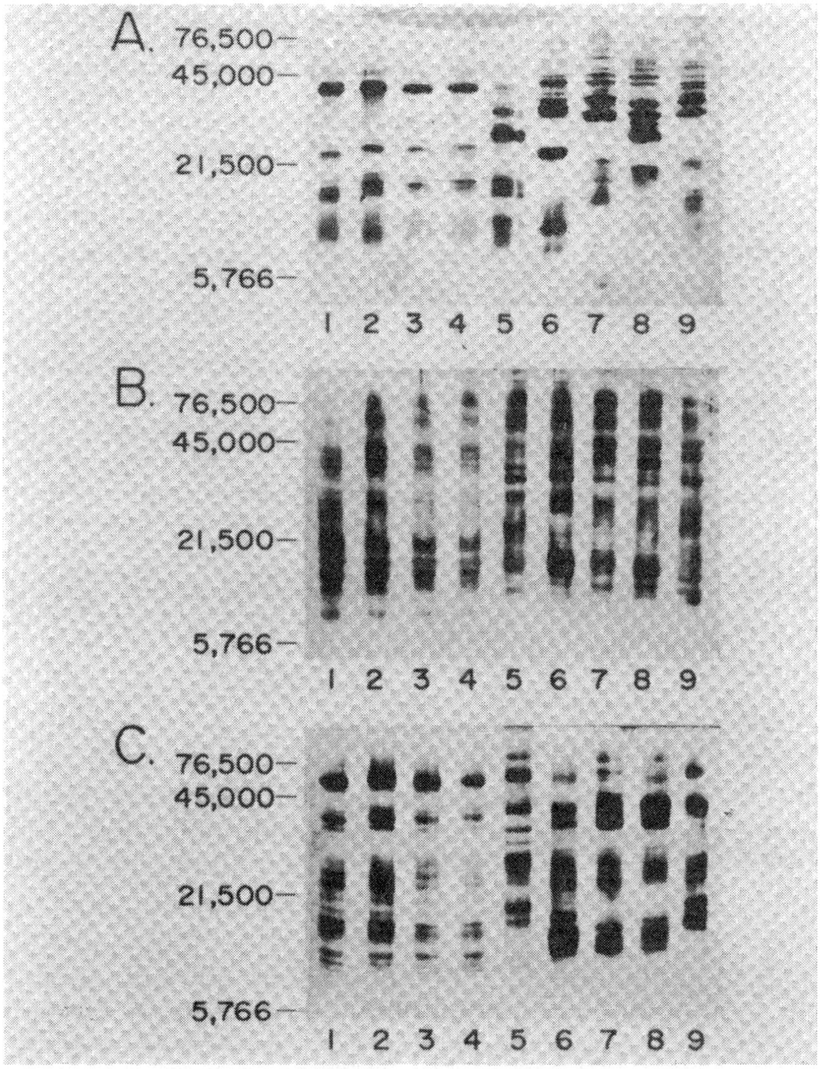

Fig. 8 Peptide maps of purified transferrins on 15% SDS-PAGE.
A. CNBr fragments: Lanes 1, OTF; 2, TF(chicken); 3, EETF; 4, NTF; 5, TF(human); 6, TF(rabbit); 7, TF(rat); 8, TF(mouse); 9, TF(horse).
B. Chymotrypsin fragments (lanes as in A).
C. Staph Aureus V8 protease (lanes as in A).

We were particularly interested in the mechanism of the trophic or supporting effects of TF on myoblasts. We analyzed whether TF (or NTF) was a true mitogen in 2 ways: by counting mitoses in myo-blasts exposed to NTF and by counting fluorescent-labeled nuclei of myoblasts at different times of exposure to NTF. The latter was a cell-cycle kinetics study for which we utilized a fluorescent-activated cell sorter. The results of these experiments have recently been published (36). NTF, in a dose-dependent fashion from 2-30 ug/ml, increases the number of mitoses seen by up to 10-fold (Table 2). Analysis of the effects of NTF on the cell cycle indicated that NTF could shift myoblasts in G_1, the predominant cell-cycle phase of satellite cells contained in embryonic chick muscle, to G_2 + M and S phases if exposure of cultured myoblasts to NTF occurred within 18-22 hrs upon removal of dissociated cells from embryonic muscle (36). These studies reinforce the interpretation that NTF (TF) is a true mitogen for embryonic myoblasts. Whether or not this holds true for satellite cells cultured from postnatal muscle is not yet known.

TABLE 2

MITOTIC INDEX OF MYOBLASTS EXPOSED TO NTF[1]

[NTF] ug/ml	x	s	S.E.
0	33.65	20.85	5.21
2	112.18	57.53	23.49
6	292.12	112.32	79.42
10	345.51	25.59	14.77
16	388.59	97.90	56.52
20	292.56	45.08	26.03
30	301.54	39.66	22.90

[1]From Popiela et al (36), modified.

2. Muscle-elaborated, neuron-supporting agents. These are expected to be synthesized by muscle cells (or possibly other cells in muscle tissue), released, selectively taken up at nerve terminals and transported up the axon to the neuron cell body where they exert supportive roles. Thus, these would be considered retroneurocrine agents.

3. Non-specific diffusible tissue growth factors. These are agents which act rather unselectively on a wide variety of cell types to support growth, survival and/or function. The sources of these factors are a variety of tissues and cells. Hormonal and humoral factors are in this class of trophic agents.

4. Non-diffusible, extracellular matrix associated factors having supportive roles on both neuron and/or muscle cells. These factors could act to secure the connection of nerve to muscle, thus allowing the transfer of information between the two cells. They may also act to direct a variety of cellular events including division and expression of differentiated functions, via transmembrane signalling. Such modulation, probably mediated via surface receptors and cytoskele-

tal elements appear to play important roles in a variety of cells. The importance of these relatively insoluble factors at the neuromuscular junction is suggested by the requirement for collagen in myogenesis, the dramatic specialization of the extracellular matrix of the junction and the role of the basal lamina in directing regeneration of nerve and muscle specializations (19).

AChE in body fluids

AChE has been detected in normal extracellular body fluids such as blood, cerebrospinal fluid (CSF) and in amniotic fluid. Reason for its presence, or for that matter, the presence of AChE in serum, remains unknown. What is known is that AChE is a secretory protein, as are most glycoproteins, and that secretion can occur in both health and disease. Recently, it has been suggested that one role of secreted AChE (sAChE, according to Hodgson, et al, 38) is its ability to hydrolyze neuropeptides, such as substance P (39).

AChE has been found to be increased in plasma of chick embryos and dystrophic chickens, but not in normal chickens (40). Similarly, we found that plasma of patients with amyotrophic lateral sclerosis (ALS) contained about twice the AChE activity as control plasma (41). This study was extended to include patients with other neuromuscular diseases (NMD) such as myasthenia gravis (MG), Charcot-Marie-Tooth disease (C-M-T), myotonic dystrophy (MyD) and Duchenne muscular dystrophy (DMD). Although age and sex-matching was not ideal we used as a denominator the creatine kinase (CK) activity present in the blood at the same time. The results indicated that some elevation of AChE (30-50%) occurs in several NMD when compared with normal controls. However, relative specificity of AChE/CK elevation occurs in ALS plasma (and, to a lesser extent, MG plasma) when compared to plasma of patients with C-M-T, MyD and DMD. Since MG is known to be a NMJ disorder, and ALS has been shown to have significant alterations in NMJ structure and function, release of AChE, preferentially over CK, in these 2 conditions suggests NMJ instability underlies the increase in plasma AChE (42). Confirmation of our original results (41) has recently been obtained (43) and underscores the specificity of increased plasma AChE in ALS.

AChE in brains and CSF of patients with senile dementia of the Alzheimer's type (SDAT) has been reported to be lower than normal (44). In contrast, plasma AChE in SDAT has been reported to be elevated (45) although not dramatically as in ALS patients. No reports of CSF AChE in ALS patients have appeared, as yet. It is of interest that an hypothesis, unifying underlying mechanisms of 3 prominent "degenerative" neurologic disorders, ALS, SDAT and Parkinson's disease, favors lack of putative "trophic" factors in their development (46).

Several reports have indicated the utility of measuring AChE in amniotic fluid in at-risk pregnant women for open neural tube defects

(NTD; 47-49). AChE is suggested to be a better marker for NTD than α-fetoprotein, the conventional amniotic fluid indicator, because AChE is derived from the fetal nervous system whereas α-fetoprotein is synthesized by fetal liver and yolk sac. If AChE passed from amniotic fluid to serum then it might also be used to screen serum of pregnant women for NTD.

Discussion and Summary

Mounting evidence suggests that trophic regulation exists within the neuromuscular system. It is likely that neurocrine, and retro-neurocrine, secretion is the mechanism involved in at least some interactions between nerve and muscle. Although a number of studies concerning AChE regulation in this system suggests a major role for activity, for both adult maintenance and developmental situations neurocrine trophic regulation also plays a role. A major candidate for a neurocrine factor for muscle is NTF or transferrin. It remains to be shown whether transferrin is synthesized by motor neurons, in addition to liver and salivary glands, or is actively taken up at pre-synaptic terminals for post-translational modification within motor neurons. Whether transferrin is involved in the stability of A_{12} AChE at the NMJ, and whether decreased amounts or altered activity of TF in ALS accounts for increased plasma AChE also awaits further studies. What role such mechanisms have for such diverse neurologic conditions as SDAT and open NTD, where alterations in AChE occur, remains speculative at present.

Acknowledgements

Support for some of the studies reported herein were provided by the Muscular Dystrophy Association, the ALS Society of America, the ALS Regional Research Center (KUMC/KCVAMC), the Medical Research Service of the Veterans Administration and NIH (R01NS17197-02). Mrs. Loretta Hurt expertly prepared the manuscript.

References

1. Hall, Z.W.: J. Neurobiol. 18, 333-350 (1973).
2. Vigny, M., Koenig, J., Rieger, F.: J. Neurochem. 27, 1347-1353 (1976).
3. Weinberg, C.G., Hall, Z.W.: Dev. Biol. 68, 631-635 (1979).
4. McMahan, U.J., Sanes, J.R., Marshall, L.M.: Nature 271, 172-174 (1978).
5. Massolie, J., Bon, S.: Ann. Rev. Neurosci. 5, 57-106 (1982).
6. Vigny, M., DiGianberadino, L., Courand, J.-Y., Rieger, F., Koenig, J.: FEBS Lett. 69, 277-280 (1976).
7. Bon, S., Vigny, M., Massoulie, J.: Proc. Natl. Acad. Sci. (USA) 76, 2546-2550 (1979).
8. Fernandez, H.L., Duell, M.J., Festoff, B.W.: J. Neurochem. 32, 581-85 (1979).
9. Fernandez, H.L., Duell, M.J., Festoff, B.W.: J. Neurobiol. 10, 441-54 (1979).
10. Bon, S., Massoulie, J.: Proc. Natl. Acad. Sci. (USA): 77, 4464-68 (1980).
11. Bon, S., Vigny, M., Massoulie, J.: Proc. Natl. Acad. Sci. (USA) 76, 2546-50 (1979).
12. Luco, J.V., Eyzaguirre, C.: J. Neurophysiol. 18, 65-73 (1955).
13. Lubinska, L., Niemierko, S.: Brain Res. 27, 329-42 (1971).
14. Brimijoin, S., Wiermaa, M.J.: J. Physiol. 285, 129-42 (1978).
15. DiGiamberandino, L., Courand, J.Y.: Nature 271, 170-172 (1978).
16. Fernandez, H.L., Duell, M.J., Festoff, B.W.: J. Neurobiol. 11, 31-39 (1980).
17. Festoff, B.W., Israel, R.S., Engel, W.K., Rosenbaum, R.B.: Neurology 27, 963-70 (1977).
18. Fernandez, H.L., Patterson, M.R., Duell, M.J.: J. Neurobiol. 11, 557-70 (1980).
19. Beach, R.L., Popiela, H., Festoff, B.W.: in Progress in Motor Neurone Disease, F.C. Rose, ed. Pitman, London, in press.
20. Festoff, B.W., Duell, M.J., Fernandez, H.L.: in Maturation of Neurotransmission, E. Giacobini. Am Vernadakis, Giacobini, eds., Karger, Basel, 1979 pp.
21. Chao, L.P., Kan, K.S., Angelini, C., Keesey, J.: Exp. Neurol. 75, 23-35 (1982).
22. Gainer, H., Fink, D.J.: Brain Res. 233, 404-8 (1982).
23. Popiela, H., Ellis, S.: Dev. Biol. 83, 266-277 (1981).
24. Popiela, H., Ellis, S., Festoff, B.W.: J. Neurosci. Res. 8, 547-567 (1982).
25. Popiela, H., Beach, R.L., Festoff, B.W.: in Acetylcholinesterase, M. Fardeau, ed. Raven Press, New York, in press.
26. Popiela, H., Beach, R.L., Festoff, B.W.: Cell Molec. Neurobiol, in press.
27. Smith, B.H., Kreutzberg, G.W.: Neurosci. Res. Prog. Bull. 14, 361-63 (1976).
28. Bonner, P.H.: Dev. Biol. 90, 175-84 (1982).
29. Ii, I., Kimura, I., Ozawa, E.: Dev. Biol. 94, 366-77 (1982).
30. Markelonis, G.J., Kemmever, V.F., OH, T.H.: J. Biol. Chem. 255, 8967-70 (1980).

31. Beach, R.L., Popiela, H., Festoff, B.W.: FEBS Lett. 156, 151-156 (1983).
32. Markelonis, G.J., Bradshaw, R.A., OH, T.H., Johnson, J.L., Bates, O.J.: J. Neurochem. 39, 315-20 (1982).
33. Beach, R.L., Popiela, H., Festoff, B.W.: Cell Diff., in press.
34. Cleveland, D.W., Fischer, S.G., Kirschner, M.W., Laemmli, V.K.: J. Biol. Chem. 252, 1102-06 (1977).
35. Coll, J., Ingram, V.M.: Exp. Cell. Res. 131, 173-184 (1981).
36. Popiela, H., Beach, R.L., Festoff, B.W.: J. Cell Physiol., in press.
37. Godfrey, E.W.: J. Neurochem. 41 (Suppl), S108D (1983).
38. Hodgson, A.J., Chubb, I.W., Smith, A.D.: Biochem. Soc. Trans. 6, 648-649 (1978).
39. Chubb, I.W., Hodgson, A.J., White, G.H.: Neuroscience. 5, 2065-2072 (1980).
40. Wilson, B.W., Linkhart, T.A., Walker, C.R., Nieberg, P.S.: J. Neurol. Sci. 18, 333-50 (1973).
41. Festoff, B.W., Fernandez, H.L.: Muscle and Nerve. 4, 41-47 (1981).
42. Festoff, B.W.: Med. Hypotheses 6, 121-32 (1980).
43. Rasool, C.G., Chad, D., Bradley, W.G., Connolly, B., Baruah, J.K.: Muscle and Nerve 6, 430-35 (1983).
44. Soininen, H., Halonen, J., Rickkinen, P.J.: Acta Neurol. Scand. 64, 217-224 (1981).
45. Perry, R.H., Wilson, I.D., Bober, J.J., Atack, J., Blessed, G., Tomlinson, B.E., Perry, E.K.: Lancet i, 174-5 (1982).
45. Appel, S.H.: Ann. Neurol. 10, 499-505 (1981).
46. Chubb, I.W., Pilowsky, P.M., Springel, H.J., Pollard, A.C.: Lancet i, 683-90 (1979).
47. Smith, A.D., Wald, N.J., Cuckle, H.S., Stirrat, G.M., Bobrow, M., Lagercrantz, H.: Lancet i, 685-88 (1979).
48. Report of the Collaborative Acetylcholinesterase Study: Lancet ii, 321-24 (1981).

STUDIES ON HUMAN CHOLINESTERASES IN RELATION TO GENETICS, PHARMACOLOGY AND NEUROMUSCULAR PATHOLOGY

Stefano Biagioni

Istituto di Istologia e Analisi di Laboratorio, Università di Urbino

Gianfranco Scarsella, Giovanni Toschi

Dipartimento di Biologia Cellulare e dello Sviluppo, Università "La Sapienza", Roma

Erythrocyte Acetylcholinesterase

In previous studies the molecular characteristics of the human erythrocyte AChE (EAChE) have been investigated by examining purified enzyme preparations from pooled blood (1,2,3). One highly hydrophobic, dimeric form, with sedimentation coefficient (SC) of 6.3 S and molecular weight (MW) 160,000 was identified. A monomer, of MW 80,000, was obtained by reduction of disulfide bonds. On the other hand, when native, non purified AChE preparations from the erythrocytes of individual subjects were examined, more than one form was detected (4,5). In a recent study (6) AChE was extracted from ghosts by Triton X-100 and submitted to polyacrylamide-gel-electrophoresis (PAGE). In 60% of the examined subjects two forms were present, the faster one representing about 15% of the total activity (FIG.1). Only the slower band was present in the other subjects. Electrophoretic analysis according to Hedrick & Smith (7) showed no appreciable differences in electric charge between the two forms and indicated that the fast form is approximately half the size of the slower form. In preparations that were purified by affinity chromatography, SDS-PAGE showed only one form, of approximately 135,000 MW. One peak with SC 6.3 S was detected by ultra-

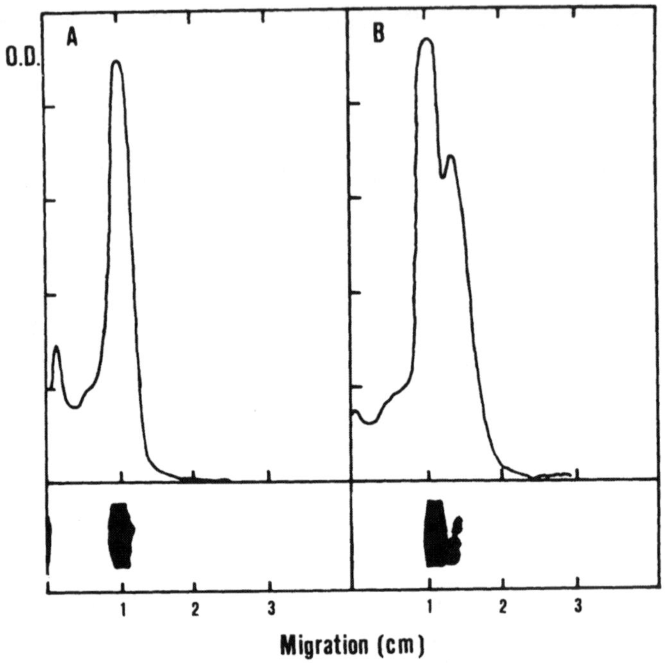

Fig.1. PAGE of human EAChE, prepared from ghosts of A) single-banded, and B) double-banded subjects. AChE revealed by the histochemical method.

centrifugal analysis. Taken together, these results indicate the presence of a major, dimeric form accompanied (in 60% of individuals) by a minor monomeric component.

In the same study (6) a similar examination of EAChE from individual rats of the same strain also revealed (in 30% of the rats) two bands with characteristics very similar to those of the human EAChE. The presence of monomeric forms in AChE preparations from tissues of other species has been reported (8).

The identity of the factors influencing the individual variation of EAChE forms is an open question. Previous studies have suggested a genetic control (4,5) but the observed variations could possibly depend on differences in the sialic acid content. It appears that this problem should be re-examined in the light of the present knowledge of the molecular forms of EAChE. Finally, it should be mentioned that a "neonatal" form of EAChE, migrating faster than the adult enzyme, has been observed in the blood of newborn babies. Its higher mobility was not due to the sialic acid content (Dr. Y. Edwards, personal communication).

Blood Serum Butyrilcholinesterase

A vast current literature deals with studies on human serum BuChE in relation to pharmacology, toxicology and pathology. In this report we will consider some studies on the genetics of this enzyme in relation to the hypersensitivity to succinylcholine (consisting in a prolonged apnea during anesthesia).

The genic and allelic constitution of this enzyme are known (9). The structural gene E_1 codes for BuChE activity and has 4 known "common" alleles; it is always expressed in 4 molecular forms, which can be separated by starch gel electrophoresis (C_1,C_2,C_3,C_4). The expression of some unusual alleles (atypical, fluoride-resistant, silent) affects the level of the enzyme activity, its kinetic properties and its sensitivity to inhibitors. A second gene, E_2, codes for a molecule that binds to one of the forms, changing its mobility and thus giving rise to a further band (C_5), present in 5 to 10% of the European population. The forms expressed by E_1 are considered size isomers (10), C_1,C_3, and C_4 being the monomer, dimer and tetramer forms, respectively, whereas C_2 appears to result from the association of C_1 with a smaller subunit. Form C_5, with a SC very close to that of C_4, is thought to result from the association of C_4 with the product of gene E_2.

The amino acid sequence of the active site region in the atypical enzyme (dibucaine-resistant) has been determined; a change in a single amino acid has been found (11).

A recent study (12) has investigated the possible correlation between serum BuChE activity and the "time of apnea" (i.e. the duration of myorelaxation induced by succinylcholine). The results show that a negative correlation (- 0.56) exists within the normal

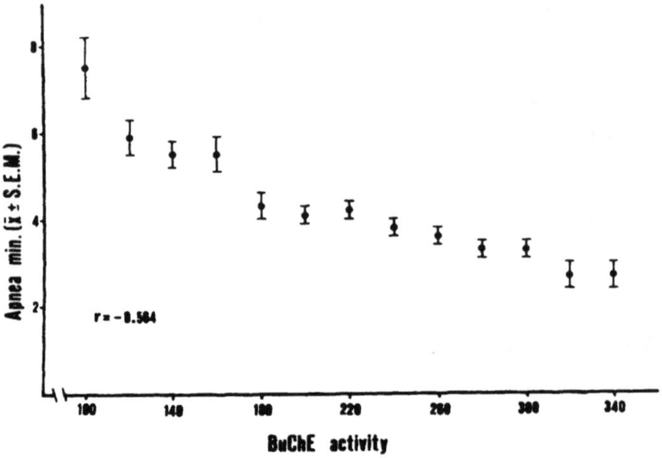

Fig.2. Relation between "time of apnea" and serum BuChE activity within the normal phenotype. BuChE activity is expressed in µmol of benzoylcholine hydrolyzed/min/100ml.

phenotype (FIG.2). Taking into account the extent to which the studied correlation is affected by experimental error and the variability in individual dosage, one can confidently assume that the individual variation in serum BuChE activity is the major determinant of the individual variation in the sensitivity to the drug. Eight dibucaine resistant subjects (heterozygotes, E_1^a, E_1^u) have been studied. As expected, they showed a reduced BuChE activity and an approximately proportional increase in the time of apnea. The high variability of these data is probably the cause of the very low correlation coefficient observed (- 0.15).

PAGE of these sera produced complex patterns of BuChE forms, with the number of bands ranging from 4 to 8 (FIG.3). Five of these bands correspond well to bands C_1 to C_5 previously described. The other bands were named C_1', C_3', C_6 and C_7 according to their relative mobilities. The examination of 260 subjects yielded 18 different patterns, resulting from combinations of these bands. Six patterns included band C_5. Two distinct patterns were present in highest frequency in both the C_5^- and C_5^+ populations. This is in line with the idea that the expression of the E_1 and E_2 genes is independent.

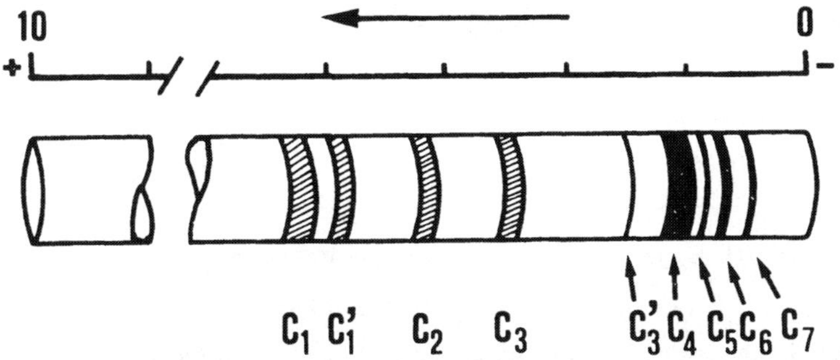

Fig.3. Schematic drawing of all serum BuChE molecular forms separated by PAGE.

When the possible correlation of the different patterns with the level of BuChE activity was examined, no significant differences in total activity were detected.

Thus it appears that the activity level has no obvious dependence on the presence of particular forms of the enzyme (at least in the C_5^- subjects). A similar analysis has shown no evident correlation of the "time of apnea" with the different patterns, either in the C_5^- or in the C_5^+ subjects. Finally, the frequency of the various patterns observed in 8 dibucaine-resistant (heterozygotic) subjects was not different from that in the normal subjects, indicating that the mutation conferring resistance does not affect the mechanism of formation of the multiple forms of the enzyme.

Cholinesterases in the Central Nervous System (CNS), Cerebrospinal Fluid (CSF) and Amniotic Fluid (AF)

In human CSF, AChE is present mainly in a soluble, globular form (G_4, a tetrameric component with a SC of about 11 S) (8). The origin and physiological significance of the AChE found in CSF are suggested by studies on various animal species which show that soluble AChE is released by nerve cells both *in vitro* and *in vivo* (13-17). Only certain forms of AChE are selectively released. It is now generally accepted that the release of AChE by nerve cells is a phenomenon of secretion that causes physiological levels of the enzyme to be present in the CSF. Therefore, changes in these levels could reasonably reflect any marked alteration of the CNS involving the AChE-secreting neurones.

Studies on humans have been rather limited to date. Brain tissue and CSF have been examined in relation to a particular disease, senile dementia of Alzheimer's type (SDAT). Both histochemical and biochemical studies have shown reduction of AChE in brain tissue (18,19). A recent study was carried out on patients for whom the diagnosis of SDAT was based on clinical and post-mortem histological data (20). Both AChE and protein concentration were found to be significantly reduced relative to age-matched controls , defined by the same criteria. The possibility of the diagnostic use of these measurements has been suggested.

The studies of AChE in CSF have provided a rational basis for a diagnostic approach to those developmental defects of the neural tube (NTD) that allow the CSF to mix with the amniotic fluid (i.e., spina bifida and anencephaly). Prenatal diagnosis is based on the determination of levels of alpha-fetoprotein (AFP) in maternal serum and amniotic fluid (AF) (together with ultrasound examinations). Certain limits in the specificity and sensitivity of the test for AFP in the AF have given rise to false positive and false negative results in a limited number of pregnancies. The examination of the AF for the presence of AChE, carried out independently by two groups (21,22) showed that the enzyme concentration was elevated in most cases of open NTD; an essential aspect of this observation is the qualitative demonstration of the presence of AChE as a distinct band (corresponding to the "secretory form" present in human CSF), separated by PAGE and characterized by the use of specific substrates and inhibitors. Since that time an extensive literature has added a mass of data (23,24,25,26) confirming the high sensitivity and specificity of this test. It has also given positive results for another fetal malformation (exomphalos) in about 50% of

the cases; in these cases AChE is probably derived from exposed nerve plexuses of the open gut wall (27).
A recent contribution to these studies has been provided by the first screening on the Italian population (28). A preliminary examination of 200 samples of AF from normal pregnancies and 8 from pregnancies which were positive for AFP test has shown that in all the fetuses with open NTDs the AChE level was significantly increased (Table I) and the gel test was positive (FIG.4). The test was also positive in one fetus with exomphalos. In normal AFs only one band of ChE was detected.

Muscle Cholinesterases

Muscle ChEs have been thoroughly investigated in various animal species, including strains that develop some genetically-determined diseases of muscle. Studies on human muscle are limited by obvious difficulties. A study on biopsies from surgical operations (29) has served to characterize the molecular forms of AChE in normal human muscle; six forms that are homologous to those of rat muscle have

TABLE I: AChE activity levels in amniotic fluid from control ($\bar{x} \pm$ S.D.) and affected pregnancies.

Case	AChE activity level
Control	2.76±1.26
Anencephaly	12.18
Multiple malformations	12.71
" "	14.65
Anencephaly	12.13
Meckel-Gruber	26.76
Anencephaly	17.94
"	19.82
Exomphalos	4.11

Values are expressed in nmoles of acetylthiocholine hydrolized/min/ml.

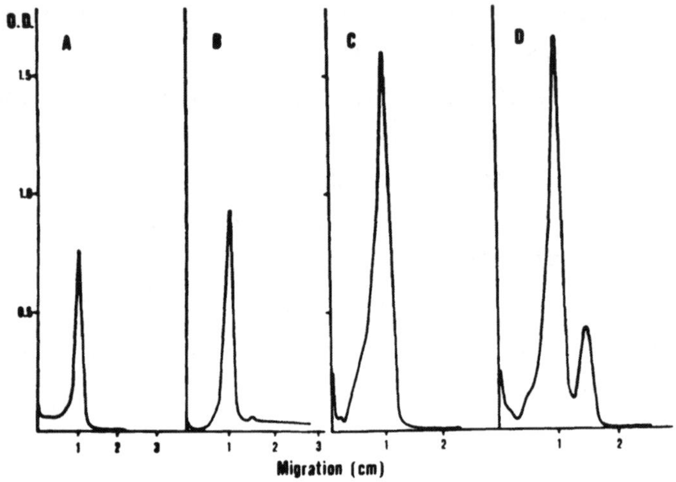

Fig.4. PAGE scanning diagrams of amniotic fluid ChEs. A and B: non-NTD pregnancy. C and D: NTD pregnancy. A and C: gel incubated with the specific inhibitor of AChE (BW 284 at 10^{-4} mol/l).

been identified. The asymmetric, collagen-tailed forms are present in areas lacking end-plates, in a higher proportion than in other species. An early histochemical study on biopsies from various human muscle disorders (30) indicated disturbances both in the regulation of AChE and in its cellular localization. Further investigations examined the level of AChE in human plasma, an approach that was suggested by studies on the inherited muscle dystrophy of chick (31). It was found that AChE is released into the blood plasma from the injured muscles of patients with a neurogenic myopathy, Amyotrophic Lateral Sclerosis (ALS) (32). Another study has been carried out by Sketely and colleagues (33) on patients with a different, non-neurogenic myopathy, the Duchenne muscular dystrophy (DMD). Plasma AChE was examined in patients at different ages and stages of the disease, as well as in normal subjects at birth and after. No difference was found between patients and controls of the same age, and there was no obvious correlation of patient age with signs of muscular damage. Taken together, these results point out an important difference between human and chicken muscular dystrophy and suggest that release of muscular AChE into blood plasma may reflect an altered nerve muscle interaction (such as that present in ALS and in denervation).

Recently a group of patients characterized by "muscular hypotony" has been examined (34). Based on clinical assessment, electromyographic evaluation, determination of serum enzymes and histological examination of biopsies from quadriceps femoris muscle, patients were divided into three categories: neurogenic myopathies (five cases), muscular dystrophies (ten) and a third form with no positive evidence of neurogenic lesion, termed "non-dystrophic myopathy" (five). Histochemical examination of biopsies indicated the absence of end-plate regions. No significant differences in the AChE levels of muscular biopsies from the three groups were detected (Table II). The molecular forms of AChE were examined by sedimentation analysis and the patterns were compared with those from normal human muscle and from muscles of patients with non-neuromuscular diseases (FIG. 5,A). Biopsies from neurogenic myopathies exhibited a marked reduction in both the heavy and medium forms (FIG.5,B); these changes are like those observed in denervated muscle and they are in agreement with the functional characteristics of the disease. In the muscle of dystrophic patients the heavy and medium forms were also reduced, the latter being particularly affected (FIG.5,C); these changes closely resemble those observed in muscles of two different

TABLE II: AChE activity levels of human muscular biopsies ($\bar{x} \pm$ S.E.M.)

Control	Neurogenic	Dystrophic	Myopathic
5.18	2.69 $\pm$ 0.64	3.04 $\pm$ 0.40	3.99 $\pm$ 1.03

Values are expressed in nmoles of acetylthiocholine hydrolized/min/mg tissue.

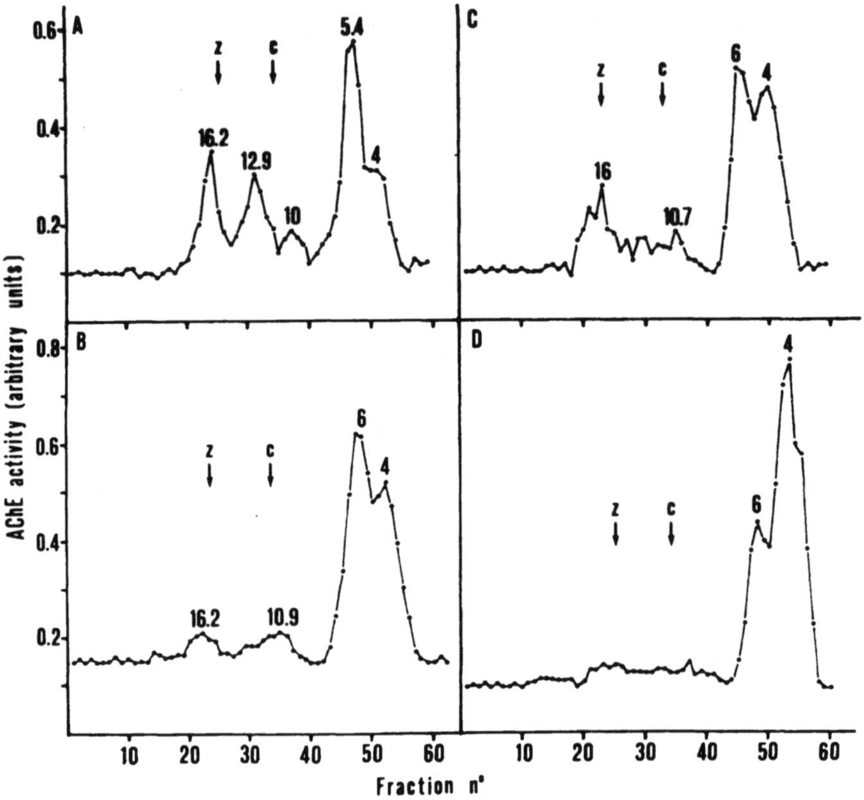

Fig.5. Sucrose gradient profiles showing the molecular forms of AChE in biopsies from (A) non-neuromuscular disease, and (B) neurogenic, (C) dystrophic, and (D) myopathic non-dystrophic patients. The arrows indicate the positions of (C) catalase 11.3 S, (Z) β-galactosidase 16 S.

strains of dystrophic mice (35,36). In the patients with "non-dystrophic myopathy" we noted the disappearance of both the high and medium forms, with all the activity concentrated in the light peak (FIG.5,D); this pattern closely resembles the profile observed in slow-tonic muscle of chicken (37), supporting the hypothesis of a defect in muscle maturation. The marked, selective loss of muscle AChE forms in all three myopathies should be compared to the abnormal levels of AChE that were found in blood plasma of patients with

ALS, but not in DMD patients. This might depend on factors such as the amount of released enzyme and the periods when the release occurs. Finally, it seems appropriate, in this occasion, to consider two open questions. One concerns the concentration of AChE in the blood plasma of normal human subjects, as the values reported in two independent studies using different substrates show wide differences (33,38). The other question concerns a critical evaluation of the various models of muscular dystrophy (chick and mouse) in relation to human myopathies.

Acknowledgements. The authors' work reported in this article was financially supported by grants from the Consiglio Nazionale delle Ricerche (no. 80.00595; 81.00366) and from the Ministero della Pubblica Istruzione (1981; 1982), and by funds for a visiting scientist (Dr. A. Longstaff) from Fidia Laboratories (Abano, Italy).

References

1. Ott, P., Jenny, B., Brodbeck, U.: Eur. J. Biochem. 57, 469-480 (1975).
2. Niday, E., Wang, C.S., Alaupovic, P.: Biochim. Biophys. Acta 469, 180-193 (1977).
3. Ott, P., Ariano, B.H., Binggeli, Y., Brodbeck, U.: Biochim. Biophys. Acta 729, 193-199 (1983).
4. Coates, P.M., Simpson, N.E.: Science 175, 1466-1467 (1972).
5. Das, P.K., Lo, E.H.M.: Enzyme 21, 304-316 (1976).
6. Biagioni, S., Scarsella, G., Settimi, L., Traina, M.E.: Mol. and Cell. Biochem. 47, 183-190 (1982).
7. Hedrick, J.L., Smith, A.J.: Arch. Biochem. Biophys. 126, 155-164 (1968).
8. Massoulié, J., Bon, S.: Ann. Rev. Neurosci. 5, 57-106 (1982).
9. Giblett, E.: Genetic markers in human blood. Blackwell, Oxford 1969.

10. Masson, P.: Biochim. Biophys. Acta 578, 493-504 (1979).

11. Yamato, K., Huang, I.Y., Muensch, H., Yoshida, A., Goedde, H. W., Agarwall, D.P.: Biochem. Genet. 21, 135-145 (1983).

12. Scarsella, G., Biagioni, S., Toschi, G., Santolamazza, C., Novelletto, A., Cermele, G., Modiano, G.: Second International Meeting on Cholinesterases (Bled, Yugoslavia) Abstracts p. 119 (1983).

13. Lazar, M., Vigny, M.: J. Neurochem. 35, 1067-1079 (1980).

14. Gisiger, V., Vigny, M.: FEBS Lett. 84, 253-256 (1977).

15. Romero, E., Smith, A.D.: J. Physiol. 301, 52P (1979).

16. Chubb, I.W., Goodman, S., Smith, A.D.: Neuroscience I, 57-62 (1976).

17. Greenfield, S.A., Smith, A.D.: Brain Research 177, 445-459 (1979).

18. Perry, E.K., Perry, R.H., Blessed, G., Tomlison, B.E.: Neuropathol. Appl. Neurobiol. 4, 273-277 (1978).

19. Davies, P.: Brain Research 171, 319-327 (1979).

20. Appleyard, M.E., Smith, A.D., Wilcock, G.K., Esiri, M.M.: The Lancet II, 452 (1983).

21. Smith, A.D., Wald, N.J., Cuckle, H.S., Stirrat, G.M., Bobrow, M., Lagercrantz, H.: Lancet I, 685-688 (1979).

22. Chubb, I.W., Pilowsky, P.M., Springell, H.J., Pollard, A.C.: Lancet I, 688-690 (1979).

23. Report of U.K. Collaborative Study on Acetylcholinesterase in relation to neutral tube defects. Lancet II, 321-324 (1981).

24. Smith, A.F.: Clin. Chim. Acta 123, 1-9 (1982).

25. Read, A.P., Fennell, S.J., Donnai, D., Harris, R.: Br. J. Obstet. & Gynaecol. 89, 111-116 (1982).

26. Coombes, E.J., Wood, P.J., Spencer, K., Batstone, G.F.: Clin. Chim. Acta 122, 249-259 (1982).

27. Wald, N.J., Cuckle, H.S., Barlow, R.D., Smith, A.D., Stirrat, G.M., Turnbull, A.C., Bobrow, M., Brock, D.J.H., Stein, S.M.: Lancet I, 1368-1369 (1980).

28. Toschi, M., Pachì, A., Biagioni, S., Scarsella, G., Troccoli, R., Ermini, M.: 23rd British Congress of Obstetrics and Gynaecology (1983).

29. Carson, S., Bon, S., Vigny, M., Massoulié, J., Fardeau, M.: FEBS Lett. 97 (2), 348-352 (1979).

30. Wilson, B.W., Taylor, R.G., Fowler jr., W.M., Patterson, G.T., Nieberg, P.A., Linkhart, S.G., Linkhart, T., Fry, D.M.: J.

Neurol. Sci. 26, 133-146 (1975).

31. Lyles, J.M., Barnard, E.A., Silman, I.: J. Neurochem. 34, 978-987 (1980).

32. Festoff, B.W.: Human Motor Neuron Disease ed. Lewis P. Rowland Raven Press, New York. 503-517 (1982).

33. Sketelj, J., Sasel, B., Zupancic, N., Brzin, M.: Exp. Neurol. in press (1983).

34. Poiana, G., Biagioni, S., Leone, F., Longstaff, A., Scarsella, G.: Second International Meeting on Cholinesterases (Bled, Yugoslavia) Abstracts p. 102 (1983).

35. Poiana, G., Biagioni, S., Giorgi, M., Leone, F., Scarsella, G., Senni, M.I.: Second International Meeting on Cholinesterases (Bled, Yugoslavia) Abstracts p. 103 (1983).

36. Stephens, H., Gisiger, V.: Second International Meeting on Cholinesterases (Bled, Yugoslavia) Abstracts p. 90 (1983).

37. Lyles, J.M., Barnard, E.A.: FEBS Lett. 109 (1), 9-12 (1980).

38. Festoff, B.W., Fernandez, H.L.: Muscle & Nerve 4, 41-47 (1981).

ACETYLCHOLINESTERASE: MULTIPLE FUNCTIONS?

Ian Chubb

Department of Human Physiology
Centre for Neuroscience
The Flinders University of South Australia
Bedford Park, South Australia 5042.

To propose that AChE has functions other than in cholinergic neurotransmission is to suggest nothing original or new. The question of whether all the functions of AChE are known has been discussed for almost as long as there have been studies of the cholinesterases. The first demonstration of choline ester-splitting activity in vivo showed that there was an active enzyme in blood (1). At the time it was reasonable to suppose that the blood-borne enzyme could play a significant role in the destruction of ACh, but it is now widely accepted that the spillover of ACh into the circulation is slight, even in animals whose AChE is completely inhibited (2,3). There is therefore no satisfactory explanation for the presence of cholinesterases in blood, whether it be in plasma, erythrocytes, platelets or other cellular material (4). While the role of AChE in the blood cells is unknown, ideas so abound that AChE seems to be "as much associated with red herrings as red blood cells" (4). Similar remarks may be directed at some studies of other sites where the presence of AChE activity does not correlate with equivalently high concentrations of ACh.

The uncovering of other functions of AChE may require an approach different from that used in the past; it may not be sufficient to assume that AChE acts exclusively as an esterase and that by influencing the esterase activity other functions will be revealed (4). This article presents the view that AChE is not exclusively an esterase and that consideration of other potential activities of AChE might prove a more fruitful avenue to an understanding of the ubiquitous distribution of the enzyme. Thus, it will be proposed that the distribution of AChE reflects that of all its substrates and not just ACh. It is intended to summarize those characteristics of AChE that suggest it has a broad range of naturally occurring, chemically diverse substrates. This review will therefore be limited in scope to two areas: (1) the localization of AChE and its relation to ACh; (2) novel substrates.

1. The Localization of AChE.

There are numerous reports in the early literature that cannot be easily explained if AChE is only capable of splitting ACh. The most consistent of these, and therefore the strongest single indication that AChE plays more than one role, is the lack of correspondence between the distributions of AChE and ACh in all species studied so far. These observations alone make it unlikely that the sole function of AChE is to hydrolyze released ACh at synapses. To interpret these data in terms of AChE/ACh, it would be necessary to suggest that ACh is more widely distributed than usually thought and that it has actions remote from synapses. Alternatively, AChE could have different substrate(s) according to its location.

AChE in non-neuronal tissue.

AChE evolved before neurons. The enzyme has been found in primitive cells (5) including bacteria and protozoa but the evidence that ACh is always found in the same unicellular organisms is not strong. There are, for example, reports that some bacteria can synthesize ACh (5) and that the enzyme responsible has similar properties to the one found in mammalian tissues (6). Few studies have been done to establish the role of ACh in these cells, although relatively high concentrations of anti- cholinesterases (and serotonin) inhibit their motility (6).

Certain species of protozoa contain an enzyme which, like AChE, is inhibited by low concentrations of both eserine and DFP (7). High concentrations of both (around 4mM) were able to influence the motility of whole cells (7). Whether the latter effects are in any way associated with the inhibition of AChE is doubtful. The two compounds in question readily pass through cell membranes so it must be assumed that the intracellular concentration would have been roughly 1000-fold higher than was necessary to inhibit the AChE activity in vitro.

The subject of AChE in invertebrates has been thoroughly reviewed (4,5) and, in particular, there is a lengthy and informative discussion in the work of Silver (4). In the present context, there is one aspect that requires further comment. Given that several species of unicellular organism contain AChE, the doubt about ACh, and the absence of nerve cells, the role of the enzyme in these cells is obscure. It may prove to be related to ACh, although the evidence that it does is scanty at best and seems not to be a uniform feature of the invertebrates in any case. Alternatively, it could involve other material produced by the cells since it seems unlikely that the cells would have a collection of substances waiting for a purpose to evolve with the nervous system. It is therefore pertinent that a number of peptides have recently been discovered in protozoa that have functions in the nervous system of vertebrates (8,9). Since it will be argued that AChE has the capacity to hydrolyze peptides (section 2), it is conceivable that some actions of AChE in single (and multi-) cellular organisms could be unrelated to the esterase activity but be due rather to another catalytic site, such as one involved in the hydrolysis of peptides.

AChE in the nervous system.

There is no doubt that AChE exists in tissues with no nerves even in species with well developed nervous systems (4,5). There is also good and widely accepted evidence that AChE is not distributed in parallel with ACh within the nervous system (4,10,11) although it has always been assumed that cholinergic cells (i.e. acetylcholine -secreting) inevitably contain AChE. The most recent studies using antibodies to choline acetyltransferase have confirmed that CAT and AChE always co-exist, although the relative amount of AChE is variable with some cells only weakly reactive (12). The exact relationship between the distribution of AChE and ACh will not be reviewed here. Instead, some well recognised but still unexplained aspects of the distribution will be considered, and the question of why cholinergic neurons should contain AChE will be developed later.

AChE appears very early in the developing nervous system where its activity can be demonstrated using histochemical techniques during the closure of the neural tube (13). After the neural tube has closed, the cells of the tube lose AChE activity until the neurons begin to differentiate. Meanwhile, the migrating cells derived from the neural crest continue to express AChE activity (13). These observations have been interpreted as indicating a role for AChE in cell movement, and this has been extended to include all cells on the basis of their staining for AChE activity during their migratory phase (13).

It is noteworthy that the enzyme is found in cells of the neural crest even though only a few give rise to cells that will be either ACh-containing or cholinoceptive in the mature nervous sytem. Many of these cells continue to have high activities of AChE in the adult (4,14,15,16,17,18) and some, like the sensory neurons in the dorsal root ganglia, are typical examples of cells that do not contain measurable amounts of ACh or CAT (19). Most of the cells derived from the neural crest are now known to contain physiologically active "neuropeptides" and, especially in the case of sensory neurons, these are thought to be the neurotransmitters (55).

Not all neurons contain AChE and so it is not a protein essential for some undefined but crucial metabolic process in all nerve cells. Furthermore, histochemical experiments indicate that there is a range of AChE activities in cells of a similar type, for example in the neurons in one ganglion (15,20,21). Until recently it may have been suggested that the different levels of AChE reflected the presence of neurons releasing different transmitters; however, it has now been shown that even neurons that contain CAT have variable AChE activity (12). This lack of correlation between AChE and CAT within a defined population of neurons brings another dimension to the discrepancies between AChE and ACh already outlined: not even cholinergic neurons have a uniform concentration of AChE. This suggests that its activity may not be linked to an intracellular metabolism of ACh essential for the normal functioning of the neurons. It should be noted that there is no indication from a mass of pharmacological and physiological data that an intracellular metabolism of ACh by AChE has functional importance (41).

Cytochemical studies have revealed that AChE-rich neurons have activity both on their surface and in the intracellular matrix. The surface AChE is associated with all parts of the neuron (4) although there is a suggestion that cells which are not cholinoceptive do not have surface AChE on the perikaryon (18). It is assumed therefore that the external AChE on the perikaryon and at the axon terminal is involved in neurotransmission. The axolemmal

AChE seems devoid of a significant (esterase) function although this has also been the subject of intense speculation and investigation over a number of years (26). The possible roles of extracellular AChE at sites not normally associated with the release of ACh will not be reviewed here; although it is noteworthy that some, such as the axon, may be sites of release of the enzyme (14,27).

Localization of intracellular AChE. The intracellular enzyme in neuronal perikarya is found chiefly in the rough endoplasmic reticulum whether the cells are cholinergic (22,23,25), non-cholinergic but a specified transmitter type (15,16,25), unknown transmitter type (24) or non-neuronal but polypeptide secreting cells (14,28). The Golgi apparatus also frequently shows high activity (15,16,22,25) with AChE included in the vesicle-like structures budding off from these membranes. There is little doubt that the neuronal cell bodies are the major sites of synthesis of AChE and that some perikarya are able to release soluble AChE into the extracellular fluid (16,18,22,29). Polypeptide secreting cells also secrete AChE activity (43).

In axons, the major location of axoplasmic AChE appears to be membrane limited particles which frequently have the appearance of elements of smooth endoplasmic reticulum (14,15,27). These tubules seem to be involved in both the transport of AChE from the cell body to the periphery and in the release of enzyme from the axon (27).

A proportion of the AChE in the axon is transported rapidly towards the terminals (30) and it has been estimated that as much as 0.7-2.0 times the cell body content is transported down the axon each day (31). It has also been found that if transport is blocked there is no accumulation of AChE in the perikaryon (31), unlike a number of other transported molecules (32). This suggests the metabolism of at least some forms of AChE is closely regulated (31,33).

AChE in nerve terminals. A thorough search of the literature up to 1974 (4) established that there were just two convincing references to the presence of AChE within nerve terminals. There have since been few other demonstrations of even very limited AChE activity in nerve terminals (42), although we in particular have made special efforts to determine whether the activity exists. In only one of several hundred synaptic terminals examined in routine experiments did we see a single structure that contained AChE activity (15), while in experiments where the incubation of the sections was deliberately prolonged, the few reactive structures that were seen gave every appearance of pinocytotic vesicles (16). Thus, despite the numerous demonstrations of both rapid and slow transport of AChE towards the nerve terminal, it seems improbable that active enzyme arrives there.

The fate of the AChE is not known, but if as much as twice the cell body content of AChE is funnelled into the axon each day (31), then an accumulation of AChE in the terminals would be expected. There is clear evidence of an accumulation of rapidly transported and neurotransmitter associated proteins in all the neurons that have been studied so far (34).

In summary, AChE exists in membranous structures within the cytoplasm of neurons. These include the rough endoplasmic reticulum and Golgi apparatus in perikarya and smooth endoplasmic retciculum in the axons. No clear demonstration of significant AChE activity in the nerve terminals has yet been provided despite the acknowledged transport of significant quantities of AChE away from the cell body. The reason why there is no accumulation is not known, although there are a number of explanations that could be considered: (i) the enzyme may be released from the neuron prior to arriving in the terminals; (ii) its esterase activity could be inhibited; (iii) since the enzyme is packaged in structures where peptide processing is likely to occur (28), it could itself be metabolized.

The function of intracellular AChE, and why it should be confined to structures like the endoplasmic reticulum and the Golgi apparatus is puzzling. It is specially obscure in cholinergic neurons where it has been estimated that the AChE concentration is 10-fold higher than in other cells (36). There is no obvious role for a hydrolytic enzyme like AChE inside the same cell as its (major) substrate. Either the relationship between AChE and ACh must be extremely subtle, the activity of the enzyme closely regulated or strictly compartmentalised, or the enzyme has another substrate even in cholinergic neurons.

2. Novel Substrates for AChE.

The question of another function for AChE revolves around whether it functions as an esterase with any of a number of substrates, or whether it has other catalytic activities. The first option is possible because, and it cannot be emphasised too strongly, AChE is not an enzyme with absolute substrate specificity (see 4). It is strategically located at synapses, and because it has an affinity for ACh it can play its important role in certain cholinergic transmission. Whether it has only the one role even at cholinergic synapses is not absolutely clear (4). The second option is also viable because there is evidence that AChE has the capacity to hydrolyze a number of non-ester substrates. It is also recognized that there are peripheral sites on the AChE molecule that allosterically regulate the esterase activity and occupation of which can alter the substrate specificity (35).

The regulation of AChE activity. There are several studies showing that a variety of multi-valent cations can either inhibit or enhance the activity of AChE (37,38,39,40). In each case the ion binds to one of a number of peripheral sites and so influences the esterase activity. These sites seem to be different from those to which organic cations can bind (44), and they appear to be numerous (38). There are also binding sites for β-endorphin on one molecular form of AChE (45). Occupation of these sites by β-endorphin inhibits the esterase activity, and the effect can be prevented by co-incubation with naloxone even though the latter drug has no effect on its own. It was also found that [met]-enkephalin was a weak inhibitor of AChE activity (45). Again, there was a selectivity in the action because not all forms were inhibited. These results indicate that AChE may have binding sites for some naturally occurring peptides but the relationship between these sites and the esterase centre is not known. Intriguingly, there is a report that [met]-enkephalin applied locally to the hippocampus results in diminished AChE activity (48).

In addition to the metal ions and peptides, a wide range of chemicals are capable of inhibiting AChE activity. Most of these are widely accepted anticholinesterase compounds and have well described modes of action (4). A particular characteristic of AChE is its inhibition by excess amounts of its substrate. This distinguishes the enzyme from other cholinesterases and is a characteristic of the enzyme from many sources (see 4). The ACh begins to inhibit at concentrations around 5mM (47), but complete inhibition is rarely achieved even with concentrations in excess of 50mM. The mechanism of the substrate inhibition is thought to be caused by an allosteric change induced by the binding of excess ACh to peripheral sites (46).

In addition to the increasingly diverse chemical nature of the molecules that influence AChE activity, often by an interaction with peripheral, allosteric, binding sites, AChE has been shown to hydrolyze several novel substrates. Thus the enzyme has amidase

(49), aryl acylamidase (50) and peptidase activity (51).

The aryl acylamidase activity is associated with AChE from human erythrocytes, sheep basal ganglia and electric tissue from electric eel; the activity from all sources was inhibited by serotonin (50; note: serotonin, like some anticholinesterases, has been reported to reduce the motility of bacteria that have AChE activity; 7). The aryl acylamidase activity was also inhibited by ACh and BW284C51 so that the evidence for its association with the AChE molecule is overwhelming. Because of the constant ratios of the specific activities and the parallel inhibition by a range of compounds, the two activities are likely to be properties of one active centre.

The peptidase activity is the most recently discovered activity believed to be associated with the AChE molecule. The naturally occurring peptides so far found to be substrates include the two enkephalins (51) and substance P (52). The possibility that peptidase contaminants were present in the AChE preparations has been considered and largely dismissed. It was concluded that AChE purified from sources as diverse as whole brain, adrenal glands, electric tissue, serum and more recently from specific brain and spinal cord regions (unpublished) had the capacity to hydrolyze peptide bonds. Significantly, the peptidase activity was inhibited by 10-20mM ACh but inhibitors of AChE activity that were directed towards the esterase centre were without effect. These experiments with inhibitors strongly suggest that the peptidase activity is due to another catalytic site in the AChE molecule (51).

The nature of the natural peptide substrate is unknown. It must be emphasised that the enkephalins have been used as substrates because they allow the study of a unique peptidase activity: AChE hydrolyzes both the amino- and carboxy-terminal amino acids from either enkephalin (51) and so the effect of different conditions of incubation on both activities can be readily studied. Whether the enkephalins are the natural peptide substrates for AChE remains to be determined.

Whatever eventually proves to be the natural peptide substrate(s) for AChE, its distribution must be seen in a new light. If the enzyme has the capacity to hydrolyze peptides as well as esters, then there is no reason to expect that its distribution should follow exclusively its ester substrate(s), or any one peptide. The discrepancy between the distributions of ACh and AChE have already been mentioned and the problems this wrought have been highlighted. Too premature a view of the peptide specificity would foster similar problems.

It is not possible to predict whether the AChE/peptidase would act chiefly outside or inside cells. Because AChE has a dual localization, it could have an extracellular role in, say, the destruction of peptides released into synaptic clefts, or an intracellular metabolic role. The first possibility has not been tested directly since the traditional inhibitors of AChE activity would be without effect on the peptidase activity except at very high concentrations; ACh is the only established inhibitor of the peptidase but its own physiological actions probably preclude its use as an inhibitor of the enzyme. The second option can be tested and we have recently demonstrated that incubation of fixed tissue sections with AChE prior to the immunohistochemical detection of enkephalins and substance P markedly <u>increases</u> the immuno-reactivity (53,54). It is therefore possible that AChE can generate small peptides from larger precursor molecules. Whether generation or degradation predominates would depend on conditions that are not yet defined. It may be pertinent, however, that AChE activity disappears from the neurons as it is transported towards the terminals. If the loss of esterase activity reflects a loss of protein and peptidase activity as well, the metabolism of AChE during processing could protect the generated peptide from degradation.

In conclusion, there are many features of AChE that are still enigmatic. The search for another role has occupied a large number of researchers for a considerable period of time, but the possibility that the enzyme might have catalytic activities distinct from its esterase activity is worthy of further investigation. While the establishment of the AChE/peptidase relationship should be relatively straightforward, the extraction and identification of the natural peptide substrate(s) is akin to a fishing expedition; but I am now confident that there will be more than red herrings at the end of the line.

References

1. Dale, H.H.: J.Pharmacol. Exptl. Therap. 6, 147-190 (1914).

2. Dudley, H.W.: J. Physiol. 79, 249-254 (1933).

3. Douglas, W.W., Paton, W.D.M.: J. Physiol. 115, 71-72p (1951).

4. Silver, A.: The Biology of Cholinesterases. North Holland, Amsterdam & Oxford. 1974.

5. Rama Sastry, B.V., Sadavongvivad, C.: Pharmacol. Rev. 30, 65-132 (1979).

6. White, H.L., Cavillato, C.J.: J. Neurochem. 17, 1579-1589 (1970).

7. Seaman, G.R., Houlihan, R.K.: J. Cell Comp. Physiol. 37, 309-321 (1951).

8. LeRoith, D., Shiloach, J., Roth, J., Lesniak, M.A.: Proc. Natl. Acad. Sci. U.S.A. 77, 6184-6188 (1980).

9. LeRoith, D., Liotta, A.S., Roth, J., Shiloach, J., Lewis, M.E., Pert, C.B., Krieger, D.T.: Proc. Natl. Acad. Sci. U.S.A. 79, 2086-2090 (1982).

10. Silver, A.: Int. Rev. Neurobiol. 10, 57-109 (1967).

11. Shute, C.C.D.: In: The Hypothalamus. (L. Martini, M. Motta, L. Franchini eds.) pp 167-179. Academic Press, N.Y. 1970.

12. Levey, A.I., Wainer, B.H., Mufson, E.J., Mesulam, M.-M.: Neuroscience 9, 9-22 (1983).

13. Drews, U.: Prog. Histochem. Cytochem. 7, 1-52 (1975).

14. Somogyi, P., Chubb, I.W., Smith, A.D.: Proc. R. Soc. Lond. B. 191, 271-283 (1975).

15. Somogyi, P., Chubb, I.W.: Neuroscience 1, 413-421 (1976).

16. Jessen, K.P., Chubb, I.W., Smith, A.D.: J. Neurocytol. 7, 145-154 (1978).

17. Brzin, M., Tennyson, V.M., Duffy, P.E.: J. Cell Biol. 31, 215-242 (1966).

18. Lewis, P.R., Schon, F.E.G.: J. Anat. 120, 373-385 (1975).

19. Hebb, C.O., Silver, A.: J. Physiol. 134, 718-728 (1956).

20. Koelle, G.B.: J. Pharmacol. Exptl. Therap. 114, 167-184 (1955).

21. Koelle, G.B.: In: Cholinesterases and anticholinesterase agents. (G.B. Koelle ed.) Handb. exp. Pharmak. Suppl. 15, pp187-298. Springer-Verlag, Berlin. 1963.

22. Kreutzberg, G.W., Schubert, P., Toth, L., Rieske, E.: Brain Res. 62, 399-404 (1973).

23. Kreutzberg, G.W., Toth, L.: Naturwissenschaften 61, 37, (1974).

24. Tennyson, V.M., Brzin, M., Duffy, P.: Prog. Brain Res. 29, 41-62 (1968).

25. Henderson, Z.: J. Comp. Neurol. 197, 185-196 (1981).

26. Nachmansohn, D.: In: Neurochemistry, (K.A.C. Elliot, I.H. Page, J.H. Quastel eds.) pp. 522-557. Thomas, Springfield, Illinois. 1962.

27. Kasa, P.: Nature 218, 1265-1267 (1968).

28. Pearse, A.G.E.: J. Histochem. Cytochem. 17, 303-313 (1969).

29. Greenfield, S.A., Cheramy, A., Leviel, V., Glowinski, J.: Nature 284, 355-357 (1980).

30. Brimijoin, S., Wierma, M.J.: J. Physiol. 285, 129-142 (1978).

31. Sinicropi, D.V., Michels, K., McIlwain, D.L.: J. Neurochem. 38, 1099-1105 (1982).

32. Ljungdahl, A., Hokfelt, T., Nilsson, G.: Neuroscience 3, 861-943 (1978).

33. Carter, J.L., Brimijoin, S.: J. Neurochem. 36, 1018-1025 (1981).

34. Jeffrey, P.L., Austin, L.: Prog. Neurobiol. 2, 205-255 (1973).

35. Barnett, P., Rosenberry, T.L.: J. Biol. Chem. 252, 7200-7206 (1977).

36. Wallace, B.G.: Brain Res. 219, 190-195 (1981).

37. Tomlinson, G., Mutus, B., McLennan, I.: Can. J. Biochem. 59, 728-735 (1981).

38. Marquis, J.K., Lerrick, A.J.: Biochem. Pharmacol. 31, 1437-1440 (1982).

39. Changeux, J.-P.: Mol. Pharmacol. 2, 369-392 (1966).

40. Tomlinson, G., Mutus, B., McLennan, I., Mooibroek, M.J.: Biochim. Biophys. Acta 703, 142-148 (1982).

41. Birks, R.I., MacIntosh, F.C.: Can. J. Biochem. Physiol. 39, 787-827 (1961).

42. Davis, R., Koelle, G.B.: J. Cell Biol. 88, 581-590 (1981).

43. Chubb, I.W., Hodgson, A.J.: In: Trends in Autonomic Pharmacology (S. Kalsner ed.) pp 61-82. Urban & Schwarzenberg, Baltimore, Munich. 1982.

44. Berman, H.A., Becktel, W., Taylor, P.: Biochemistry 20, 4803-4810 (1981).

45. Haynes, L.W., Smith, M.E.: Neuroscience 7, 1007-1013 (1982).

46. Niday, E., Wang, C.-S., Alaupovic, P.: Biochem. Biophys. Acta 612, 67-72 (1980).

47. Augustinsson, K.-B.: Acta Physiol. Scand. 15, Suppl 52, 1-182 (1948).

48. Grigoreva, O.N., Gusel, V.A., Kozhenikova, N.I., Vlasov, G.P.: Biull. Eksp. Biol. Med.:95, 36-38 (1983).

49. Moore, D.E., Hess, G.P.: Biochemistry 14, 2386-2389 (1975).

50. George, S.T., Balasubramanian, A.S.: Eur. J. Biochem. 111, 511-524 (1980).

51. Chubb, I.W., Ranieri, E., White, G.H., Hodgson, A.J.: Neuroscience in press.

52. Chubb, I.W., Hodgson, A.J., White, G.H.: Neuroscience 5, 2065-2072 (1980).

53. Chubb, I.W.: Neuroscience Letts. Suppl 11, s6-s7 (1983).

54. Millar, T.J., Chubb, I.W.: Submitted for publication.

55. Hokfelt, T., Johansson, O., Ljungdahl, A., Lundberg, J.M., Schultzberg, M.: Nature 284, 515-521 (1980).

V. ANTICHOLINESTERASES: TOXICOLOGY AND STRUCTURE-FUNCTION RELATIONSHIP OF INHIBITORS AND ANTIDOTES

INTRODUCTION TO SESSION V

V. Vojvodić

Military Medical Academy, 11002 Belgrade, Yugoslavia

The papers concerning toxicology and structure-function relationship of anticholinesterases and antidotes presented at the Meeting were mainly devoted to the mechanism of action, storage depot, bioactivation and detoxification of these compounds, as well as to the mechanism of action of ChE reactivators.

In connection with the mechanism of action, it has been lately repeatedly shown that single administration of AChE inhibitors produced myopathies characterized by complete but localized necrosis of affected muscle fibers, which, as suggested by Dettbarn, were mainly due to the inhibition of the 16 S molecular form of the enzyme. From the data presented in poster session about ChE reactivators of mono- and bis-pyridinium types, it can be concluded that they are efficient in antagonizing the skeletal muscle fiber necrosis induced by organophosphorus antiChEs.

AntiChEs aimed at the use as chemical warfare agents were reviewed by J. Dacre. Several aspects of these agents deserve further studies, such as the effect of chronic exposure, possibilities of mutagenic screening, teratology and delayed neuropathic effects.

While an increasing number of data indicates the existence of significant depots for nerve agents in the body, for soman in particular (Bošković et al., van Helden et al.), their true nature, beyond BuChE and tributyrinase is, however, still little understood.

As reviewed by Casida, organophosphorus compounds are metabolicaly activated either by reactions at or near the phosphorus atom, or by oxidations at sites more distant from it, e.g. by sulfoxidation of thioethers and

N-demethylation of dimethylamides. On the other hand, organophosphorus compounds are detoxified by methylene hydroxylation and cleavage of P-O-CH_2, P-N-CH_2 and possibly P-S-CH_2 substituents and aryl hydroxylation, and methylcarbamate insecticides by hydroxylation of aryl and *N*-methyl and O-ethyl substituents or by sulfoxidation.

Two possible ways of detoxification of soman in mammals were reported by Sterri and Fonnum. Soman is either bound to plasma aliesterases or rapidly cleared from blood passing through the liver by being efficiently degraded by phosphorylphosphatases. The effective concentration in body fluids of soman responsible for inhibition of AChE in tissues, is therefore considerably decreased by these mechanisms representing a kind of natural resistance to organophosphorus agents.

EFFECTS OF SARIN, SOMAN AND TABUN ON PLASMA AND BRAIN ALIESTERASE ACTIVITY IN THE RAT

Bogdan Bošković, Milan Jokanović, Matej Maksimović

Military Technical Institute, Katanićeva 15,
11000 Belgrade, Yugoslavia

Introduction

The interest in aliesterase (tributyrinase /TBE/, B-type esterase) (1) in poisoning by chemical warfare nerve agents began with the finding of Myers (2) that DAM (diacetylmonoxime) greatly enhanced the destruction of sarin in the rat by a cyclic process of TBE inhibition by the organophosphate and its subsequent reactivation by DAM. Later results of the other authors (3, 4, 5) confirmed the proposed biochemical mechanism (2) and established that rat plasma proteins to which the radioactivity of ^{32}P-sarin was attached were identical with TBE.

It has been repeatedly shown in the last several years that TOCP (tri-o-cresyl phosphate), an irreversible inhibitor of rat plasma (3) and brain TBE (6), as well as CBDP (2-/o-cresyl/-4 H-1:2:3-benzodioxa phosphorin-2 oxide), its active metabolite (7), markedly increased the toxicity of sarin, soman or tabun in several species of animals (8, 9, 10, 11). It was accordingly suggested that the nerve agents mentioned, soman in particular, were stored *in vivo* in some sort of depot comprising plasma TBE (12, 13), adipose tissue, low density lipoproteins and or/albumin (14), from which they were gradually released. In order to further evaluate the importance of TBE as the part of the nerve agents depot, we examined the rates of inhibition and recovery of plasma and brain TBE and the influence of TOCP pretreatment on sarin, soman and tabun toxicity and the protective effects of antidotes in the rat.

Methods

Materials. The following drugs were used in this study: AChJ, AThCh, BuThCh, atropine sulphate, diazepam, HI-6, TMB-4, tributyrin, heparin, sarin, soman, tabun and TOCP. The purity of the nerve agents was 97-98%.

TBE determinations. TBE activity was assessed by the pH-stat method using tributyrin as the substrate. Tributyrin (10 ml of 0.2% solution) in CO_2-free 0.9% saline was added to the reaction vessel and titrated (at 25°C) to pH 7.9 with 0.01 N NaOH by a Radiometer titragraph. Either 0.2 ml of plasma or 0.8 ml of brain homogenate (1:3 w/v prepared in CO_2-free saline) was added to start the reaction. The addition of 0.01 N NaOH from the first to fifth min was used in determining the reaction rate. The reaction was linear over this time period.

ChE determinations. RBC AChE activity was determined by the pH-stat method using AChJ (final conc. = 2.44 mM) as the substrate. Ten ml of 0.9% CO_2-free saline and 0.3 ml of rinsed erythrocytes were added to the reaction vessel and titrated to pH 7.6 with 0.01 N NaOH by a Radiometer titragraph. ChE activities in plasma and brain of the rats were determined according to the procedure of Ellman et al (15).

Toxicology. Male Wistar rats (160 - 200 g) were used in this study. All drugs were injected in a volume of 1% of body weight.

Results

1) The results in Table 1 demonstrate that plasma TBE was about 10 times more sensitive to tabun than plasma ChE, while the sensitivity of both enzymes to sarin and soman was of the same order. Concerning the activity of the brain enzymes, ChE was 60, 2.500 and 2.000 times more sensitive to tabun, sarin and soman than TBE, respectively.

TABLE 1. Effect of in vitro incubation of rat plasma and brain homogenate with tabun, sarin and soman on tributyrinase and cholinesterase activity

Treatment	pI_{50}, (37°C, 30 min)			
	Plasma		Brain	
	ChE[a]	TBE[b]	ChE[b]	TBE[c]
Tabun	6.0	7.1	7.9	6.1
Sarin	6.4	6.5	8.3	4.9
Soman	6.6	6.6	8.7	5.4

[a]Plasma + 0.9% saline (1:1) containing the inhibitor.

[b]Diluted (1:10) with 0.9 saline containing the inhibitor.

[c]Homogenate diluted with 0.9% saline (1:3) containing the inhibitor.

2) The activity of TBE in plasma <u>in vivo</u> 30 min after s.c. injection of 0.25, 0.5 and 0.75xLD_{50} of tabun, sarin and soman, respectively (taken to represent the

maximum degree of inhibition) was the following: 9.8, 0 and 0; 24, 0.8 and 1.5; 61.8, 37.5 and 11.3, expressed as percentage of the control value (747 ± 63 nmoles tributyrin/ml/min taken as 100). On the contrary, the brain TBE in vivo (Table 2) was much less sensitive to the toxic agents studies, especially so in the cases of sarin and soman.

TABLE 2. Effect of tabun, soman and sarin on the <u>in vivo</u> activity of brain tributyrinase in the rat[a]

Multiple of LD_{50}	Tributyrinase activity, % of control[b]		
	Tabun	Soman	Sarin
0.5	84.6	-	-
0.75	54.8	100	100
1.5	54.5	89	-
4.0	-	61	92.6
6.67	53.5	57.3	-
10.0	-	56.1	85.8

[a]Animals were sacrificed 30 min after s.c. injection of the toxic agents.

[b]Control activity = 1.119 ± 115 (nmoles tributyrin hydrolyzed/g tissue/min).

(-) = not determined

At the same time, the activity of ChEs in poisoning by $0.25xLD_{50}$ of tabun in RBC, plasma and brain amounted to 15.6, 42.2 and 72.6% of the control, whereas the brain ChE activity in poisoning by $0.75xLD_{50}$ of tabun and soman was 3.5 and 47.2% of the control, respectively. The inhibitory effect of $0.75xLD_{50}$ of soman and sarin on plasma ChE activity was approximately equal to their corresponding effects on the plasma TBE activity.

When DAM (50 mg/kg, s.c.) was injected 60 min after the $0.75xLD_{50}$ of the toxic agents and the activity of the plasma TBE determined 60 min later, it has been found that the activity increased from 30 to 100% in sarin, from 14.7 to 65 in soman and from 5.9 to 6.5% of the control value in tabun poisoning, respectively.

TABLE 3. Renewal of plasma and brain tributyrinase activity in rats given sarin, soman and tabun

Treatment	t/2, hr[a]	
	Plasma[b]	Brain[c]
Sarin	2.1	-
Soman	17.1	32.8
Tabun	43.7	41.8

[a]Half-time for return of tributyrinase activity after s.c. injection of the toxic agents.

[b]After $0.75xLD_{50}$ of the toxic agents.

[c]After $6.67xLD_{50}$ of soman or tabun. Five min before the injection of the toxic agents, rats were given atropine (14 /umoles/kg i.m.), oxime (HI-6, 400 /umoles/kg, i.m. in soman or TMB-4, 50 /umoles/kg i.m. in tabun poisoning) and diazepam (8.78 /umoles/kg, i.p.).

(-) = not determined

In contrast to the brain TBE (Table 2), the brain ChE activity was almost completely inhibited by up to $4xLD_{50}$ of the toxic agents given after the pretreatment of the animals with antidotes.

3) The most rapid recovery of TBE activity <u>in vivo</u> (Table 3) was observed in the plasma of the rats poisoned by sarin (t/2 = 2.1 hr), followed by soman and tabun, which had t/2 rates of 17.1 and 43.7 hr, respectively. In the brain, the longest period of recovery was observed in tabun poisoning (t/2 = 41.8 hr). Due to the low degree of inhibition, even by $10xLD_{50}$, t/2 of recovery of sarin inhibited TBE activity could not be determined.

TABLE 4. The rate of the *in vivo* plasma and brain cholinesterase and tributyrinase activity inhibition by sarin, soman and tabun in the rat

Enzyme	t/2, min[a]		
	Sarin	Soman	Tabun
RBC AChE[b]	1.9	1.6	2.7
Plasma ChE[c]	2.9	4.7	3.2
Plasma TBE	0.9	4.8	1.5
Brain ChE[d]	3.7	13.4	7.9
Brain TBE	-	-	31.2

[a]Half-time required for the inhibition of 50% of the enzyme activity after s.c. injection of $0.75xLD_{50}$ of the toxic agents.

Control activity: b = 1.069 ± 308 nmoles ACh/ml/min; c = 111 ± 15 nmoles BuThCh/ml/min; d = 9.426 ± 882 nmoles AThCh/g/min.

(-) = No inhibition.

4) The results in Table 4 demonstrate that the shortest t/2 rates of the enzyme activity inhibition were observed in plasma TBE by sarin (0.9 min) and tabun (1.5 min), followed by RBC AChE inhibition with soman (1.6 min). The most rapid inhibition of the brain ChE activity was observed in soman poisoning, whereas the brain TBE activity was the least affected, being inhibited only by tabun, but not by sarin and soman.

TABLE 5. The influence of TOCP on subcutaneous toxicity of soman, tabun and sarin in male rats and the protective effects of atropine and oximes

Treatment	LD_{50}, μmoles/kg $\pm$ SE		Relative potency[c]
	Untreated animals	Atropine + oxime[b]	
Soman	0.38 $\pm$ 0.02	1.37 $\pm$ 0.1	3.6
TOCP[a] + soman	0.075 $\pm$ 0.004	0.23 $\pm$ 0.01	3.1
Tabun	1.17 $\pm$ 0.08	6.1 $\pm$ 0.6	5.2
TOCP + tabun	0.48 $\pm$ 0.02	3.7 $\pm$ 0.3	7.7
Sarin	0.64 $\pm$ 0.06	107.1 $\pm$ 14	167
TOCP + sarin	0.19 $\pm$ 0.005	46.4 $\pm$ 0.5	241

[a]TOCP (270 μmoles/kg) was given s.c., 24 hr prior to the toxic agent administration.

[b]Atropine (14 μmoles/kg) and oximes (HI-6, 265 μmoles/kg in soman and sarin and TMB-4, 50 μmoles/kg in tabun poisoning) were given together i.m., immediately after the toxic agent administration.

[c]LD_{50} with treatment LD_{50} without treatment. LD_{50} values, based on 24 hr mortalities were calculated by the method of Miller and Tainter (16).

5) The findings in Table 5 show that the acute toxicity of soman, tabun and sarin in TOCP pretreated rats was increased 5, 2.4 and 3.4 times, respectively, whereas the protective effect of antidotes varied related to the control. It was lower in soman, and higher in sarin and tabun pretreated animals.

Discussion

The results of our experiments have shown that sarin, soman and tabun were strong inhibitors of rat TBE plasma activity in vitro and in vivo, whereas the corresponding sensitivity of the brain enzyme was much lower. When sarin, soman (17) or tabun were given s.c. to rats, they simultaneously reacted with the plasma TBE and ChE, as well as with RBC AChE (Table 4), thus preventing them from inhibiting vital tissue AChE. At the same time, the pretreatment of the animals with TOCP resulted in marked potentiation of the toxicity of the nerve agents studied.

That the plasma TBE plays an important part in modifying the toxicity of soman and similar organophosphorus compounds is shown by its two opposite effects: the potentiation of their toxicity in TOCP or CBDP pretreated animals (8, 9, 10, 11, 17, 18) and their reduction by the increase of liver and plasma TBE activity (19).

The next question concerns the ratio of the brain TBE to ChE activity. Except tabun, very high doses of the other two toxic agents (from 4 to $10xLD_{50}$) were required for partial inhibition of brain TBE activity, especially in the case of sarin poisoning (Table 2), whereas any dose equal to or higher than $1.5xLD_{50}$ of sarin, soman or tabun completely inhibited the brain ChE activity. This might be attributed either to the aliesterase isoenzymes non sensitive to the toxic agents studied, or to their strong affinity and binding to some other non-specific sites representing the yet unidentified nerve agents depot (20). Likewise, the differences in the degree of soman, sarin and tabun toxicity potentiation (Table 5, ref. 8) point to the existence of some other factors beyond TBE which modify their toxicity.

While the lowest toxicity of tabun and the highest one of soman (out of the three agents tested) in control animals (1.17 : 0.38 µmoles/kg) might, at least partly, be attributed to their differences in the pI_{50} (Table 1), the ratio (Table 2) and the rate (Table 4) of TBE activity inhibition, the differences in the protective effects of antidotes in soman and sarin poisoning in control versus TOCP pretreated animals is difficult to explain at the present.

Summary

Sarin, soman and tabun strongly inhibited the rat plasma TBE activity _in vitro_ and _in vivo_, the intensity of which was comparable with the corresponding plasma and RBC ChEs activities inhibition, whereas the sensitivity of the brain TBE was much lower, especially in sarin poisoning. Strong inhibition of the brain ChE activity by sarin and soman and low inhibition of TBE activity by the two agents, might be attributed either to insensitive isoenzymes of the latter, or to the existence of other binding sites in CNS for the toxic agents. The differences in the degree of soman, sarin and tabun toxicity potentiation in TOCP pretreated animals, as well as in the protective effects of antidotes in these poisoning, also speak in favour of the presence of some additional sites which, beyond TBE, may serve as a depot for the nerve agents.

References

1. Aldridge, W.N.: Biochem. J. 57, 692-702 (1953).
2. Myers, D.K.: Biochem. Biophys. Acta 34, 555-557 (1959).
3. Polak, L.R., Cohen, M.E.: Biochem. Pharmacol. 18, 813-820 (1969).
4. Polak, L.R., Cohen, M.E.: Biochem. Pharmacol. 19, 877-881 (1970).
5. Cohen, E.M., Christen, P.J., Mobach, E.: The inactivation by oximes of sarin and soman in plasma from various species. I. The influence of diacetylmonoxime on the hydrolysis of sarin. J.A. Cohen memorial issue. North-Holland publishing company - Amsterdam, London, 113-131 (1971).
6. Manno, M., Rigoni, F., Bartolucci, G.B., Bianchi, M., Mazzota, M.: Brit. J. Ind. Med. 36, 153-156 (1979).
7. Casida, J.E., Eto, M., Baron, R.L.: Nature 191, 1396 (1961).
8. Bošković, B.: Arch. Toxicol. 42, 207-216 (1979).
9. Clement, J.G., Filbert, M.: Life Sci. 32, 1803-1810 (1983).
10. Sterri, S.H.: Acta pharmacol. et toxicol. 49, suppl. V, 67-71 (1981).
11. Benschop, H.P., Van den Berg, G.R., Van Hooidonk, C., De Jong, L.P.A., Kientz, C.E.: J. Med. Chem. 22, 1306-1313 (1979).
12. Sterry, S.H., Lyngaas, S., Fonnum, F.: Acta pharmacol. et toxicol. 49, 8-13 (1981).
13. Clement, J.G.: Biochem. Pharmacol. 31, 4085-4088 (1982).
14. Maliwal, B.P., Guthrie, F.E.: Mol. Pharmacol. 20, 138-144 (1981).
15. Ellman, G.L., Cortney, K.D., Andres, V., Featherstone, R.M.: Biochem. Pharmacol. 7, 88-95 (1961).
16. Miller, L.G., Tainter, M.L.: Proc. Soc. Exp. Biol. Med. 57, 261-264 (1944).
17. Fonnum, F., Sterri, S.: Fundam. Appl. Toxicol. 1, 143-147 (1981).
18. Bošković, B.: Fundam. Appl. Toxicol. 1, 203-213 (1981).
19. Clement, J.G.: Biochem. Pharmacol. 32, 1411-1415 (1983).
20. Wolthuis, O.L., Benschop, H.P., Berends, F.: Eur. J. Pharmacol. 69, 379-383 (1981).

ON THE EXISTENCE OF A SOMAN DEPOT

Herman van Helden, Frits Berends, Otto Wolthuis
Medical Biological Laboratory TNO,
P.O. Box 45, 2280 AA Rijswijk, The Netherlands

Henk Benschop
Prins Maurits Laboratory TNO,
P.O. Box 45, 2280 AA Rijswijk, The Netherlands

Introduction

The therapy of soman intoxication is hampered by at least three factors, slow reactivation of the phosphorylated cholinesterase by oximes, rapid dealkylation of this molecule which makes it even more oxime resistant and a predominant central action of the organophosphate which makes it necessary for an oxime to pass the blood brain barrier in order to be effective. The study of soman therapy, moreover, is encumbered by the existence of marked differences in oxime-effectiveness between the usual laboratory animals and man (for review see 1). In addition, with the arrival of new effective oximes like HI-6 it was shown that persistence of soman in the body poses a new problem in the therapy. It appeared that after a seemingly successful therapy, a subsequent autoinfusion with residual soman again threaten life (2, 3). It was demonstrated that the persistence of soman could be influenced by soman-simulators, i.e. compounds that resemble soman in both chemical structure and lipophilicity but are devoid of anticholinesterase activity. The results indicated that at least part of the soman persisting in the body is reversibly bound to sites other than cholinesterase which henceforth will be called "the depot". The depot sites showed specificity when the structure of the simulator was varied. At least part of this depot appeared to be localized in muscle tissue (4). Administered prophylactically, i.e. before soman and subsequent oxime therapy, several of these simulators could prevent death. The data suggested that the efficacy depended on the structural similarity to soman. The objective of this paper is to discuss these findings.

I. Evidence for soman-storage in the body

In a previous investigation Wolthuis and Kepner (5) injected atropinized, anaesthetized rats with 4 or $6xLD_{50}$ soman and kept them alive by artificial ventilation. When one hour later these animals were treated with HI-6 and 15 min later artificial ventilation was terminated, all animals appeared to have reacted well to the therapy. However, gradually the condition of the animals poisoned with $6xLD_{50}$ soman deteriorated; they again showed symptoms of organophosphate poisoning and died after several hours (Table 1). When identically treated rats were sacrificed soon after HI-6 treatment or several hours later and the neuromuscular transmission (NMT) of their diaphragms was tested in vitro, considerable recovery was observed in muscles taken soon after HI-6, whereas NMT in preparations taken several hours after HI-6 was almost completely inhibited (figure 1).

Rapid inhibition of purified AChE injected into the bloodstream of rats one to several hours after soman poisoning and the identification of soman in bloodsamples of similarly treated rats, yielded further evidence for persistence of soman in the body (see II).

These results suggested that intact soman can persist in the body for several hours in sufficient amounts to cause a lethal reinhibition of oxime-reactivated acetylcholinesterase (AChE). Such a persistence of soman in the body was quite unexpected in view of the reported fast degradation of soman in blood and in other organs (6, 7). It was postulated that part of the administered amount of soman was stored in a kind of depot where it would be protected against degradation. Subsequent release from this depot would then be responsible for reinhibition of AChE. This view was strengthened by the finding that repeated HI-6 injections could delay death (unpublished data).

Table 1. Number of survivors and median survival times of non-survivors in groups of atropinized rats poisoned with soman and treated by HI-6 60 min later.*

i.v. injections		No. survivors/group of 12 rats at 24 h	Mean time to death of non-survivors (h)
t = o	t = 60 min		
saline	HI-6(210 μmol/kg)	12	-
$4xLD_{50}$	"	10	12.6
$6xLD_{50}$	"	1**	4.8
$4xLD_{50}$	HI-6(150 μmol/kg)	12	-
$6xLD_{50}$	"	1**	5.8

* Immediately following the injection of soman or saline the rats received artificial respiration (A.R.) via a tracheal intubation. The intubation was removed 15 min after HI-6 administration. During A.R. the animals were kept in hexobarbital anaesthesia. Note that non-survivors died after several hours. A control group only received HI-6.

** Significantly different ($p<0.05$, two-tailed) from the control group and from animals injected with $4xLD_{50}$ soman.

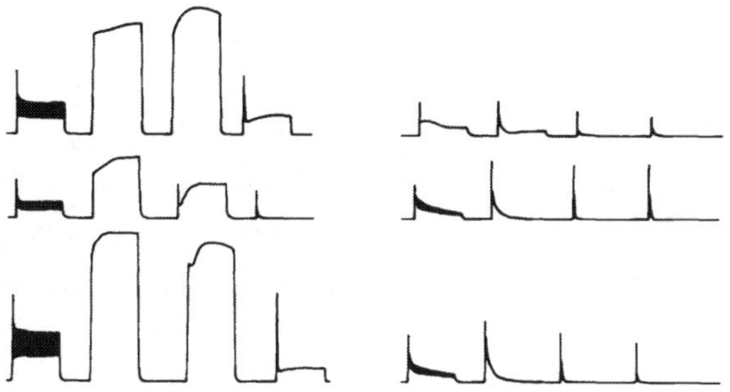

Fig. 1. Recordings of NMT of 6 rat diaphragm preparations. Three diaphragms (left row) were obtained 15 min after HI-6 (150 μmol/kg, i.v.) treatment (i.e. 75 min after $6xLD_{50}$, soman i.v.) and the other three (right row) were obtained 3.5 hours later. Note that after initial recovery, failure of neuromuscular transmission occurred.

II. Kinetics of soman

In order to verify the depot-hypothesis it was examined whether several hours after an intoxication with soman, sufficient amounts of the inhibitor are still available for inhibition of AChE. To detect anticholinesterase activity in intact animals, purified electric eel AChE was injected into the bloodstream of atropinized and anaesthetized rats at various time intervals after soman poisoning, and AChE-inhibition was determined in blood samples taken from these animals. The results are shown in figure 2 (2, 3). During the first few hours after soman, a fast progressive AChE-inhibition was observed, the rate of which depended on the time span between the injections of soman and enzyme. This inhibition was not due to soman already present in blood, since AChE added *in vitro* to blood samples from identically treated rats was hardly inhibited. So it appeared that *in vivo* an anticholinesterase, most likely soman itself, was leaking back into the bloodstream. In order to show that the anticholinesterase activity in the bloodsamples was due to soman itself, a gas-chromatographic procedure was developed by dr. L.P.A. de Jong et al. (Prins Maurits Laboratory TNO). Soman was identified and could be detected up to 90 min after poisoning. Bloodlevels up to that moment were in reasonable agreement with the apparent soman concentrations calculated from the AChE-inhibition in earlier experiments in which electric eel enzyme was injected into the bloodstream (3).
The influence of HI-6 on the inhibition of administered AChE *in vivo* was studied in identically treated rats which were injected with HI-6 in stead of saline (figure 2). Shortly after HI-6 injection, the oxime appeared to protect the enzyme to a large extent against reinhibition. In the subsequent hours the protection diminished ($t\frac{1}{2}$ of HI-6 = 18 min) and $2\frac{1}{4}$ hrs after HI-6 injection the effect had virtually disappeared.

III. Soman-simulator (som-sim) and the toxicokinetics of soman

Soman released from the depot may seriously complicate the therapy (Wolthuis and Kepner (5)). The question arose whether it would be possible to block the depot, or to chase soman from it, with a compound similar to

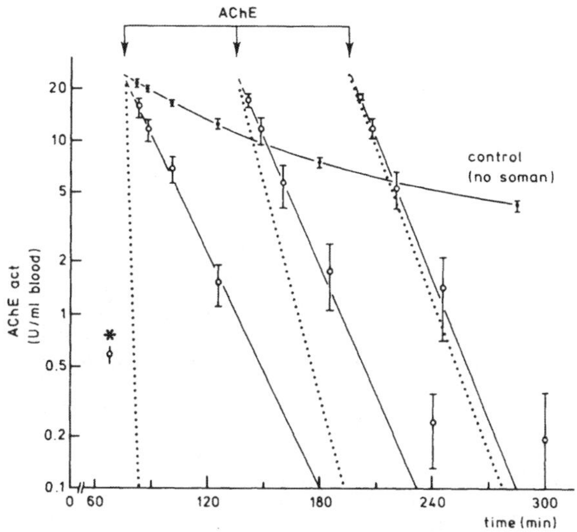

Fig. 2. Inhibition of electric eel AChE administered (i.v.) to rats at 75, 135 or 195 min after soman intoxication (6xLD_{50}, i.v., at t = 0). At t = 60 min, saline (....) or HI-6 (210 µmol/kg, i.v.)(————) was injected. * endogenous AChE activity in blood samples of control animals (= 0 in soman treated rats).

soman in chemical structure and lipophilicity but devoid of anticholinesterase activity. Such a compound was called a soman-simulator, and the first compound was nicknamed "som-sim" (3, 1). In the chemical structure of the first simulator synthesized, the fluorine atom of soman is replaced by an ethoxy group (see compound II, table 3). The LD_{50} of som-sim is 52 mg/kg, i.v. and higher than 500 mg/kg, i.p. The influence of som-sim on the course of inhibition of administered AChE into the bloodstream of soman-intoxicated rats is shown in figure 3. When som-sim was injected some time after the administration of AChE, the rate of inhibition of the enzyme increased almost instantaneously, presumably because soman was displaced from the depot. From this result it was concluded that som-sim competes with soman for the reversible binding sites, which are considered as the depot for soman. In view of the rapidity of the effect of som-sim, this depot appears to be readily accessible to the simulator.

Som-sim administration before soman caused an approximately 10-fold de-

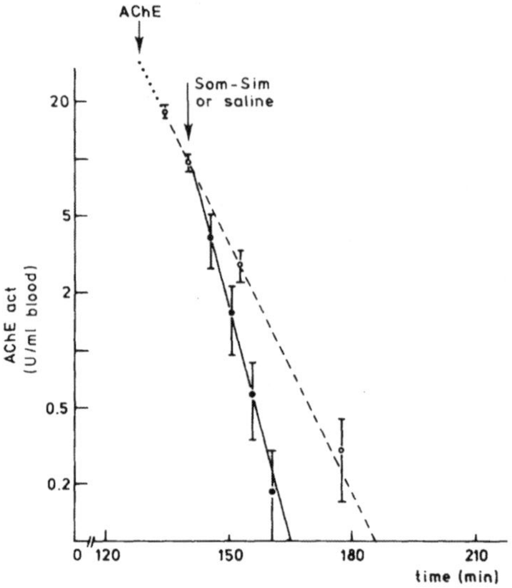

Fig. 3. Effect of som-sim (27 µmol/kg, i.v.) on the course of inhibition of i.v.-injected electric eel AChE in rats previously intoxicated with $6xLD_{50}$ soman (2.7 µmol/kg, i.v.). AChE is injected 135 min after soman. Thirteen min later saline (-----) or som-sim (————) was added to the bloodstream. The animals were kept alive with artificial ventilation.

crease in the rate of inhibition of AChE injected 75 min after the intoxication, whereas the inhibition of AChE injected one hour later proceeded approx. 6 times as slowly as in the absence of som-sim (fig. 4). Evidently, som-sim can occupy a significant part of the soman-depot. Consequently, a substantial amount of soman has to remain in circulation in stead of being protected in the depot. This may lead to a more rapid elimination.

IV. Improving effect of som-sim on the therapy against soman

On the basis of the results so far it would be expected that som-sim administration just before or soon after soman intoxication and subsequent HI-6 treatment, would lead to a beneficial effect on survival because in that case soman could not occupy the depot or would be expelled from it while sufficient amounts of HI-6 are still present to protect or reacti-

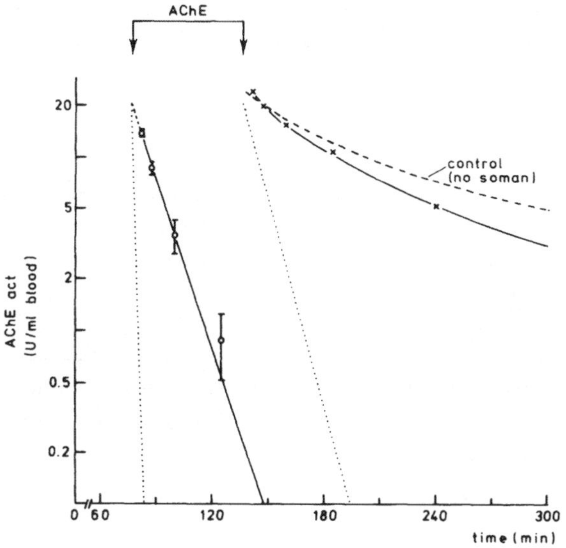

Fig. 4. Effect of som-sim (27 µmol/kg, i.v.), given 10 min before soman ($6xLD_{50}$, i.v.), on the course of inhibition of injected electric eel AChE in rats which were kept alive by artificial ventilation. AChE was injected 75 min or 135 min after soman.

vate AChE (3). In contrast, som-sim administration at a later stage after soman poisoning and subsequent oxime treatment, might cause a reduction in survival time since soman would be expelled from the depot at a time when most of the HI-6 had been eliminated. To investigate the effect of som-sim relative to the time of poisoning, anaesthetized, atropinized and artificially ventilated rats were injected with $8xLD_{50}$ soman and 15 min later with HI-6. Som-sim was given either 10 min before, 15 min after, or 75 min after soman (2). As predicted (table 2), administration of som-sim 75 min after soman caused a significant shortening of survival time. In contrast, all animals prophylactically treated with som-sim appeared in good condition. Their condition did not deterioriate during the next 24 hours nor during the week that followed. Som-sim administration 15 min after soman together with HI-6 did not significantly affect survival time, contrary to expectation.

In the absence of oxime, it would be expected that a concomitant administration of soman and som-sim, might lead to a larger lethality because

Table 2. Effect of som-sim (36 µmol/kg, i.v.) on survival time of atropinized, anaesthetized rats intoxicated with 8xLD_{50} soman (3.6 µmol/kg, i.v.) and treated 15 min later by HI-6 (210 µmol/kg, i.v.)*

Treatment	Mean (± S.E.M.) survival time (h) after soman	n
saline, 15 min after soman	6.5 ± 0.6	12
som-sim, 75 min after soman	4.6 ± 0.5**	12
som-sim, 15 min after soman	7.3 ± 0.6	12
som-sim, 10 min before soman	>24**	12

* Artificial ventilation was supplied during the first 30 min after soman. In the different groups som-sim or saline was injected at different times as indicated.

** Significantly different ($p<0.05$, two-tailed) from control groups.

more soman remains available to contribute to the acute toxicity. However, attempts to demonstrate such an effect failed. The lethality of an LD_{10} of soman was not increased by som-sim.

V. Localisation of the soman-depot

Several attempts to discover the localisation of the soman-depot in various parts of the body, a.o. by the use of radioactively labelled som-sim, yielded disappointing results. In recent experiments, however, isolated diaphragms taken from soman-poisoned rats treated with HI-6, were studied for neuromuscular transmission (NMT) during incubation in medium. They showed a gradual failure of NMT (fig. 5). This finding suggested that at least part of the soman was stored in the muscle tissue from which it was released in sufficient amounts to inhibit neuromuscular function almost completely (4). This inhibition could only be prevented to a slight degree by repeated washings of the muscle preparations, indicating that

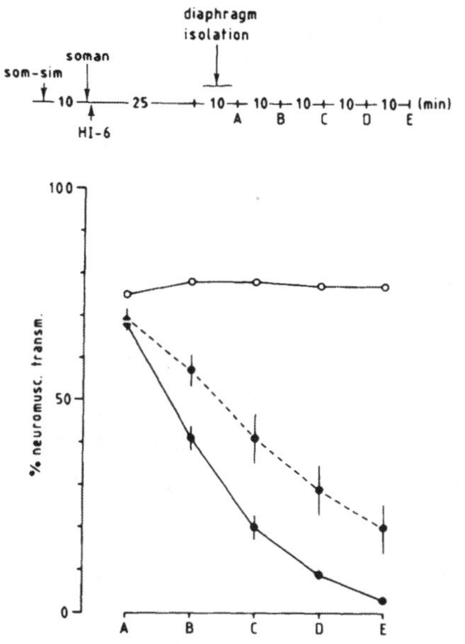

Fig. 5. Neuromuscular transmission (NMT) in rat diaphragm preparations expressed in % of NMT of 25 untreated control preparations. As indicated at the top of the figure the treated preparations originated from anaesthetized atropinized rats, decapitated 25 min after administration of $8xLD_{50}$ soman (3.6 µmol/kg, i.v.) and HI-6 (150 µmol/kg, i.v.). Five animals had been pretreated with som-sim (O), eleven were not (●). Six preparations from the latter group were subjected to repeated washing (see broken line). Every 10 min after decapitation NMT in the diaphragms was tested (A, B, C, D and E). Som-sim pretreatment prevented the gradual decrease of NMT. Repeated washing had only a small effect. Vertical bars indicate S.E.M., in the som-sim treated group they were too small to be drawn.

most of the soman was not just absorbed in the tissue. In vivo pretreatment of the animals with som-sim prevented NMT-failure in vitro, which suggested specific binding of soman in the muscle tissue at non-cholinesteratic sites and again indicated that the observed NMT-failure was not merely a reflection of soman aspecifically absorbed in the tissue.

VI. Structural specificity of the depot for soman-simulators

So far, the results indicated that the accumulation of soman in its depot can be influenced by som-sim. The question arose whether analogues of som-sim would be effective and whether structure-activity relationships could be observed. Several analogues of som-sim were synthesized and tested for their efficacy to prevent death and re-appearance of NMT-failure after soman intoxication and oxime treatment (8). Upon pretreatment with these simulators (figure 6), re-appearance of NMT-failure could be prevented to various degrees. When R was O-alkyl (Table 3; compounds I-IV), a good effect was observed when the alkyl group either was methyl (I) or ethyl (II)(som-sim), but it decreased markedly upon chain lengthening (III) or branching (IV). Substitution of the O-alkyl chain by a methyl group or by hydrogen (V and VI respectively), resulted in a pre-

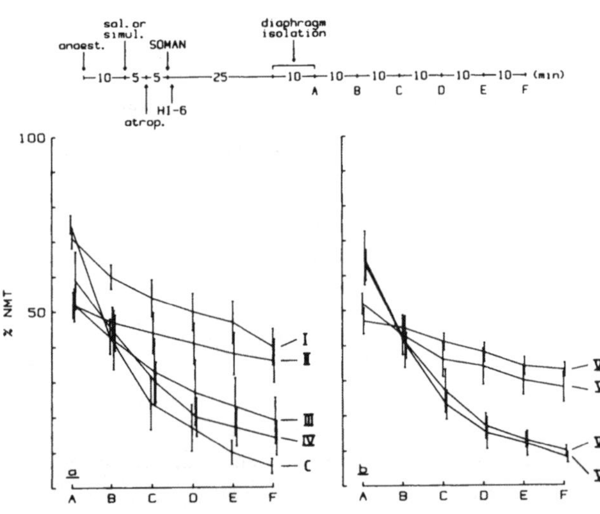

Fig. 6. Mean (± S.E.M.) neuromuscular transmission (NMT) in rat diaphragm preparations expressed as a percentage of the NMT determined separately in 20 untreated control preparations. Each experimental group consisted of 5 animals and the control group (C) of 9 animals. From each animal 2 diaphragm strips were tested. The soman dosage was $8xLD_{50}$ (3.6 µmol/kg, i.v.), whereas the HI-6 dose was 150 µmol/kg, i.v. The structures of compounds I-VIII are shown in table 3. The time schedule is shown at the top of the figure. Note that pretreatment with various simulators (I-VIII) prevented the gradual decrease of NMT to different degrees.

vention of NMT-failure comparable to the effect of I or II. Simulators structurally unrelated to soman (VII and VIII), were ineffective.
With regard to survival, the same trends were visible (table 3) in that pretreatment with I, II, V or VI resulted in a significantly better survival than that of control animals and tended to be better than that of animals pretreated with III or IV. Prophylaxis with V even saved all animals. Compounds VII and VIII were ineffective as before.
These findings suggest that the simulators have to meet certain requirements in order to block the binding sites in the depot effectively. Replacement of the fluorine atom of soman by small groups led to effective simulators, whereas replacement by larger groups rendered them ineffective. Hence, these results indicate the presence of reversible, specific binding sites in the depot.

TABLE 3.

Effects of prophylaxis with soman-simulators (I-VIII, 36 µmol/kg, i.v.) on survival (times) of anaesthetized atropinized (50 mg/kg, i.p.) rats poisoned with 6 x LD50 soman (2.7 µmol/kg i.v.) and subsequently treated with HI-6 (150 µmol/kg i.v.). In soman R = fluorine. The time schedule of the experiment - shown at the top of the table - is comparable to that of experiment A (see figure). * = significantly different from control animals.

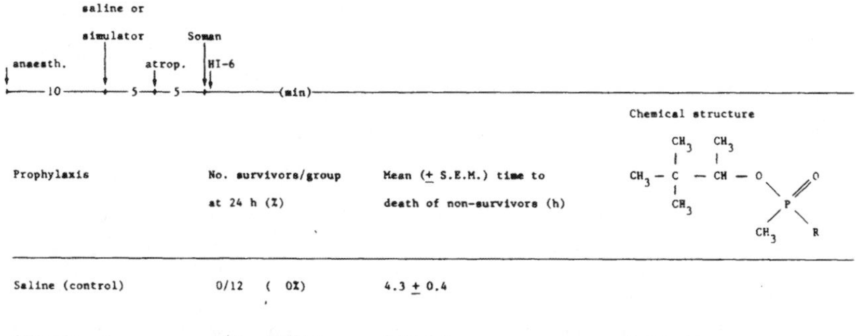

Chemical structure

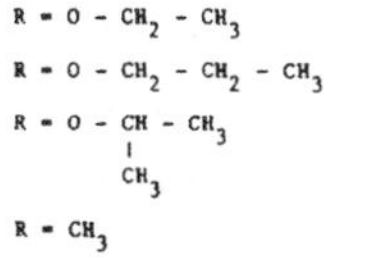

Prophylaxis	No. survivors/group at 24 h (%)	Mean (± S.E.M.) time to death of non-survivors (h)	Chemical structure
Saline (control)	0/12 (0%)	4.3 ± 0.4	
Compound: I	9/12 (75%) *	3.3 ± 2.6	$R = O - CH_3$
II	9/12 (75%) *	2.6 ± 1.8	$R = O - CH_2 - CH_3$
III	6/12 (50%) *	4.0 ± 1.7	$R = O - CH_2 - CH_2 - CH_3$
IV	4/12 (30%)	0.7 ± 0.1*	$R = O - CH(CH_3) - CH_3$
V	15/15 (100%) *		$R = CH_3$
VI	7/12 (58%) *	5.8 ± 2.6	$R = H$
VII	2/12 (16%)	4.2 ± 1.4	$[(CH_3)_2CHO]_3\ P = O$
VIII	0/12 (0%)	3.3 ± 0.3	$(CH_3CH_2CH_2O)_3\ P = O$

VII. Discussion

Complete inhibition of purified electric eel AChE injected into the bloodstream several hours after soman poisoning, led to the conclusion that soman was released from a depot into the bloodstream. This auto-infusion with soman was held responsible for enzyme reinhibition at the motor-endplate, the re-appearance of NMT failure and subsequent death (1, 2, 3). Later results indicated that a significant part of soman is stored at sites in muscle tissue, presumably in the vicinity of the motor-endplate (4).

It is unknown whether muscle tissue contains the only storage site of soman, but since about 45% of the body mass of the rat consists of muscle, a large storage capacity is potentially available. It is unlikely that a significant part of persistent soman is present in the blood of the rat, since AChE added to blood samples derived from soman poisoned animals 75 min after the intoxication of the animal, did not undergo the inactivation observed in vivo (1). The suggestion by Clement (9) that aliesterase in blood may act as a depot, is hard to understand since after disruption of the covalent bond between soman and the enzyme, soman has lost its potency to inhibit AChE. His findings can only be explained if soman is bound to aliesterase in a releasable form, for which there is no evidence. At any rate, if aliesterase binds soman in an unknown way and acts as a depot it is a depot quite different from the one described here, since the time scales for soman release do not fit and since it cannot be influenced by som-sim (Clement, personal communication). As the amount of soman released into the bloodstream may be only a small part of the total amount of depot-soman, it is not surprising that Sterri et al. (10) found very little storage of soman in the organism after injection of sublethal doses. It may very well be that administration of smaller amounts of soman will not lead to a significant storage. This would fit in with the finding that som-sim did not increase lethality after an LD_{10} of soman. However, care should be excercised in extrapolating data about a soman-depot in the rat to other species; Clement used mice and Sterri et al. used guinea pigs.

Although attempts failed to increase the toxicity of the LD_{10} of soman in rats by a pretreatment 10 min prior to soman with som-sim (7.5 mg/kg, i.v.), Talbot et al. (11) recently reported a 25% enhanced sensitivity of rats by pretreatment with this simulator (15 mg/kg, i.m.), 30 min prior to soman.

In conclusion, the findings reported in this paper are indicative of the existence of a soman-depot which complicates the therapy of soman poisoning. At the same time, however, they show that the concept of using non-toxic simulators, competing for the storage site(s) of soman, may yield valuable insight and improved treatment.

VIII. Summary

Experiments in our laboratory showed that atropinized rats could initially be saved from lethal doses of soman (up to $8xLD_{50}$) by HI-6 treatment. In the hours that followed, however, the condition of the animals deteriorated and they died showing symptoms of organophosphate poisoning. Shortly before death neuromuscular function failed, death could be postponed by repeated HI-6 injections.

Purified electric eel acetylcholinesterase (AChE), injected i.v., 75, 135 or 195 min after poisoning with $6xLD_{50}$ soman, was rapidly inhibited, presumably by a gradual release of soman from a depot. The rate of inhibition of injected AChE was decreased by HI-6 injected 60 min after soman intoxication.

The hypothesis of a depot was supported by the results obtained with a soman-simulator (som-sim), a non-toxic organophosphate structurally similar to soman but devoid of anticholinesterase activity. The evidence indicated that som-sim can expel soman from the depot or, given prophylactically, can prevent soman accumulation in the depot.

At least part of the soman-depot appeared to be localized in muscle tissue.

In vivo pretreatment with various soman-simulators prevented re-appearance of NMT failure *in vitro* and improved the survival to different degrees. These results give evidence for reversible binding of soman at the depot site(s), in which structural specificity is involved.

Keywords: soman-depot soman-simulators structural specificity organophosphate HI-6 oxime

Acknowledgement

The authors are grateful to mrs. H.J. van der Wiel and mrs. E. Mobach of the Medical Biological Laboratory TNO and to mr. G.R. van den Berg of the Prins Maurits Laboratory TNO for their expert technical assistance.

References

1. Wolthuis, O.L., Berends, F., Meeter, E.: Fundam. Appl. Toxic. 1, 183-193 (1981a).
2. Wolthuis, O.L., Benschop, H.P., Berends, F.: Eur. J. Pharmacol. 69, 379-383 (1981b).
3. Benschop, H.P., Berends, F., De Jong, L.P.A.: Fundam. Appl. Toxic. 1, 177-183 (1981).
4. Van Helden, H.P.M., Wolthuis, O.L.: Eur. J. Pharmacol. 89, 271-274 (1983).
5. Wolthuis, O.L., Kepner, L.A.: Eur. J. Pharmacol. 49, 415-425 (1978)
6. Christen, P.J., Van der Muysenberg, J.A.C.M.: Biochim. Biophys. Acta 110, 217-227 (1965).
7. Frederiksson, T.: Acta Dermato-Venereol. 49, 490-498 (1969)
8. Van Helden, H.P.M., Benschop, H.P., Wolthuis, O.L.: J. Pharm. Pharmacol. (in press).
9. Clement, J.G.: Biochem. Pharmacol. 31, 4085-4089 (1982).
10. Sterri, S.H., Kloster, Ø., Valdal, G.: Acta Pharmacol. Toxicol. 50, 326-331 (1982).
11. Talbot, B.G., Heyl, W.C., Kindell, C., Lennot, W.J., Green, M.D., Braun, R.A., Harris, L.W.: Fed. Proc. 42, 890 (1983).

DETOXIFICATION OF ORGANOPHOSPHORUS COMPOUNDS

Sigrun H Sterri and Frode Fonnum

Norwegian Defence Research Establishment, Division for Environmental Toxicology
2007 Kjeller, Norway

Introduction

It is well established that highly toxic organophosphorus compounds are detoxificated through hydrolysis catalyzed by phosphorylphosphatase(s) which are widely distributed in the body (1, 2, 3, 4). Moreover, detoxification may also result from covalent binding of organophosphorus compounds to serine hydrolases other than AChE, i.e. BuChE and aliesterases (= carboxylesterase) (5, 6, 7).

In the present paper we will summarize our results concerning the significance of aliesterase and phosphorylphosphatase for detoxification of soman and sarin in rodents. This has been evaluated by studying the effect of repetitive administration of sublethal doses in rat, guinea-pig and mouse (8, 9, 10, 11), by perfusion of rat liver with soman solutions (12), by inhalation experiments with soman in rat (13), and by the use of aliesterase inhibitors. Also, two different substrates for aliesterase have been studied and indicates the presence of heterogeneity among this class of enzymes.

Materials and Methods

Organophosphorus compounds, soman [O-(1, 2, 2-trimethylpropyl)-methyl-fluorophosphonate], sarin (isopropyl-methyl-fluorophosphonate) and tri-o-cresyl phosphate (TOCP), were obtained and handled as described (8, 9, 10, 12, 13). Methyl-[1-^{14}C]-butyrate (0,41 Ci/mole), purer than 99%, was synthesized in our laboratory. Animals were purchased from the National Institute of Public Health, Oslo.

Tissues were collected and prepared as described (8, 9, 12). For aliesterase measurement in lung, or to compare two different substrates, the animals were etheranaesthesized and perfused with 40 ml saline through the heart ventricles before dissection. This removed the contamination of blood in the tissues.

ChEs were determined by the radiochemical method of Sterri and Fonnum (14), with 0,1 mM ethopropazine to inhibit BuChE in the assay mixture for AChE.

Aliesterase was determined by three methods:

A. By the Warburg technique with 15,7 mM tributyrine as the substrate (15, 9).

B. Spectrophotometrically mostly as described by Ljungquist and Augustinsson (16) with 1,9 mM p-nitrophenyl butyrate as the substrate.

C. By the radiochemical method of Sterri et al (to be published) with 1,9 mM methyl-[1-^{14}C]-butyrate as the substrate (Fig. 1).

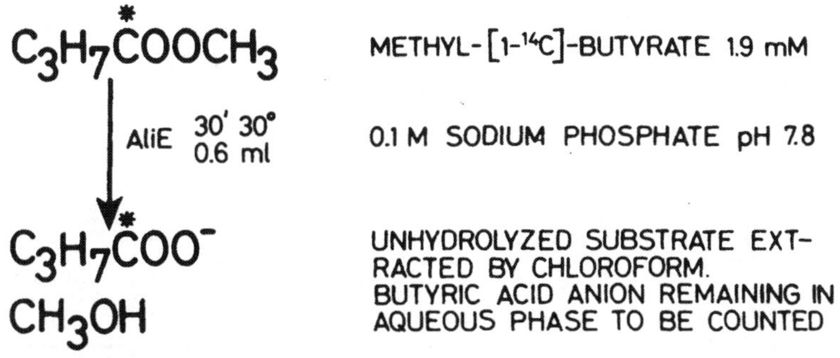

Fig. 1 Radiochemical method for aliesterase measurement

Results

Repetitive injection of 0,4-0,6 acute LD_{50} of soman or sarin in several groups of rats, guinea-pigs or mice at several constant time intervals led to different cumulative LD_{50}, which increased when the time interval between doses increased (Table 1). In some cases 50% mortality was not reached even after a total exposure of 4-6 times the acute LD_{50}.

A linear relationship was found between the cumulative LD_{50} and the same divided by the dosing regimen (= the single doses given divided by the time interval between them) (Fig. 2). The linearity existed for each species and for both intraperitoneal (i.p.) and subcutaneous (s.c.) route of administration. The slope of the lines gives the rate of detoxification, and the intercept is the acute LD_{50}.

In both rats and guinea-pigs pretreated with TOCP, an alieste-

Table 1. LD_{50} of soman in rat and guinea-pig

Species and route	Acute LD_{50} (µg/kg)	Cumulative LD_{50} (µg/kg) Time between injections 4 hrs	8 hrs	12 hrs	24 hrs
Rat i.p.	200	245	430	480	not reached
Guinea-pig s.c.	26	59	78	143	not reached

Soman doses at time intervals indicated were 75 µg/kg (rat) and 13 µg/kg (guinea-pig). Data extracted from Sterri et al (8, 9).

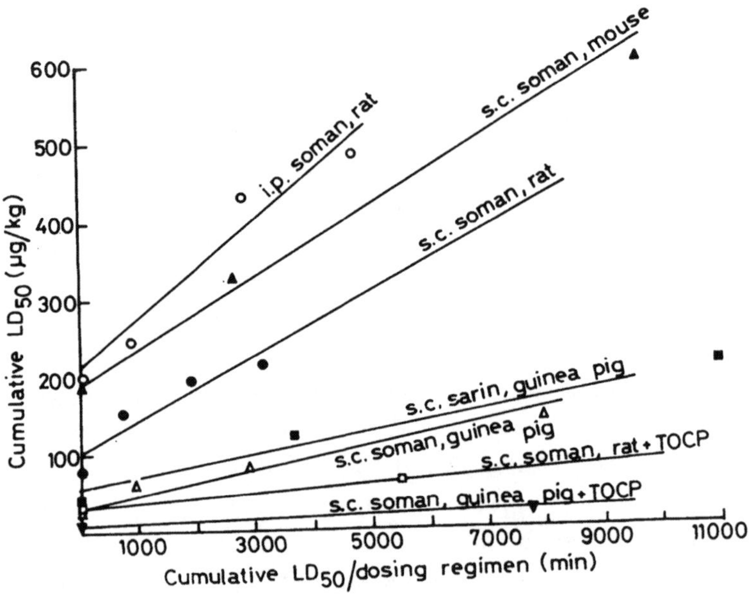

Fig.2 Linear regression analysis of cumulative LD_{50} of soman and sarin in repetitive injection experiments. Data, except soman + TOCP in rat, extracted from Sterri et al (8, 9, 10)

rase inhibitor (17), the acute LD_{50} of soman was one third and the rate of detoxification was one seventh of that without TOCP pretreatment (Fig. 2). Esterase measurements before repetitive injection experiments showed that TOCP treatment did not lead to any significant reduction in ChE activities (Table 2).

Esterase measurements in animals (without TOCP) throughout repetitive injection experiments showed that several injections of soman were needed for extensive inhibition of AChE in brain and diaphragm, whereas ChEs in blood were strongly inhibited after one injection (Table 2). Aliesterase in plasma, but not in liver, was highly reduced after one injection, but recovered within 24 hrs (Table 2).

Table 2. Esterase activities in rat and guinea-pig after administration of TOCP or soman

Compound species x injection	Time after injection (hrs)	Esterase activity (% of control) AChE			ChE		Aliesterase	
		Erythrocytes	Brain	Diaphragm	Plasma	Liver	Plasma	Liver
TOCP								
rat	20	-	100	-	91	87	4	3
guinea-pig	20	-	98	-	93	-	10	-
Soman								
rat	24	15	97	99	-	102	-	-
x4	24	2	80	65	-	99	-	-
x11	24	3	31	20	-	-	-	-
Soman								
guinea-pig	1	14	100	98	12	-	35	89
x2	1	2	100	102	11	-	27	76
x2	24	6	-	-	43	-	95	98
x11	1	2	35	20	10	-	32	77

TOCP dose = 100 mg/kg s.c.
Soman dose = 75 µg/kg i.p. (rat) or 13 µg/kg s.c. (guinea-pig)
Time between soman injections 24 hrs
Aliesterase = tributyrinase
Data on soman extracted from Sterri et al (8, 9)

Like the aliesterase activity, also the ChE activity in liver was only inhibited to a small extent in the repetitive injection experiments (Table 2). This low inhibition of aliesterase and ChE in liver was confirmed by perfusion experiments with low concentration (4 μM) of soman through rat liver (Fig. 3).

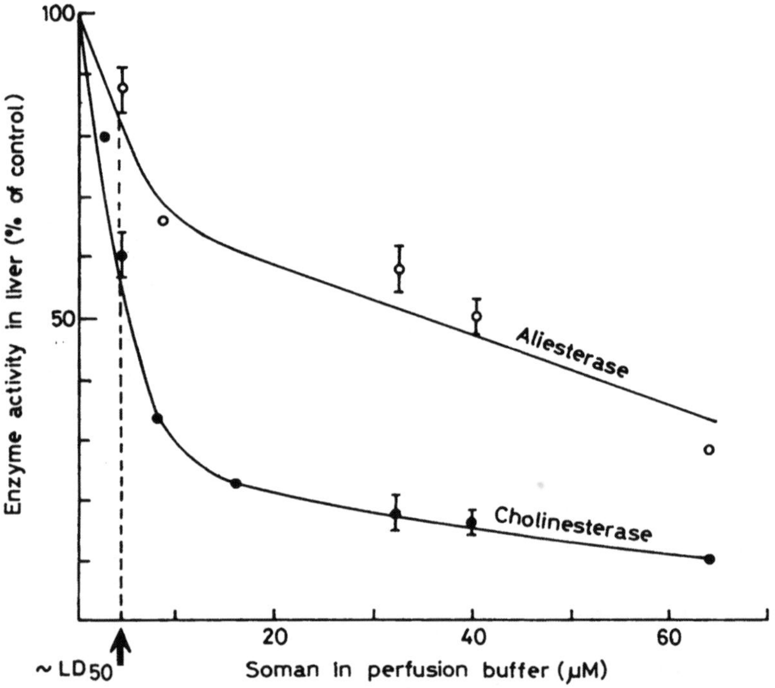

Fig. 3 Esterase activities in rat liver after perfusion with 50 ml Krebs-Ringer containing soman. Aliesterase = tributyrinase (From Sterri et al (12))

However, the inhibition of the two enzymes increased with stronger concentration of soman in the perfusion buffer (Fig. 3). The liver perfusion experiments also demonstrated that liver possess a high capacity of soman detoxification. Thus, 80-90% of soman was detoxificated during a single pass through the liver, even of an amount corresponding to 8 times the i.p. LD_{50} (Table 3). At this concentration of soman the aliesterase and ChE activities were inhibited 40% and 80% respectively (Fig. 3).

Table 3. Soman in rat liver and perfusate after perfusion with Krebs-Ringer containing 228 μg soman (= 100%) ≈ 8 x i.p. LD_{50}

Rat no	Soman (%) Liver	Perfusate
1	6	14
2	6	9
3	8	1
4	7	3

Data extracted from Sterri et al (12)

Table 4. Esterase activities in rat following inhalation of soman

Soman mgmin/m^3	Esterase activity (% of control) Bronchi		Lung		Plasma		Liver		Brain
	AliE	ChE	AliE	ChE	AliE	ChE	AliE	ChE	AChE
Lethal 520	23	3	53	3	13	6	99	90	2
207	41	38	72	27	87	43	-	-	75

AliE = aliesterase, methylbutyrate was the substrate

The aliesterase and ChE activities in liver were not inhibited following lethal exposure of rats to inhalation of soman, whereas the enzymes in bronchi and lung were inhibited to a similar extent as the plasma enzymes (Table 4).

Some measurements were performed, with the substrates methyl butyrate and p-nitrophenyl butyrate used in parallel, to investigate the distribution of aliesterase in different organs. With selected inhibitor compounds in vitro (30 min) it was found that both substrates are fairly good for aliesterase in different organs, except brain (Table 5). There was only minor hydrolysis due to ChE and no hydrolysis by arylesterase (Table 5). Interestingly, however, the ratio between aliesterase activities in various organs as measured with methyl butyrate was quite different from that with p-nitrophenyl butyrate, except for the liver/lung ratio (Table 6).

Table 5. Effect of inhibitor compounds on aliesterase activities in vitro

Substrate	Inhibitor (M)	Activity (% of control)				
		Rat				Guinea-pig
		Plasma	Liver	Lung	Brain	plasma
Methyl-butyrate	BPNPP 10^{-4}	30	3	1	46	1
	Physost 10^{-5}	95	90	97	92	96
	EDTA 10^{-4}	102	95	97	102	97
p-nitro-phenyl-butyrate	BPNPP 10^{-4}	38	18	4	81	1
	Physost 10^{-5}	95	83	91	89	90
	EDTA 10^{-4}	99	100	98	111	104

BPNPP = bis-p-nitrophenyl phosphate = aliesterase inhibitor (18)
Physost = physostigmine = ChE inhibitor (19)
EDTA = arylesterase inhibitor (20, 21)

Table 6. Ratio of aliesterase activities

Substrate	Rat: Liver/Plasma	Rat: Liver/Lung	Rat: Liver/Brain	Guinea-pig plasma/Rat plasma
Methyl-butyrate	1750	3	1550	20
p-nitrophenyl-butyrate	80	3	34	5

Discussion

The results show that rodents can tolerate several fold the acute LD_{50} of soman or sarin when they are exposed over a long period (Table 1, Fig. 2). This effect of repetitive injection of sublethal doses should not be due to any specific reactivation of functional AChE in the diaphragm (8). Neither should it be due to any induction of phosphorylphosphatase hydrolyzing soman in the liver (8).

The results indicates, however, that the effect may be due to binding of soman and sarin to aliesterase and subsequent recovery of that enzyme. Thus, 80-90% of the repetitively administered soman was detoxificated through binding to TOCP sensitive sites, which may be considered as aliesterase (Fig. 2, Table 2). Further, the recovery of plasma aliesterase within 24 hrs (Table 2), correlated well with the time interval between doses which did not lead to any cumulative LD_{50} (Table 1).

Therefore, plasma aliesterase may act as a scavenger and remove soman and sarin circulating in the blood stream before they reach the target organs (brain and diaphragm). This is consistent with the fact that AChE activities in brain and diaphragm were not extensively inhibited until several injections had been performed (Table 2).

Large amounts of sarin and DFP are known to combine with plasma aliesterase from rat and guinea-pig (22, 23, 24, 25). At the moment, however, it is uncertain whether binding to plasma aliesterase alone may account for the large proportion (80-90%) of soman found to be detoxificated through binding to TOCP sensitive sites during the repetitive injection experiments.

Based on activity measurements, the aliesterase in liver does not seem to have any important significance in detoxification of soman (Table 2, Fig. 3, Table 4). The high capacity of soman detoxification in liver during perfusion (Table 3) may mostly be due to the action of phosphorylphosphatase (3), since neither aliesterase nor ChE was fully inhibited until large concentrations of soman were used in the perfusion buffer (Fig. 3).

The aliesterase in lung tissue may be able to bind soman to a similar extent as the ChEs in lung based on activity measurements (Table 4). At the moment, however, it does not seem to constitute any barrier for soman to reach the blood stream during inhalation (Table 4).

Aliesterase is a very unspecific enzyme (or a group of unspecific enzymes or isoenzymes), several substrates can therefore be used for activity measurements (see 26, 27, 28 for review). The results indicate that both methyl butyrate and p-nitrophenyl butyrate are good substrates for aliesterase in plasma, liver and lung (Table 5). However, it seems to be two different groups of aliesterase which are measured with the two substrates (Table 6). Whether these groups of aliesterase may also have different affinity for soman in different tissues is a matter of further investigation in our laboratory.

References

1. Mazur, A.: J. Biol. Chem. 164, 271-289 (1946).

2. Augustinsson, K.-B., Heimbürger, G.: Acta chem. scand. 8, 753-761 (1954).

3. Mounter, L.A., Dien, L.T.H., Chanutin, A.: J. Biol. Chem. 215, 691-697 (1955).

4. Adie, P.A.: Can. J. Biochem. Physiol. 36, 15-20 (1958).

5. Aldridge, W.N.: Biochem. J. 53, 110-117 (1953).

6. Aldridge, W.N., Davison, A.N.: Biochem. J. 55, 763-766 (1953).

7. Jansz, H.S., Posthumus, C.H., Cohen, J.A.: Biochim. Biophys. Acta 33, 396-403 (1959).

8. Sterri, S.H., Lyngaas, S., Fonnum, F.: Acta pharmacol. et toxicol. 46, 1-7 (1980).

9. Sterri, S.H., Lyngaas, S., Fonnum, F.: Acta pharmacol. et toxicol. 49, 8-13 (1981).

10. Sterri, S.H.: Acta pharmacol. et toxicol. 49, Suppl. V 67-71 (1981).

11. Sterri, S.H., Kloster, Ø., Valdal G.: Acta pharmacol. et toxicol. 50, 326-331 (1982).

12. Sterri, S.H., Valdal, G., Lyngaas, S., Odden, E., Malthe-Sørenssen, D., Fonnum, F.: Biochem. Pharmacol. 32, 1941-1943 (1983).

13. Fonnum, F., Aas, P., Sterri, S.H., Helle, K.B.: Fundam. Appl. Toxicol. (1983) in press.

14. Sterri, S.H., Fonnum, F.: Eur. J. Biochem. 91, 215-222 (1978).

15. DuBois, K.P., Kinoshita, F.K., Frawley, J.P.: Toxicol. Appl. Pharmacol. 12, 273-284 (1968).

16. Ljungquist, Å., Augustinsson, K.-B.: Eur. J. Biochem. 23, 303-313 (1971).

17. Mendel, B., Myers, D.K.: Biochem. J. 53, xvi (1953).

18. Heymann, E., Krisch, K.: Hoppe-Seyler's Z. Physiol. Chem. 348, 609-619 (1967).

19. Myers, D.K., Mendel, B.: Proc. Soc. Exptl. Biol. Med. 71, 357-360 (1949).

20. Marton, A.V., Kalow, W.: Biochem. Pharmacol. 3, 149-154 (1960).

21. Augustinsson, K.-B.: Ann.N.Y.Acad.Sci. 94, 844-860 (1961).

22. Myers, D.K.: Science 115, 568-570 (1952).

23. Goutier, R.: Biochim. Biophys. Acta 19, 524-534 (1956).

24. Christen, P.J., Cohen, E.M.: Acta physiol. pharmacol. Neerlandica 15, 36-37 (1969).

25. Polak, R.L., Cohen, E.M.: Biochem. Pharmacol. 19, 877-881 (1970).

26. Krisch, K.: In "The Enzymes" (ed. Boyer, P.D.) 5, 43-69 (1971).

27. Junge, W., Krisch, K.: Crit. Rev. Toxicol. 3, 371-434 (1975).

28. Heymann, E.: In "Enzymatic Basis of Detoxication" (ed. Jakoby, W.B.) 291-323, Academic Press (1980).

CONSEQUENCES OF ACETYLCHOLINESTERASE INHIBITION IN FAST AND SLOW MUSCLE OF RAT

Wolf-D. Dettbarn

Department of Pharmacology
Vanderbilt University School of Medicine
Nashville, Tennessee 37212, U.S.A.

Introduction

The structural integrity of skeletal muscle depends on the presence and normal function of neuromuscular transmission. Dysfunction may lead to changes in the development, maintenance, and integrity of the endplate and muscle fiber. Acetylcholinesterase (AChE), a constituent of the membranes at the synapse, plays an essential role in the removal of acetylcholine (ACh) from the synaptic cleft by hydrolyzing ACh to choline and acetic acid. Inhibition of AChE profoundly modifies neuromuscular transmission. This was shown by electrophysiological analyses, by studies of the muscle response to nerve stimulation and by observations on spontaneous muscular activity in the intact animal. Reports from several laboratories have shown that some of the reversible as well as irreversible AChE inhibitors induced myopathies (1-7). Injection of these agents produced a progressive myopathy in skeletal muscle. The earliest lesions noted were focal areas of abnormality close to the surface of the muscle fibers. These focal changes progressed to a generalized breakdown of fiber architecture, characterized by a loss of staining quality followed finally by phagocytosis. Longitudinal sections indicated that the early changes in a focal necrosis affected only a small segment of fiber lengths. The later stages affected progressively greater lengths of muscle fibers. Ultrastructural studies of motor nerve terminals showed varying degress of change within 30 minutes to 2 hours after AChE inhibition (4). Some nerve terminals appeared relatively normal with the exception of slightly swollen mitochondria. More severely affected nerve terminals displayed myelin figures, membrane enclosures, and an increase in the number of large coated vesicles. More obvious changes were seen in the subsynaptic area and the surrounding muscle fiber. Soman, paraoxon and neostigmine initiated the formation of vesicular structures in the primary and secondary subsynaptic cleft (8, 4, 7). Occasionally some of these were seen in the sarcoplasm. Many of the cleft vesicles were similar in density and size to synaptic vesicles but with considerable variation in diameter. The severity of lesions in the subsynaptic folds varied even within the same muscle. Normal subsynaptic clefts with few cleft vesicles were seen side by side with subsynaptic clefts with many cleft vesicles and a widening of the cleft itself. In addition to the changes seen in the region of the endplate, AChE inhibitors caused changes in the muscle fibers themselves. Muscle surrounding the motor endplate showed a disruption of cytoarchitectural organization. Initially the first changes were in the mitochondria which showed swelling, leading to lysis of the central cristae. Myelin figures beneath the endplate were frequently observed while the region more distal to the endplate was less affected. The nucleoli of the muscle cell nucleus were enlarged and moved to the periphery of the nucleus. There was an increase in the number of sarcoplasmic ribosomes, the sarcoplasmic reticulum became dilated followed by a loss of striation of the myofibrils, and later total destruction of the myofilaments and fragmentation of the Z bands occurred. The role of AChE inhibition as the triggering factor leading to excessive ACh mediated hyperactivity in muscle and nerve is strongly supported by the observation that 2-PAM prevented the necrosis (5). The possibility exists, however, that the AChE inhibitors may have a direct action, unrelated to AChE on the postsynaptic membrane and along the muscle fiber. Functional recovery took place at a much faster rate than that of enzyme activity, which also varied between the muscle types and inhibitors used. Little evidence is available in rat muscle, beyond measurements of overall AChE activity on the fine dynamics of enzyme recovery after regaining functional control (9, 10). Metabolic characteristics among the various molecular forms of AChE could be responsible for the observed differences after irreversible inhibition. Further analysis appeared therefore desirable. Although the general importance of AChE in neuromuscular transmission is well established, the possible physiological role of the individual molecular weight forms remained unclear. Recently, differences in molecular species distribution of AChE were observed in rat skeletal muscle following denervation (11). A study of the multiple forms of AChE (16S, 12S, 10S, and 4S) and their distribution in endplate and non-endplate regions, indicated that the 4S and 10S forms are mainly found in non-endplate regions while the 16S and 12S forms are highly but not exclusively concentrated in the endplate region (12, 13). Two irreversible inhibitors, the tertiary phospholine and the quaternary phospholine, were used to investigate the localization of the AChE critical to the development of the necrosis. The quaternary phospholine form is poorly lipid soluble and should inhibit only the extracellularly localized AChE. The tertiary phospholine is highly lipid soluble and should inhibit AChE whether intracellularly or extracellularly located. In addition we have studied the rate of recovery of the individual forms after irreversible inhibition. Changes in the relative proportions of the various forms during prolonged recovery provided insight into the biosynthetic process of AChE.

Methods

Male Sprague-Dawley rats maintained on a 12 hr light/dark cycle were used for all studies. Drugs were dissolved in saline and administered subcutaneously (0.1 ml/100g/b. wt.). The duration and degree of enzyme inhibition and myopathic severity were studied in muscles from animals injected with paraoxon (0.23 mg/kg), tertiary phospholine (0.2 mg/kg) and quaternary phospholine (0.08 mg/kg). The rats were sacrificed 60 minutes-14 days after drug administration for biochemical analyses or 24 hours-7 days after drug administration for histochemical analyses.

For biochemical analyses the left hemidiaphragm, soleus (SOL), and extensor digitorum longus (EDL) muscles were removed. The tissue was weighed, minced and homogenized in phosphate buffer. AChE activity was determined according to previously published procedures (11).

For the analysis of molecular weight forms SOL and EDL were homogenized in velocity sedimentation buffer and prepared for linear gradient centrifugation (11, 12, 13). Histochemical analysis: The muscles were removed, cleaned and frozen in isopentane cooled in liquid nitrogen, mounted with Ames OCT compound and 10 um sections were cut in a cryostat and stained with trichrome as an indicator of fiber necrosis. Five muscle regions were selected from each slide with 16X objective and photographed. Only those regions with grouped lesions (two or more/field) were considered to be indicative of the localized myopathy. Normal muscles were used as control. The total number of fibers per field were counted and analyzed quantitatively as previously described (9). Results were expressed as number of lesions per 1000 fibers.

Results

To determine the role of the various molecular forms of AChE in the muscle necrosis, animals were injected with phospholine iodide, a quaternary organophosphate with limited lipid solubility, thought to inhibit only externally localized AChE such as the 16S form, mainly localized in the endplate. Other animals were injected with phospholine oxalate, the tertiary form of the organophosphate. This compound, being highly lipid soluble, has access to the internally located molecular forms of AChE as well and thus inhibits external as well as internal localized enzyme. As Table I shows, both compounds caused lesions in the muscles tested.

While SOL was equally vulnerable to either of the inhibitors used, however, in the EDL, tertiary phospholine caused a significantly higher number of lesions than the quaternary form. It is also apparent that the quaternary compound had better access to the enzyme in SOL than in EDL, since overall activity of AChE was reduced to less than 40% in SOL while in EDL the remaining AChE activity was as high as 70% of control. In order to determine the distribution of the molecular forms of AChE in these muscles and their accessibility to the two forms of the inhibitor used, both muscles were removed one hour after injection of the inhibitor to be determined, and muscle extracts were applied to sucrose gradients. As can be seen from Fig. 1B, in SOL the quaternary phospholine reduced all molecular forms to less than 40% including the 4S form, which has been postulated to be intracellular, while the tertiary compound (Fig. 1A) inhibited the activity of all molecular forms to less than 10% of control activity. In the EDL (Fig. 2B), the quaternary inhibitor had little effect on the 4S form, while the activity of the 16S and that of the 10S forms were reduced to 50% of control. The tertiary phospholine (Fig. 2A) reduced AChE activity of all forms to less than 10%, as was also seen in the SOL (Fig. 1A). The effects of a single dose of paraoxon (0.23 mg/kg s.c.) on recovery AChE activity and on the relative contributions of individual molecular weight forms are presented in Tables II and III. One hour after injection maximal inhibition was seen in both

TABLE I

NUMBER OF LESIONS FOLLOWING EXPOSURE TO TERTIARY OR QUATERNARY PHOSPHOLINE*
CONTROL ACHE ACTIVITY IS EXPRESSED AS μM ACH/g/hr

	PHOSPHOLINE			
	TERTIARY		QUATERNARY	
TIME PAST INJECTION	EDL	SOL	EDL	SOL
CONTROL ACHE	0 120.90±0.18 (100%)	0 64.23±2.97 (100%)	0 124.68±2.51 (100%)	0 57.59±0.99 (100%)
1 DAY	28±3 (4%)	2±1 (6%)	18±3 (71%)	2±1 (38%)

*AChE activity in % of control in brackets, 10 animals were used in each experiment ± S.E.

muscles. At this time the contribution of the heavier molecular weight forms to the overall activity was reduced while that of the 4S form was increased. This was still apparent until the third day. By day seven a normal relationship had been established in SOL, with an increase in activity of all forms above control activity. In EDL, recovery did not occur as rapidly as in SOL since overall activity had not reached control values after seven days.

The effect over time of a single non-lethal dose of organophosphate on the rate of AChE recovery is presented in Table IV. The data are given as half-time rate of recovery in days. It is apparent that, depending on the muscle tested, different half-time values were observed. The fastest rate of recovery was seen in SOL with all of the inhibitors tested, followed by diaphragm and EDL. These muscles also varied in

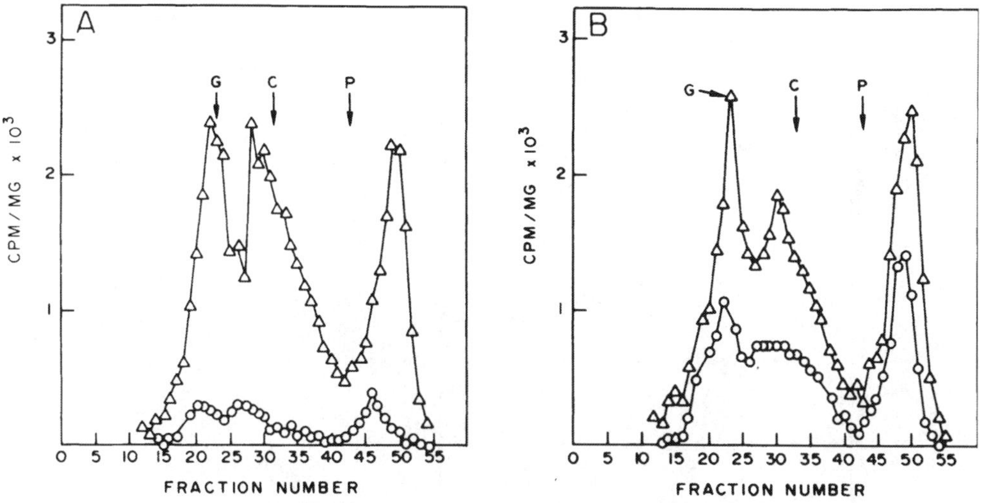

FIG. 1 Velocity sedimentation gradient separation of AChE molecular forms in SOL muscle 60 min after in vivo injection of A tertiary phospholine (0.2 mg/kg s.c.) and B quaternary phospholine (0.08 mg/kg s.c.). Δ-----Δ = control, o-----o = experimental muscle. AChE activity is expressed in cpm/mg protein x 10^{-3}. The position of proteins with known sedimentation such as alkaline phosphatase 6.1S (P), catalase 11.1S (C) and B-galactosidase 16.0S (G) are indicated with arrows.

their sensitivity to the various inhibitors used, which is most obvious with EDL in regard to soman and with the SOL in regard to DFP.

Discussion

The organophosphate and carbamate inhibitors induced a progressive, dose related necrosis in skeletal muscle fibers. The severity of the myopathy depended upon the speed with which a critical decrease in AChE activity was reached as well as on the duration of inhibition. These events resulted in repeated transmitter-receptor

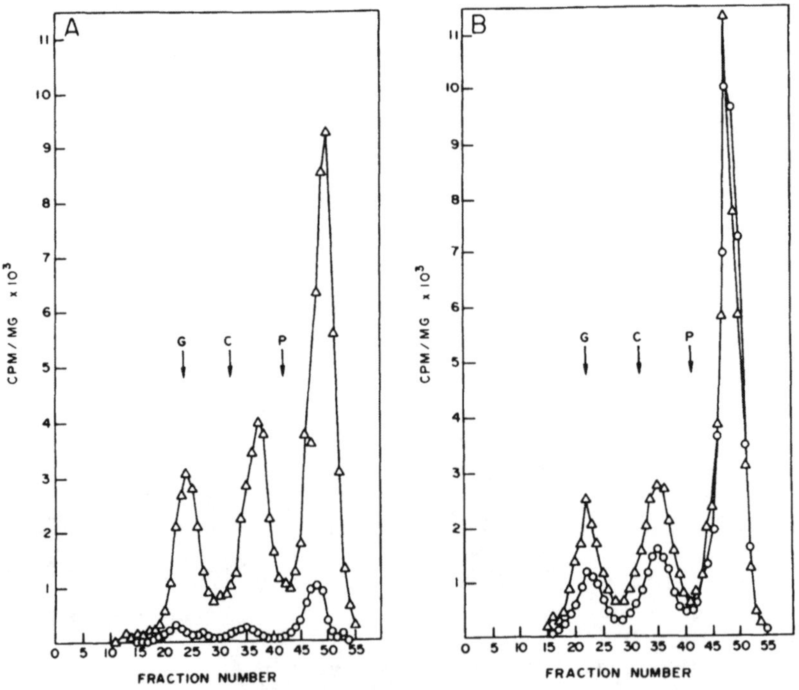

FIG. 2. Velocity sedimentation gradient separation of AChE molecular forms in EDL muscle 60 min after in vivo injection of A tertiary phospholine (0.2 mg/kg s.c.) and B quaternary phospholine (0.08 mg/kg s.c.). Δ-----Δ= control, o-----o = experimental muscle. See Fig. 1 for further explanation.

interactions, and a consequent increase in muscle activity. We suggest that with the increased duration of muscle activity as seen in fasciculations, Ca^{++} uptake into the muscle may become so excessive that a significant fall in glycogen, ATP and creatine phosphate occurs. Under these conditions muscle function and structural integrity cannot be maintained, because the high energy pool becomes exhausted. Thus the defect may be caused by the inability of the sarcoplasmic reticulum to sequester the sudden increase in Ca^{++}. Recent in vitro studies (15) have demonstrated increased Ca^{++} uptake into the endplate region of muscle when stimulated by high concentrations of carbamylcholine, an agonist of ACh. The presence of Ca^{++} activated proteases could explain the loss of the Z disc from myofibrils near the endplate, if prolonged ACh-receptor interactions elevates sarcoplasmic Ca^{++} levels sufficiently (16). The extreme vesiculation and disrupted

TABLE II

RECOVERY OF THE MOLECULAR FORMS OF ACHE IN FAST AND SLOW MUSCLE AFTER PARAOXON
EXPRESSED AS PERCENT OF CONTROL

TIME AFTER INHIBITOR	SOLEUS 4S	SOLEUS 10S	SOLEUS 12S	SOLEUS 16S	EXTENSOR DIGITORUM LONGUS 4S	EXTENSOR DIGITORUM LONGUS 10S	EXTENSOR DIGITORUM LONGUS 12S	EXTENSOR DIGITORUM LONGUS 16S
0 Time	100	100	100	100	100	100	-	100
60 Minutes	26	12	18	17	17	24	-	11
24 Hours	91	51	56	51	64	24	-	24
3 Days	109	104	77	120	79	63	-	33
7 Days	110	129	126	112	75	64	-	83

Comparisons of the enzyme activity of each molecular form after paraoxon. Activities of the individual forms from experimental muscles were compared with those from control muscles and the rate of recovery was calculated. Values are given in percent of control. Between three to five determinations were made for each period, and there were three muscles for each group. Values are the mean.

sarcoplasmic reticulum under the endplate, as well as the swollen mitochondria, may reflect an overloading of the muscle Ca^{++} binding capacity which could result in high sarcoplasmic Ca^{++} levels.

An indirect action of ACh itself is suggested by the findings that proteolytic enzymes were released from muscles treated either with ACh or neostigmine, which induced changes at the endplate and the muscle (17).

Ongoing studies have shown that there exists a special relationship between a given inhibitor and the muscle itself. While diaphragm, SOL and EDL were sensitive to all inhibitors tested, they vary in their vulnerability to given inhibitors. The metabolic pathways a muscle uses to obtain its energy is related to the function it must perform. Changes in activity pattern can modify energy utilization and thus

TABLE III

ACTIVITIES OF THE MOLECULAR FORMS OF ACHE
EXPRESSED AS PERCENT OF TOTAL ACTIVITY AT DIFFERENT PERIODS AFTER PARAOXON

	SOLEUS				EXTENSOR DIGITORUM LONGUS			
TIME AFTER PARAOXON	4S	10S	12S	16S	4S	10S	12S	16S
0 Time	31	18	25	26	60	22	-	19
60 Minutes	48	15	19	18	70	20	-	10
24 Hours	45	13	23	19	73	23	-	10
3 Days	39	16	19	26	67	22	-	7
7 Days	28	19	27	26	66	16	-	28

Activities of molecular forms of AChE are calculated as percent of total AChE activity at different periods after inhibition with paraoxon. Three determinations were made for each time period. Three muscles for each group. Values are the mean.

TABLE IV

LINEAR REGRESSION ANALYSIS OF RECOVERY OF ACHE ACTIVITY IN SOLEUS, EXTENSOR DIGITORUM LONGUS AND DIAPHRAGM MUSCLE AFTER INHIBITION BY ORGANOPHOSPHATE

	ACHE ACTIVITY IN μM/g/hr	SLOPE	REGRESSION COEFFICIENT	HALFTIME RATE OF RECOVERY IN DAYS
		SOLEUS		
CONTROL	54.86±2.59			
SOMAN	16%	7.2	0.98	5.5
DFP	27%	5.0	0.96	6.7
PARAOXON	19%	5.1	0.82	5.5
		EDL		
CONTROL	138.75±3.21			
SOMAN	32%	2.32	0.87	12.0
DFP	21%	3.37	0.93	11.0
PARAOXON	20%	4.66	0.91	7.4
		DIAPHRAGM		
CONTROL	101.07±5.18			
SOMAN	16%	4.85	0.95	7.7
DFP	23%	5.32	0.95	7.1
PARAOXON	20%	5.29	0.96	7.0

Numbers are expressed as percent of control AChE activity remaining 60 min after injection of inhibitor. 10 animals were used in each experiment.

resistance to fatigue. Differences, in recruitment of fibers during AChE inhibition, in their energy production, such as being glycolytic or oxidative, or in their capacity for rapid metabolic recovery after stimulation may determine the differences in sensitivity of these muscle fibers.

The use of the quaternary phospholine to study the involvement of molecular forms in the development of the myopathy clearly indicated differences in the distribution or accessibility of the molecular forms between SOL and EDL. In SOL all major forms such as the 4S, 10S, 12S and 16S forms were inhibited to a much larger degree than those of the EDL where the 4S form was protected against inhibition. This may indicate that in SOL the enzyme forms are more extracellularly located than was the case in EDL. Greater inhibition of enzyme activity as seen with the tertiary inhibitor did not increase the number of lesions in SOL. This suggests that the 50% inhibition of the 16S and 12S forms is enough to trigger the mechanisms that lead to the necrosis. The differences seen in EDL between the two forms of the inhibitor may indicate that more of the enzyme is intracellularly located. 2-PAM, which is poorly lipid soluble, when given 10-30 min after the inhibitor protected the muscles against the necrotizing action of AChE inhibitors, thus supporting the idea that the extracellular enzyme is important for the development of the myopathy (5).

The recovery studies (Table IV) are in general agreement with other reports of half-time rates after organophosphates (18, 19, 20). The shorter half-time rate seen in SOL when compared to that of other muscles is also seen during denervation and reinnervation indicating that AChE synthesis is under a special control in this muscle. Half-time rates when determined after irreversible inhibition with organophosphates, however, are not true indicators for turnover rates of AChE, since the organophosphates are known to stimulate protein synthesis (21) and therefore do not represent true turnover rates.

As far as the changes in relative proportions of molecular forms are concerned one can assume that the lower molecular weight forms are the initial step in the synthesis of the other forms. There also may be different conversion rates from low to medium to heavy weight forms or different rates of transport in a muscle which could explain the differences between muscles, a suggestion also made for AChE in brain after recovery from inhibition with DFP (22).

In conclusion, AChE inhibitors induced a progressive, dose related necrosis in skeletal muscle fibers. The severity of the myopathy depended upon a rapid critical reduction of AChE activity lasting over a critical time period. This inhibition triggers neurally mediated events, including increased neurotransmitter release and antidromic nerve activity resulting in repeated transmitter-receptor interactions with a subsequent increase in skeletal muscle activity. It is suggested that the cause for the lesions is the loss of ATP and creatine phosphate adding to changes in membrane properties resulting in an increase in intracellular Ca^{++} concentration. A rise in Ca^{++} may activate intracellular proteases leading to the observed necrosis.

References

1. Laskowski, M.B., Olson, W.H., Dettbarn, W-D.: Exp. Neurol. 47, 290-306 (1975).

2. Laskowski, M.B., Dettbarn, W-D.: J. Pharmacol. Exp. Ther. 194, 351-361 (1975).

3. Laskowski, M.B., Dettbarn, W-D.: Ann. Rev. Pharmacol. Toxicol. 17, 387-409 (1977).

4. Laskowski, M.B., Olson, W.H., Dettbarn, W-D.: Exp. Neurol. 57, 13-33 (1977).

5. Wecker, L., Kiauta, T., Dettbarn, W-D.: J. Pharmacol. Exp. Ther. 206, 97-104 (1978).

6. Tiedt, T.D., Albuquerque, E.X., Hudson, C.S., Rash, J.H.: J. Pharmacol. Exp. Ther. 205, 326-339 (1978).

7. Hudson, C.S., Rash, J.H., Tiedt, T.N., Albuquerque, E.X.: J. Pharmacol. Exp. Ther. 205, 340-356 (1978).

8. Preusser, J.H.: Z. Zellforsch. Mikrosk. Anat. 80, 436-457 (1967).

9. Wecker, L., Dettbarn, W-D.: Exp. Neurol. 51, 281-289 (1976).

10. Wecker, L., Dettbarn, W-D.: Exp. Neurol. 57, 94-101 (1977).

11. Groswald, D.E., Dettbarn, W-D.: Exp. Neurol. 79, 519-533 (1983).

12. Hall, Z.: J. Neurobiol. 4, 343-361 (1973).

13. Massoulie, J.: Trends in Biochem. Sci. 5, 160-164 (1980).

14. Dettbarn, W-D.: Fundamental Toxicol., in press (1983).

15. Leonard, J., Salpeter, M.M.: J. Cell Biol. 82, 811-819 (1979).

16. Fenichel, G.M., Kibler, W.B., Olson, W.H., Dettbarn, W-D.: Neurology 22, 1026-1033 (1972).

17. O'Brien, R.A.D., Osterberg, A.J.C., Vrbova, G.: Neuroscience 5, 1367-1379 (1980).

18. Glow, P.J., Rose, S., Richardson, S.: Austral. J. exp. Biol. med. Sci. 44, 73-86 (1966).

19. Kiauta, T., Brzin, M., Dettbarn, W-D.: Exp. Neurol. 56, 281-288 (1977).

20. Grubic, Z., Sketelj, J., Klinar, B., Brzin, M.: J. Neurochem. 37, 909-916 (1981).

21. Welsch, F., Dettbarn, W-D.: J. Comp. Biochem. and Physiol. 38B, 393-403 (1971).

22. Michalek, H., Meneguz, A., Bisso, G.M.: Neurobehavioral Toxicology and Teratology 3, 303-312 (1981).

Acknowledgements

This work was supported by NIH Grants EHS 02028, NINCDS 12438, and a grant from the Air Force 82-0310.

TOXICOLOGY OF SOME ANTICHOLINESTERASES USED AS CHEMICAL WARFARE AGENTS - A REVIEW

Jack C. Dacre

U.S. Army Medical Bioengineering Research and Development Laboratory, Fort Detrick, Frederick, Maryland, U.S.A.

The anticholinesterases considered in this review are those compounds used as chemical warfare agents. They are among the most potent synthetic toxic agents known since they are lethal to mammals in submilligram quantity. The toxicology of six of these chemical agents will be reviewed. They fall into two groups; the G agents which are derivatives of phosphoramidocyanidic or methylphosphonofluoridic acid, i.e. they have cyano or fluoro groups attached to phosphorus, and the V agents which are derivatives of methylphosphonothioic acid, i.e. they have sulfur attached to the phosphorus of the molecule. The identification of these compounds is given in Table 1.

TABLE 1. IDENTIFICATION OF THE CHEMICAL WARFARE AGENTS

GA, Tabun	EA 1205	CAS 77-81-6
GB, Sarin	EA 1208	CAS 107-44-8
GD, Soman	EA 1210	CAS 96-64-0
VM	EA 1664	CAS 21770-86-5
VX	EA 1701	CAS 50782-69-9
Vx	EA 1699	CAS 20820-80-8

EA - Edgewood Arsenal Number
CAS = Chemical Abstracts Service Registry Number

The chemical structure of these six agents is set out in Figures 1-6.

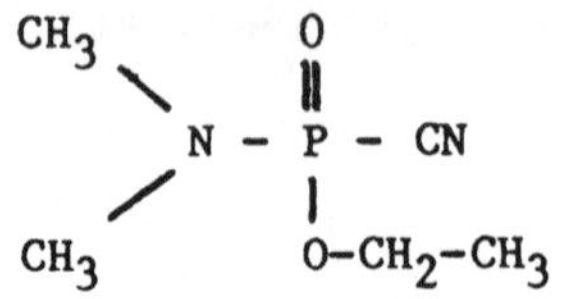

Phosphoramidocyanidic Acid, Dimethyl-, Ethyl Ester

Figure 1. Chemical Structure of GA - Tabun.

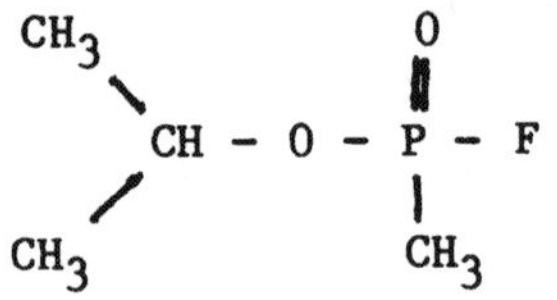

Phosphonofluoridic Acid, Methyl-, 1-Methylethyl Ester

Figure 2. Chemical Structure of GB - Sarin.

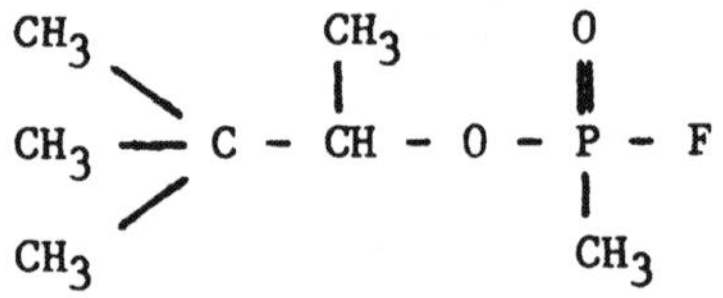

Phosphonofluoridic Acid, Methyl-,1,2,2-Trimethylpropyl Ester

Figure 3. Chemical Structure of GD - Soman

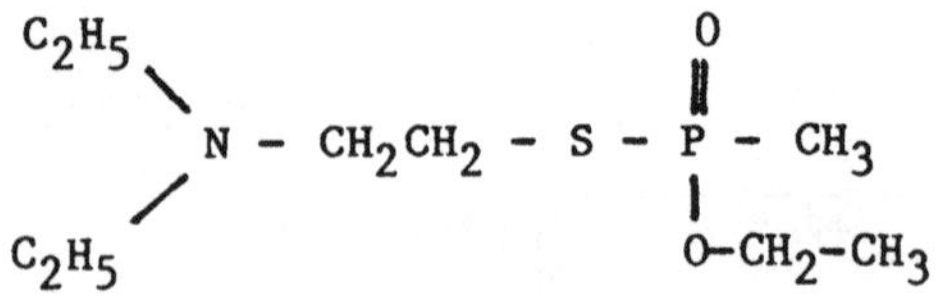

Phosphonothioic Acid, Methyl-, S-[2-(Diethylamino)Ethyl]
O-Ethyl Ester

Figure 4. Chemical Structure of VM.

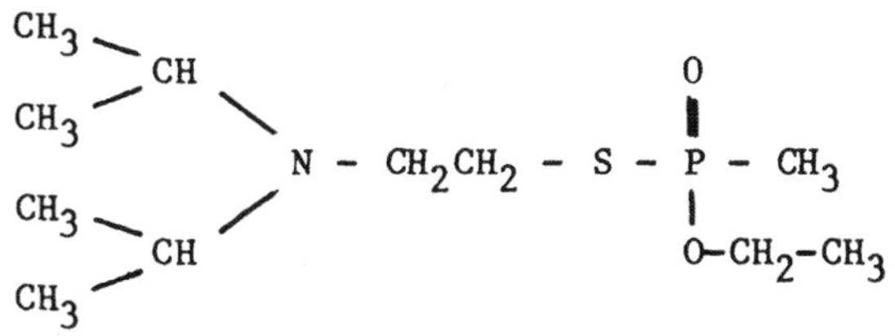

Phosphonothioic Acid, Methyl-, S-[2-(Bis[1-Methylethyl]amino)Ethyl] O-Ethyl Ester

Figure 5. Chemical Structure of VX

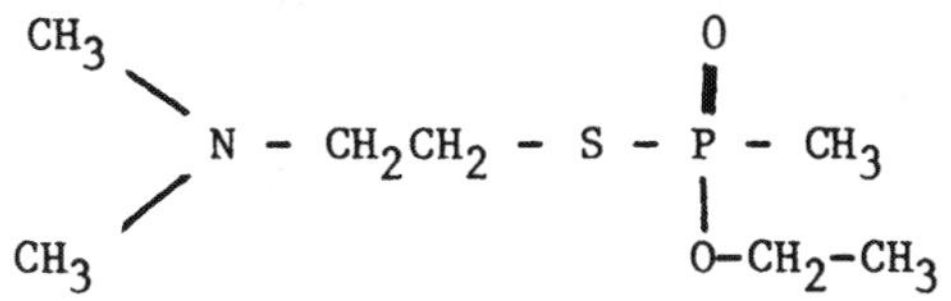

Phosphonothioic Acid, Methyl-, S-[2-(Dimethylamino)Ethyl] O-Ethyl Ester

Figure 6. Chemical Structure of Vx

The chemical purity of experimental samples of these agents has not been well defined. Most investigators did not report analytical data, although in many cases laboratory samples of high purity were used. Table 2 gives a comparison of the purity of laboratory and plant samples of five of the agents studied.

TABLE 2. PURITY RANGE (%) OF THE CHEMICAL AGENTS

	Laboratory Sample	Manufacturing Plant Sample
GA	88-97	-
GB	90-99	94-96
GD	85-99	93-96
VM	94-96	83-87
VX	86-98	94-96

When used in warfare the agents may be stabilized to prevent hydrolytic degradation by the addition of chemical stabilizers. In general, two stabilizers are used; they are dicycyclohexylcarbodiimide and diisopropylcarbodiimide (DICDI). Their use pattern is given in Table 3 and their chemical structure is given in Figure 7.

TABLE 3. IDENTIFY OF THE STABILIZERS USED FOR THE CHEMICAL AGENTS

Agent	Stabilizers
GA Tabun	None
GB Sarin	Tributylamine (Type I) DICDI (Type II)
GD Soman	Dicyclohexylcarbodiimide DICDI
VX	Dicyclohexylcarbodiimide DICDI
VM	Carbodiimides (?)

Little is known of the toxicological properties of these compounds used as stabilizers and they will not be considered or discussed here.

1. Tributylamine

   N,N′-Dibutyl-1-Butanamine (CAS 102-82-9)

   $(CH_3CH_2CH_2CH_2)_3N$

2. DICDI

   N,N′-Diisopropylcarbodiimide (CAS 693-13-0)

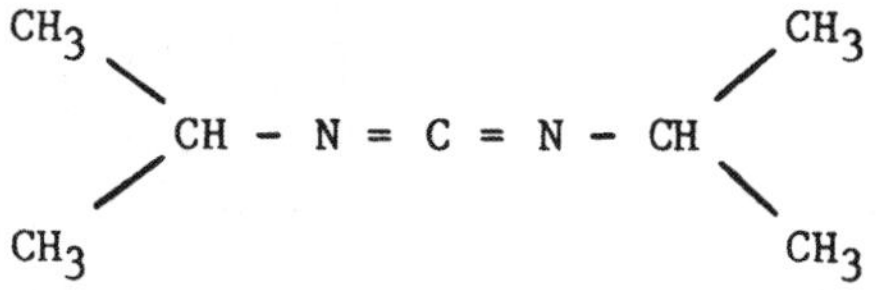

3. N,N′-Dicyclohexylcarbodiimide (CAS 538-75-0)

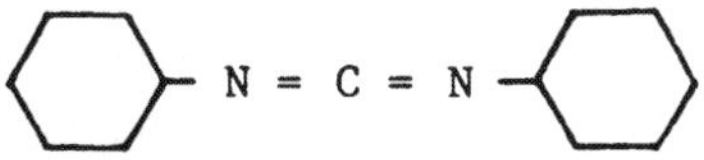

Figure 7. Chemical Structure of the Stabilizers.

A review of the toxicological literature of the nerve agents indicates a vast literature on their anticholinesterase inhibitor properties and on the determinations of acute lethal data, especially LD50, and LCt50, in a wide range of experimental animal models. The anticholinesterase properties of these and related compounds, particularly those used as insecticides, have been extensively reviewed elsewhere and will not be considered here.

However, a comparison of the toxic potencies as inhibitors of acetylcholinesterase, the pI_{50} values, for several representative nerve agents is given in Table 4. The larger the value, the more potent is the agent.

TABLE 4. POTENCY AS AN INHIBITOR OF ACETYLCHOLINESTERASE

Agent	pI_{50}
GA	8.6
GB	8.9
GD	9.2
VM	9.5
Vx	8.8
DFP	6.6

It is quite clear from a survey of the acute toxicity data for these chemical agents that they are among the most toxic substances known to man. A comparison of their relative toxicities with those of some naturally occurring toxins is presented in Table 5.

TABLE 5. RELATIVE ACUTE TOXICITIES OF SOME CHEMICAL AND BIOLOGICAL TOXINS COMPARED WITH SARIN

	1,000	= Sarin (GB) =	1,000	
Tabun (GA) Physostigmine Methyl Fluoroacetate, Strychnine	10^3–10^4	Decreasing Toxicity ↓	10^3–10^2	Russell Viper Venom Amanitine d-Tubocurarine
Hydrogen Cyanide Mustard Gas Parathion Phosgene Arsine	10^4–10^5	Increasing Toxicity ↓	10^2–10	Ricin, Saxitoxin Curare, Abrin
			10 – 1	Batrachotoxin
			10^{-2}–10^{-3}	Tetanus Toxin
Chlorine	10^5–10^6			
			10^{-3}–10^{-4}	Botulinus Toxin

Adapted from Beswick (Human Toxicol., 1983, 2, 250).

Further comparisons of the acute toxicity of these chemical agents is given in Table 6 for the intraperitoneal, subcutaneous, and intravenous routes of administration.

TABLE 6. COMPARATIVE ACUTE TOXICITY IN LABORATORY ANIMALS (Acute LD50, µg/kg)

	Mice			Rats	Rabbits
	ip	sc	iv	iv	iv
GA	600	270	150	70	63
GB	283-420	271		63	17
	590	200	100	45	14
GD	225	125	57-64		
	620	160	75	50	9-11
VM	20-40	22	<20	<20	9
		35			
VX	50				
	33-43.9	13-19.3	11.9-15.5	6.9-10.1	7.1-9.9
Vx	50	25	17		

The acute oral LD50's are given in Table 7 and the acute LCt50's are given in Table 8 for various animal species.

Comprehensive summaries of the lethal dose data for GA, GB, GD, and VX can be found in the "Registry of Toxic Substances, 1980 Edition" (see Selected References).

TABLE 7. COMPARATIVE ACUTE TOXICITY IN LABORATORY ANIMALS (Oral LD50, mg/kg)

	Rat	Rabbit	Dog
GA	3.7	16	5 (LDLo)
GB	1.06 0.87 (starved)	2.5	
GD	0.40	0.35-0.47	
VX	0.077-0.128		
Vx	0.122		

TABLE 8. COMPARATIVE ACUTE TOXICITY IN LABORATORY ANIMALS (Acute LCt50, $mg/min/m^3$)

	Rats	Rabbits	Dogs	Monkeys	T
GA	450	960	320	187	10
GB	220	120	60	74	10
GD	230 279	160			10
VM	11	ca 30	13		1
VX (Aerosol)	9[a]	25[a]	15[a]		10

a. Head exposure only.

A review of the literature has indicated only a limited number of other toxicological studies on some of these compounds. These are outlined in Table 9. In most of these studies, no harmful toxicological effects were reported in dogs and rats exposed to some vapor levels of GB. The reproductive system of rats with respect to dominant lethal mutation, reproductive performance, fetal toxicity, and teratogenesis were not affected. Low-level exposures of VX vapor for 5 and 10 days in mice, rats, guinea pigs, and rabbits did not produce significant lesions or changes that could be attributable to the exposures.

TABLE 9. OTHER REPORTED TOXICOLOGICAL STUDIES OF CHEMICAL AGENTS

GB
Inhalation of GB vapor in dogs (5 days)
Inhalation of GB vapor in dogs (6 months)
Chronic exposures of GB vapor in rats (Reproductive performance effects, testicular atropy effects)
VX
Subacute exposures of VX in mice, rats, guinea pigs, rabbits

The US Army Medical Research and Development Command is initiating and supporting extensive animal toxicologic studies on three of these agents. The studies that are currently in progress are listed in Table 10. Results of the mutagenicity screening studies on VX so far reported indicate that this agent is not mutagenic.

TABLE 10. STUDIES IN PROGRESS ON CHEMICAL AGENTS

GB	Teratology in rats and rabbits
GD	Teratology in rats and rabbits
VX	Mutagenicity - Ames assay - Saccharomyces assay - Mouse lymphoma
	Teratology in rats and rabbits
	Dominant lethal in rats
	Reproduction (3 generation) in rats
	Subchronic (90 day) oral in rats
	Delayed neuropathy in chickens

Recommendations for additional research on the six chemical agents considered here are presented in Table 11. Besides identifying the target organ for toxicity or lethality, the data will be used to derive both environmental and occupational exposure criteria values necessary for protecting the environment and the health of all persons who might be exposed to these highly toxic compounds.

TABLE 11. RECOMMENDATIONS FOR TOXICOLOGICAL STUDIES OF THE CHEMICAL AGENTS

	GA	GB	GD	VM	VX	Vx
Mutagenesis						
Ames assay	+	+	+	+		+
Mouse lymphoma	+	+	+	+		+
Dominant lethal rats	+		+	+		+
Teratology rats/rabbits	+			+		+
Reproduction (X3) rats	+	?	+	+		+
Subchronic rats						
Oral	+	?	+	+		+
Inhalation	+	?	+	+		+
Delayed Neuropathy						
Chickens	+	+	+	+		+
Toxicokinetics	+	?	+	+	+	+
Metabolism						
Rats/rabbits	+	?	+	+	+	+

+ = requirement for additional data

In summary -

The toxicology of six of the commonly used chemical agents has been reviewed. The available literature indicated extensive studies involving their anticholinesterase activities as well as determinations of acute lethal data in many animal species. Only limited studies in other toxicological areas have been reported. Studies in progress supported by US Army Medical Research & Development Command were listed and recommendations for additional mammalian toxicological research were presented.

SELECTED REFERENCE MATERIAL

Health Aspects of Chemical and Biological Weapons, Report of a WHO Group of Consultants. World Health Organization, Geneva, 1970.

The Problem of Chemical and Biological Warfare, Volume II CB Weapons Today. Stockholm International Peace Research Institute, Stockholm: Almquist & Wiksell, N.Y.: Humanities Press, 1973.

Chemical Agent Data Sheets, Volume 1. Edgewood Arsenal Special Report, EO-SR-74001, Department of Army, Headquarters, Edgewood Arsenal, APG, MD, December 1974.

Toxicology of War Gases. V. Vojvodic. Belgrade: Military Publishing House, Institute for Military Medical Information and Documentation, 1981.

Registry of Toxic Effects of Chemical Substances, 1980 Edition - Volumes 1 and 2. Edited by R.J. Lewis, Sr. and R.L. Tatken. National Institute for Occupational Safety and Health, US Department of Health and Human Services, Washington, D.C.: US Government Printing Office, February 1982.

Possible Long-Term Health Effects of Short-Term Exposure to Chemical Agents. Volume 1 Anticholinesterases and Anticholinergics. National Academy of Sciences, Washington, DC: National Academy Press, June 1982.

OXIDATIVE BIOACTIVATION OF ACETYLCHOLINESTERASE INHIBITORS WITH EMPHASIS ON S-ALKYL PHOSPHOROTHIOLATE PESTICIDES

John E. Casida

Pesticide Chemistry and Toxicology Laboratory
Department of Entomological Sciences
University of California, Berkeley, California 94720 USA

Introduction

The effectiveness of organophosphorus (OP) and methylcarbamate (MC) insecticides depends on initial stability to reach the target organism and nerve and ultimate reactivity with AChE, a combination of properties often made possible by using a propesticide undergoing metabolic activation. The ultimate AChE inhibitor is usually formed by one or more oxidation steps and is quite reactive or unstable. Oxidation is also a major detoxification mechanism for OP and MC insecticides. Alternative activation and detoxification sites may contribute to selective toxicity. This review supplements earlier treatises (1-4) by considering recent advances on oxidative bioactivation and detoxification of AChE inhibitors with emphasis on *S*-alkyl phosphorothiolate pesticides.

Oxidative Bioactivation

Recognition and Assay. Oxidative bioactivation can be recognized in any one of several types of *in vivo* studies and in *in vitro* experiments with the microsomal mixed-function oxygenase (MFO) system (1-4). Oxygenase inhibitors (5), *e.g.*, piperonyl butoxide and SV-1, may reduce the toxicity or delay the action of toxicants undergoing oxidative bioactivation.

They may also protect against in vivo AChE inhibition from bioactivated OP compounds.

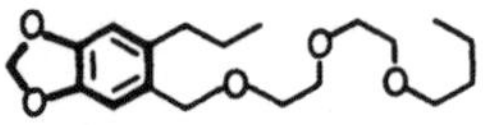

piperonyl butoxide

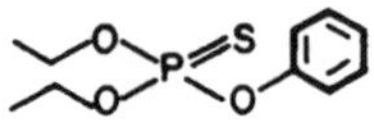

SV-I

In vivo AChE inhibition more severe than anticipated from in vitro inhibitory potency suggests possible activation. MFO-enhanced esterase inhibition provides direct evidence for activation. The metabolite mixture can be generated and then assayed directly or following separation, such as by thin-layer chromatography (6). An improved procedure involves co-incubation of the metabolite generation system [microsomes + reduced nicotinamide-adenine dinucleotide phosphate (NADPH)] and the detection system (AChE) allowing recognition of even unstable, activated intermediates (7, 8).

Enzymes Involved. The oxidative bioactivations result from oxidation at carbon, nitrogen, sulfur and phosphorus (phosphite) substituents. The enzymes involved include cytochrome P-450-dependent and flavin-adenine dinucleotide (FAD)-dependent monooxygenases (E.C. 1.14.13.8) of mammalian microsomes (9-11) and peroxidases of plants (12). The cytochrome P-450-dependent enzymes are generally more important than the FAD-dependent monooxygenase but the latter oxidizes both thioethers to sulfoxides (9, 10) and desulfurates certain phosphonothionates (11). Most studies have been conducted with rat or mouse liver or housefly microsomes often following treatment of the animals with inducers of oxygenase activity. Other species are also used and the preparations are purified or modified to various degrees to remove or inhibit detoxifying enzymes. Mechanism studies are facilitated by the use of oxygenases purified to homogeneity, e.g., FAD-dependent monooxygenase (9-11) and the cytochrome P-450 enzyme reconstituted from purified components (13).

Examples of Bioactivated Organophosphorus Esters. The most important bioactivation reaction (A) is thionophosphorus (1) desulfuration that proceeds with retention of configuration for the chiral isomers (13, 14). The S-oxide (2) or phosphooxathiiran intermediate (3) either loses sulfur in a singlet state to form the oxon (4) or cleaves to the thiophosphorus (5), phosphorus (6) and non-phosphorus acid fragments. Substituent effects importantly influence the course of these reactions (13-15). The liberated sulfur atom probably forms a hydrodisulfide linkage with the side chain of a cysteine in the cytochrome P-450 molecule with accompanying loss of oxygenase activity (13).

A

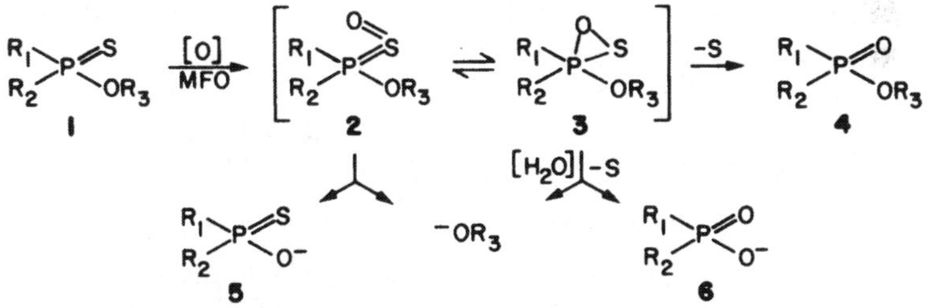

Dimethylphosphoramides (7) are bioactivated in a process initiated by carbon or nitrogen oxidation (16, 17), in the latter case possibly via an N-oxide (8) that rearranges to the N-methylol compound (9) or the P-dimethylaminooxyphosphonous derivative (10) (18) (Reaction B). The established enzymatic products are the monomethylphosphoramide (11) and formaldehyde (16, 17) but the metabolic reactions should be reexamined with current analytical techniques (18).

B

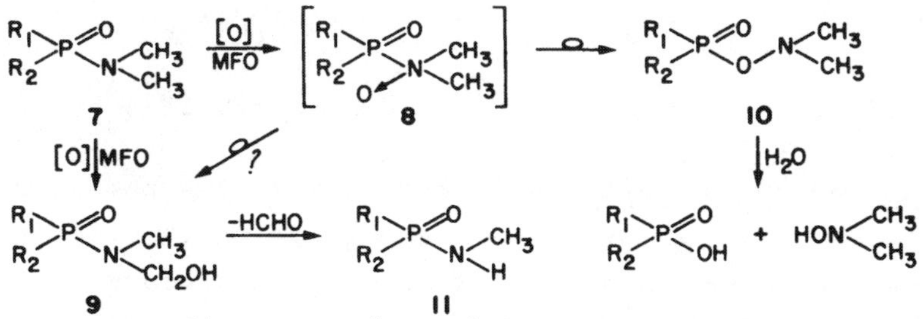

There are many other examples of OP compounds suspected or established to undergo oxidative bioactivation reactions (19,

20). Insecticidal phosphoramidothiolates can be converted to a variety of proinsecticides with suitable *N*-acyl (21) or *N*-(alkoxycarbonyl)(alkylamino)thiol (22) substituents instead of the replaceable hydrogen. The oxidative activation of phosphorothiolates is considered later.

Examples of Bioactivated Methylcarbamates. Methylcarbamates undergo a variety of biooxidation reactions at substituents other than the carbamyl moiety (6, 23). Several compounds are under development involving substitution of the carbonyl nitrogen atom with a variety of functionalizing groups, for example (22, 24-26) (abbreviations used are Me = methyl, Et = ethyl, Pr = propyl, Bu = butyl, Ph = phenyl and Ar = aryl):

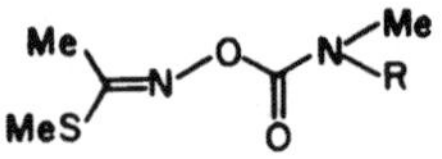

methomyl R = -H
larvin
R = -SN(Me)C(O)ON=C(Me)SMe
U-56,295 R = -S

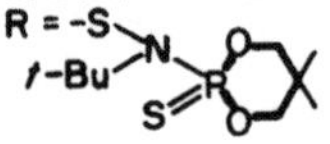

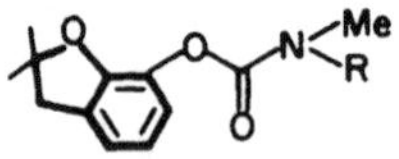

carbofuran R = -H
carbosulfan
R = $-SN(Bu\text{-}n)_2$
CGA 73,102
R = -SN(Me)C(O)OBu-*n*

On a more general basis the R substituent can be alkyl- or arylthio, thiocarbamate, dialkylaminothio, and many different *N*-sulfinyl derivatives. These compounds are susceptible to chemical and enzymatic N-S cleavage and oxidation, regenerating the parent AChE inhibitor (22-27). Their selectivity is improved by the derivatizing group due to different balances of reaction pathways in insects compared to mammals, *i.e.*, activation vs detoxification, and differences in their physical properties.

S-Alkyl Phosphorothiolate Pesticides and Toxicants

Examples of Structure-Activity Relationships. The phosphorothiolate substituent is present in about 15% of the commercial insecticides and in many nematocides, fungicides and herbicides. Examples are as follows:

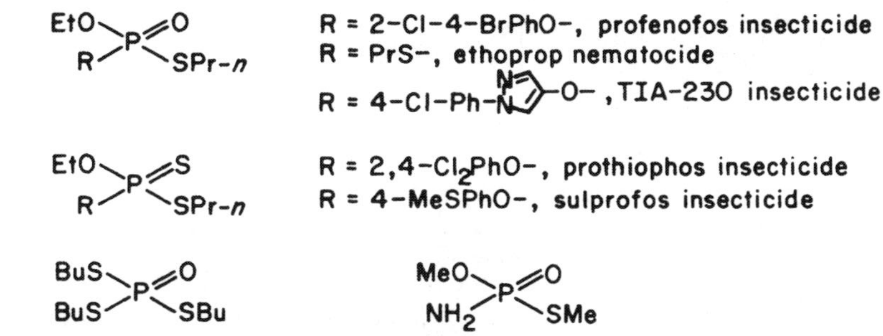

DEF cotton defoliant   methamidophos insecticide

With the exception of methamidophos these compounds have at least two P-S-alkyl substituents or a P-S-alkyl plus a P-O-aryl substituent, both linkages with potential reactivity as phosphorylating agents. *O*-Aryl *O*-ethyl *S*-propyl phosphorothioates and phosphorodithioates (two of the types above) generally have low acute toxicity to mammals and excellent activity on strains of lepidopterous larvae and housefly adults resistant to other OP insecticides (20, 28, 29). The aryl group can be widely varied but the optimal combination of alkyl groups is usually *O*-ethyl and *S*-propyl (28, 29). Discovery that these compounds have high insecticidal activity was very surprising, especially on finding that they are rather weak *in vitro* AChE inhibitors (7, 30, 31). The structure-activity relationships and pattern of biological activity were distinctly different than those of earlier OP compounds.

Chiral Isomers: Preparation and Toxicity. The chiral isomers of profenofos were obtained by treating the individual diastereoisomers of *O*-(4-bromo-2-chlorophenyl) *N*-[(2*S*)-2-(carboxyethyl)-pyrrolidinyl] *S*-propyl phosphorothioamidate with 1 M sulfuric acid in ethanol at 55°C for 48 h (32). Chiral enantiomers of *O*-ethyl *S*-propyl methylphosphonothioate (EPMP) and related compounds were prepared from the optically active thio acids and alkyl bromides (33). The absolute configurations for the profenofos isomers are tentatively suggested to be $(R)_P$-(-) and $(S)_P$-(+), based on nuclear magnetic resonance spectroscopy with a chiral shift reagent (32). Stereochemical assignments in the methylphosphonothioate series are $(R)_P$-(+) and $(S)_P$-(-) (33).

(-)-Profenofos is 4-23-fold more toxic than (+)-profenofos to insects, birds and mammals (7, 32). It was therefore intriguing to find that the (+)-isomer is 2- to 48-fold more potent than the (-)-isomer as an _in vitro_ esterase inhibitor (7, 32). Again with EPMP (but not with related _O_-alkyl S-alkyl phosphonothiolates) the chiral isomer of highest toxicity (+) is the less potent inhibitor of AChE _in vitro_ (33). These findings from both series prompted the suggestion that the more toxic isomer may undergo metabolic activation (32, 33), possibly by sulfoxidation (32).

Peracid Oxidation of _S_-Alkyl Phosphorus Derivatives

Oxidative Activation as Phosphorylating Agents. m-Chloroperoxybenzoic acid (MCPBA) readily oxidizes a variety of sulfur substituents in thiophosphorus pesticides and sometimes serves as a useful biomimetic model (4). With sulprofos the relative ease of sulfur oxidation, shown by numbers in the figure, decreases in the sequence thioether to sulfoxide and sulfone and then phosphorodithioate to phosphorothiolate prior to any phosphorothiolate oxidation (34).

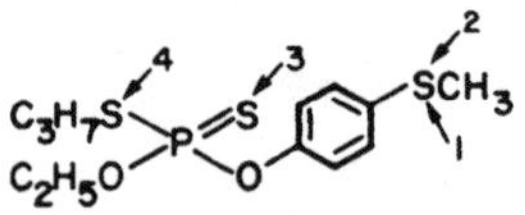

With the _S_-alkyl thiophosphorus compounds, the rate is dependent on the R substituents, i.e.: phosphorotrithiolates > phosphoramidothiolates >> phosphonothiolates > phosphorothiolates (34-38). The balance of products (Reaction _C_) is dependent on the substituents (R_1, R_2 and R_3), the ratio of MCPBA to OP compound, and the reaction solvent. The presumed sulfoxide (_13_) is very short lived and has not been isolated, synthesized or identified based on its spectral features.

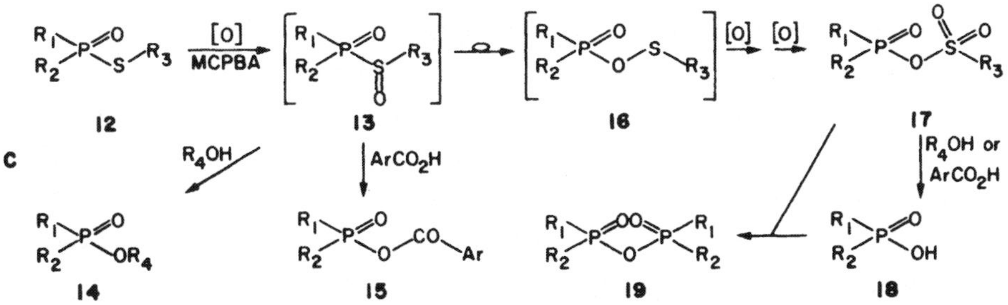

The proposal that it exists as a transitory intermediate is based on the products obtained on oxidizing 12 in alcohols as opposed to solvents without hydroxy substituents. In each case it appears that the rate-limiting step is the oxidation of 12 to 13 rather than any subsequent reaction with the solvent or various degradation products. The conversion of 12 to 14 with excess MCPBA is essentially quantitative in primary alcohols (R_4 = Me, Et or *n*-Pr), ~50% in secondary alcohols (R_4 = *i*-Pr or *s*-Bu) and ~5% in a tertiary alcohol (R_4 = *t*-Bu) (37). The reaction of intermediate 13 with alcohols is therefore sterically controlled depending mainly on the bulkiness of the alcohol and less upon the phosphorus substituents (37). Racemization does not occur prior to the nucleophilic displacement at the phosphorus in the sulfoxide intermediate, which is assumed to proceed with inversion of the configuration (36). It appears that the sulfoxide is formed with retention of configuration (36) and is an extremely reactive intermediate with the -S(O)R substituent being one of the best known leaving groups attached to phosphorus (37).

Rearrangement of Proposed Phosphorothiolate S-Oxide Intermediates. Conversion of 12 to 17-19 is rationalized as proceeding via 13 and 16 (Reaction C). Phosphoric-benzoic anhydride 15 is a major product from phosphonothiolates (36). In contrast, phosphorothiolates give phosphinyloxysulfonates (17) in high yields on MCPBA oxidation in dry acetone, chloroform or benzene (34, 35). The phosphorothiolate *S*-oxides (13) and their phosphinyloxysulfenate rearrangement products (16) are probable intermediates in forming sulfonic-phosphoric anhydride 17. Attempts to directly observe 16 or the sulfinate intermediate have thus far been unsuccessful. The transformation of 13 to 16 appears to proceed via a phosphoranoxide as the transition state rather than via separate ion-pairs or dissociation to radicals and recombination based on studies with optically active 12 (R_1 = Me, R_2 = i-PrO, R_3 = Et) (36). Phosphinyloxysulfonate 17 lacks phosphorylating activity and reacts with R_4OH (or H_2O) to liberate the phosphoric acid (18) which in turn reacts with 17 to yield the pyrophosphate 19; the sulfur fragment is released primarily as the mixed anhydride ($R_4OSO_2R_3$) (34-36). These studies with MCPBA show that the phosphorylation vs rearrangement rates are strongly dependent on the nature of the nucleophile. They also serve as a potential biomimetic model for metabolic activation or detoxification, respectively.

Analogous Reactions of S-Alkyl Thiocarbamates. Some analogies can be made between the MCPBA oxidation of S-alkyl thiophosphorus derivatives (Reaction C) and of S-alkyl thiocarbamates (22) and dithiocarbamates (20) (Reaction D), with the advantage in the latter case that the oxygenated intermediates are sufficiently stable for direct examination (39, 40). The thion-S-oxide predominantly desulfurates in the thiophosphorus series (2, Reaction A), whereas deoxygenation is favored over desulfuration for 21 in the thiocarbamate series (Reaction D). The thiocarbamate S-oxide 23 is either oxidized to the sulfone (24) or, if an S-(2-chloroallyl) derivative, it undergoes a spontaneous [2,3] sigmatropic rearrangement to give the S-O-sulfenate ester (25) which is further oxidized to the sulfinate (26) and sulfonate (27) esters. In contrast, the sulfoxide in the phosphorus esters rearranges to the P-O-S-C rather than the P-S-O-C derivative analogous to the product in the thiocarbamate series, but in each case the sulfenate ester is further oxidized to the sulfonate ester (35, 39). The thiocarbamate sulfoxides and sulfones (23 and

24, R = n-Pr, R' = Et) inhibit chymotrypsin (41) analogous to the phosphorothiolate S-oxides as AChE inhibitors as discussed below.

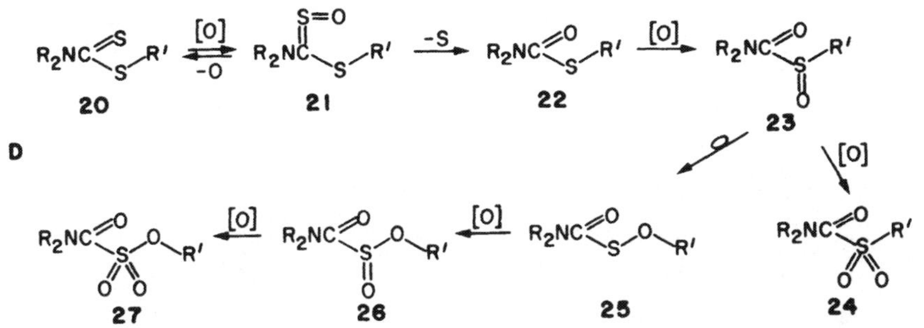

Oxidative Bioactivation of S-Alkyl Phosphorus Derivatives

Oxidative Metabolism. S-Propyl phosphorothiolates undergo extensive P-S-C cleavage in rats administered the oxygen analog of prothiophos (42) or ethoprop (43) and in the MFO system incubated with ethoprop (43) or profenofos (7, 8). These cleavage reactions probably occur in the most part via the corresponding sulfoxides.

Influence of S-Substituent on Bioactivation. Several phosphorothiolates with a C_2 to C_6 S-alkyl substituent undergo metabolic activation to more potent AChE inhibitors, i.e., two compounds with S-Et substituents, five compounds with S-n-Pr substituents, and one each with S-i-Pr, -n-Bu, -t-Bu, -n-pentyl and -cyclohexyl substituents (7, 8, 38, 44). No activation was evident for two compounds each with S-Me, S-benzyl or S-Ph substituents and phosphorothiolates with a variety of other thiol substituents; in addition phosphoramidothiolates were not converted to more potent AChE inhibitors (7, 8). (-)-Profenofos and O,S-diethyl O-phenyl phosphorothioate undergo in vivo activation as evidenced by lessened chick brain AChE inhibition after pretreatment with piperonyl butoxide (7, 8). Moreover, piperonyl butoxide delays the onset of tremors in chicks administered (-)-profenofos, which also indicates a protective effect (7). Phosphorothiolate S-oxides are the probable phosphorylating agents formed on both MCPBA and MFO oxidations.

Influence of Chirality at Phosphorus. The bioactivation reaction (E) is stereospecific for the chiral isomers of profenofos (28, Ar = 2-Cl-4-BrPh): the more toxic (-) isomer becomes a 34-fold better inhibitor of AChE in vitro, whereas the less toxic (+) isomer is detoxified by a factor of 2 (7). The reversal of chiral specificity in the bioactivation system may be due to differences in rates of oxidation or, more probably, in the enantiomeric selectivity for AChE inhibition. The AChE reacts preferentially with the nonoxidized form of (+)-profenofos and the oxidized form of (-)-profenofos (29). This may indicate a change in the leaving group, i.e., cleavage of the P-O-Ar linkage for (+)-profenofos (30) and of the activated P-S-Pr linkage for (-)-profenofos (31) (7, 8, 45). Spontaneous rearrangement of S-oxide 29 to phosphinyloxysulfenate 32, if it occurs in vivo, constitutes a detoxification mechanism. Ethoprop is a prochiral compound and following bioactivation the phosphorothiolate S-oxide is a mixture of chiral isomers which may vary in their stereospecificity for AChE inhibition, ultimately giving the same two isomers of aged enzyme (33) involved with profenofos.

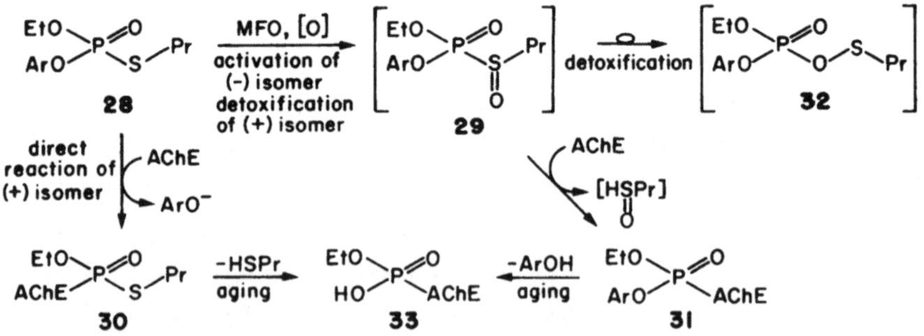

Antidotes, Reactivation and Aging. The LD_{50} of profenofos is increased up to 7-fold in chicks and 4-fold in mice on coadministration of atropine with eserine, pyridinium oximes or the bis-pyridinium but non-oxime compound SAD-128 (45). Atropine and the oximes are less effective as profenofos antidotes, indicating that profenofos-inhibited AChE may undergo rapid aging (45). Brain AChE from chicks poisoned with profenofos is not reactivated by 2-PAM though it is with methamidophos poisoning. It appears that the action of eserine and possibly SAD-128 is due to protecting AChE or cholinergic receptors from profenofos or bioactivated profenofos and that oximes may act in the same way rather than as reactivators due to rapid aging of the inhibited AChE (45).

Electric eel AChE inhibited *in vitro* by bioactivated (-)-profenofos or several other bioactivated phosphorothiolates does not reactivate spontaneously or with 2-PAM in contrast to that inhibited by non-bioactivated profenofos or methamidophos (8, 45). Bioactivation of profenofos therefore changes the aging properties of the inhibited AChE, possibly by shifting the site of cleavage upon phosphorylation from the P-O-Ar to the activated P-S-Pr linkage. Many *S*-alkyl phosphorothiolates, even without bioactivation, yield inhibited AChE which undergoes rapid aging (33) (46). The P-O-aryl substituent is also appropriate for rapid aging reactions. The unique biological properties of the *O*-aryl *O*-ethyl *S*-propyl phosphorothioates and phosphorodithioates therefore appear to be related to oxidative bioactivation resulting in two good leaving groups and rapid aging in some cases. These features may also contribute to difficulties in antidote therapy and in the failure of insects to rapidly develop resistance to profenofos and related insecticides.

Acknowledgments. Study supported in part by National Institutes of Health Grant PO1 ES00049 and by a grant from CIBA-Geigy Corporation (Greensboro, North Carolina, USA). These studies were conducted in the most part by A. H. Glickman, I. Holden, H. Leader, Y. Segall and K. D. Wing in the Pesticide Chemistry and Toxicology Laboratory at Berkeley.

References

1. Casida, J. E.: J. Agr. Food Chem. 18, 753 (1970).
2. Nakatsugawa, T., Morelli, M. A.: in Insecticide Biochemistry and Physiology, Wilkinson, C. F., Ed., pp. 61-114, Plenum, New York, 1976.
3. Kulkarni, A. P., Hodgson, E.: Pharmac. Therap. 8, 379 (1980).
4. Casida, J.E.: in Pesticide Chemistry: Human Welfare and the Environment, Miyamoto, J., Kearney, P. C., Eds., Vol. 3, pp. 239-246, Pergamon, New York, 1983.
5. Testa, B., Jenner, P., Drug Metab. Rev. 12, 1 (1981).
6. Oonnithan, E. S., Casida, J. E.: J. Agr. Food Chem. 16, 28 (1968).
7. Wing, K. D., Glickman, A. H., Casida, J. E.: Science 219, 63 (1983).
8. Wing, K. D., Glickman, A. H., Casida, J. E.: Pestic. Biochem. Physiol., accepted (1983).
9. Hajjar, N. P., Hodgson, E.: Science 209, 1134 (1980).
10. Hajjar, N. P., Hodgson, E.: Biochem. Pharmacol. 31, 745 (1982).
11. Hajjar, N. P., Hodgson, E.: in Biological Reactive Intermediates - II, Part B, Snyder, R., Parke, D. V., Kocsis, J. J., Jollow, D. J., Gibson, C. G., Witmer, C. M., Eds., pp. 1245-1253, Plenum, New York, 1982.
12. Knaak, J. B., Stahmann, M. A., Casida, J. E.: J. Agr. Food Chem. 10, 154 (1962).
13. Neal, R. A.: Amer. Chem. Soc. Symp. Ser. 158, 19 (1981).
14. Ohkawa, H.: in Insecticide Mode of Action, Coats, J.R., Ed., pp. 163-185, Academic Press, New York, 1982.
15. McBain, J. B., Yamamoto, I., Casida, J. E.: Life Sci. 10, 947 (1971).
16. Arthur, B. W., Casida, J. E.: J. Econ. Entomol. 51, 49 (1958).
17. Jones, A.R., Jackson, H.: Biochem. Pharmacol. 17, 2247 (1968).

18. Holden, I., Segall, Y., Kimmel, E. C., Casida, J. E.: Tetrahedron Lett. 23, 5107 (1982).
19. Eto, M.: Organophosphorus Pesticides: Organic and Biological Chemistry, CRC Press, Cleveland, Ohio, 1974.
20. Fest, C., Schmidt, K.-J.: The Chemistry of Organophosphorus Pesticides, Springer-Verlag, New York, 1982.
21. Magee, P. S.: Residue Rev. 53, 3 (1974).
22. Fukuto, T. R.: in Pesticide Chemistry: Human Welfare and the Environment, Miyamoto, J., Kearney, P. C., Eds., pp. 203-212, Pergamon, New York, 1983.
23. Kuhr, R. J., Dorough, H. W.: Carbamate Insecticides: Chemistry, Biochemistry and Toxicology, CRC Press, Cleveland, Ohio, 1976.
24. Fahmy, M. A., Fukuto, T. R.: in Pesticide Chemistry: Human Welfare and the Environment, Miyamoto, J., Kearney, P. C., Eds., pp. 193-200, Pergamon, New York, 1983.
25. Drabek, J., Bachmann, F.: in Pesticide Chemistry: Human Welfare and the Environment, Miyamoto, J., Kearney, P. C., Eds., pp. 271-277, Pergamon, New York, 1983.
26. Fukuto, T. R., Fahmy, M. A. H.: Amer. Chem. Soc. Symp. Ser. 158, 35 (1981).
27. Cheng, H.-M.,Casida, J. E.: J. Agr. Food Chem. 21, 1037 (1973).
28. Drabek, J., Flück,V.: in Advances in Pesticide Science, Geissbühler, H., Ed., pp. 130-134, Pergamon, New York, 1979.
29. Kudamatsu, A., Iyatomi, A., Hayashi, A., Kano,R.: Eisei Dobutsu 29, 317 (1978).
30. Hart, G. J., O'Brien, R. D.: Pestic. Biochem. Physiol. 6, 85 (1976).
31. El-Sebae, A. H., Soliman, S. A., El-Feel, E. A. A., Galal, I., Zeid, M. I.: Med. Fac. Landbouww. Rijksuniv. Gent 45/4, 935 (1980).
32. Leader, H., Casida, J. E.: J. Agr. Food Chem. 30, 546 (1982).

33. Hall, C. R., Inch, T. P., Inns, R. H., Muir, A. W., Sellers, D. J., Smith, A. P.: J. Pharm. Pharmac. 29, 574 (1977).

34. Segall, Y., Casida, J. E.: in Phosphorus Chemistry, Quin, L. D., Verkade, J., Eds., pp. 337-340, Amer. Chem. Soc. Symp. Ser. 171, Washington, D. C., 1981.

35. Segall, Y., Casida, J. E.: Tetrahedron Lett. 23, 129 (1982).

36. Segall, Y., Balan, A., Moalem,R.: International Congress of Phosphorus Chemistry, Nice, France, September, 1983.

37. Segall, Y., Casida, J.E.: International Congress of Phosphorus Chemistry, Nice, France, September, 1983.

38. Kono, Y., Sato, Y., Okada, Y.: Abstract IIa-14, Fifth International Congress of Pesticide Chemistry, Kyoto, Japan, September, 1982.

39. Schuphan, I., Segall, Y., Rosen, J.D., Casida, J.E.: Amer. Chem. Soc. Symp. Ser. 158, 65 (1981).

40. Segall, Y., Casida, J. E.: J. Agr. Food Chem. 31, 242 (1983).

41. Toia, R., Casida, J. E.: Biochem. Pharmacol. 28, 3307 (1979).

42. Ueyama, I., Takase, I.: Pestic. Biochem. Physiol. 14, 98 (1980).

43. Iqbal, Z. M., Menzer, R. E.: Biochem. Pharmacol. 21, 1569 (1972).

44. Ardelt, B., Hollingworth, R. M.: 186th National Meeting, Amer. Chem. Soc., Washington, D.C., August, 1983.

45. Glickman, A. H., Wing, K. D., Casida, J. E.: Toxicol. Appl. Pharmacol., accepted (1983).

46. Clothier, B., Johnson, M. K., Reiner, E.: Biochim. Biophys. Acta 660, 306 (1981).

VI. ANTICHOLINESTERASES AND NEUROTOXIC ESTERASE: MECHANISM OF DELAYED NEUROTOXICITY

INTRODUCTION TO SESSION VI

Barry W. Wilson

University of California at Davis, Davis, California, USA, 95616

Research on cholinesterases and studies of the anticholinesterase organophosphate esters (OPs) have gone hand in hand for many years. There has been much less study of other esterases with serine active sites. The last four papers in the symposium are concerned in whole or in part with an esterase called "neurotoxic, or neuropathic target esterase" (1) whose inhibition is believed by some to be responsible for an important toxic action of OPs known as organophosphate induced delayed neuropathy (OPIDN).

OPIDN is an axonal neuropathy characterized by loss of motor function, flaccid paralysis, axonal degeneration and demyelination (1,2). It is caused by some OPs such as TOCP, DFP, DEF, mipafox, sarin and soman, but not by others such as parathion, malathion and VX. Symptoms appear one to two weeks following a single acute dose of a neuropathic agent "as if a fuse had been lit but the dynamite keg were a long way removed" (3). Sensitive animals include dogs, cats, chickens and humans, but not rats, mice and rabbits. Hens are probably the most common test animal. Certain classes of OPs such as phosphates, phosphoramidates and phosphonates are likely to be neuropathic. Some phosphinates, sulphonates and carbamates have been shown to protect animals from the disorder (1).

Historically, OPIDN has been a major health problem associated with OPs. For example, at least 20,000 persons were paralyzed to some extent in the southern and mid-western United States in the late 1920's and early

1930's due to the ingestion of an alcoholic extract of Jamaican ginger adulterated with TOCP, and thousands more were poisoned in Morocco in 1959 when cooking oil became contaminated with the same compound. The poisoning of three research workers from mipafox in 1953 and the subsequent paralysis of two of them signaled that TOCP was not the only OP capable of causing long-term paralysis. (See Metcalf (4) for a recent historical review.) Since 1978 OPs are required to be tested for delayed neurotoxicity in the United States before registration by the EPA (5).

The pathogenesis of the disorder is not well understood. Interruptions in axoplasmic flow (2), or in regulation of protein synthesis by abnormal phosphoproteins (6) are two of the mechanisms that have been proposed for OPIDN. Aldridge (7) suggested in 1954 that the initial biochemical event in OPIDN was phosphorylation of an esterase. There is general agreement that this hypothesized neuropathic-OP-sensitive esterase is not a cholinesterase; inhibitions of AChE and non-specific cholinesterases are not correlated with the disorder. However, in 1969, Johnson (8) first demonstrated a site of phosphorylation in neural tissue with the appropriate properties. Screening a large number of compounds, he showed that part of the hydrolysis of phenyl valerate by esterases of nervous tissue was sensitive to inhibition by neuropathic OPs; this fraction he called "neurotoxic esterase, NTE" (1). Proponents of the theory that inhibition of NTE causes OPIDN point out that greater than 80% inhibition of NTE activity in an animal almost invariably means that neuropathy will occur, and compounds that inhibit NTE activity but do not "age", that is covalently bind to the active site with loss of a "leaving group", protect the animal from contracting the neuropathy when a neuropathic OP is administered later. Skeptics of the theory (2) note that NTE activity is inhibited by neuropathic OPs in animals that do not get the neuropathy such as rodents and young chicks, and that NTE activity is present in many non-neural tissues. The enzyme or enzymes responsible for NTE activity have not yet been purified, leaving room for doubt that the paraoxon-insensitive, mipafox-sensitive activity (by definition, the NTE activity) is due to a single enzyme.

The first paper in the section is by Dr. M.B. Abou-Donia. He has studied many aspects of delayed neuropathy ranging from experiments on axoplasmic flow and enzyme alterations that accompany the disorder (2) to implicating the neuropathic OP leptophos in the death of approximately 1300 water buffalos in Egypt (9). His paper deals with DEF, an OP known to be neuropathic, yet licensed for use in the United States as a cotton defoliant, and the different effects produced by the compound depending on the route of its entry into the body. The subject is of great practical importance since laboratory animals are seldom treated dermally with agents that may gain entry through the skin of workers in the field.

The second paper is by Dr. M. K. Johnson. In it he presents the evidence that NTE activity is due to a single protein and that an aging step is essential for the production of the toxic protein. The results are the latest in his and his colleagues step by step search for the molecular basis for OPIDN.

The third paper is by Dr. R. Richardson and his colleagues. Dr. Richardson has studied many of the properties of NTE including its extractability, solubility, kinetics and its distribution in the body. For example, the finding that NTE activity is in white blood cells (10), suggests the possibility of a blood test for workers that may have contacted neuropathic compounds. The work he reports here is most appropriate for an AChE conference; he compares the distribution of NTE and AChE activities in rat and hen brains.

The last paper by Dr. B. W. Wilson and his coworkers presents research on both AChE and NTE reflecting his long-term interest in the life history of AChE in avian muscle and nerve and his more recent concern with the neuropathic actions of OPs (6). Recent experiments are presented on the regulation of AChE forms by endogenous and exogenous factors including evidence that serum factors block the assembly of AChE and that glucocorticoid therapy partly prevents changes of AChE forms that accompany denervation and dystrophy in the chicken. With respect to NTE, data is presented to show that NTE activity migrates as a 9S form on a sucrose sedimentation gradient as if it were a single, or at the least, a set of related enzymes. In closing he speculates that glucocorticoid receptors may be causally involved in both regulation of AChE and OPIDN.

References

1. Johnson, M.K. Crit. Rev. Toxicol. 3, 289-316 (1975).

2. Abou-Donia, M.B. Ann. Rev. Pharmacol. Toxicol. 21, 511-548 (1981).

3. Johnson, M.K. Neurobehav. Toxicol. and Teratol. 4,759-765 (1982).

4. Metcalf, R.L. NeuroTox. 3,269-284 (1983).

5. Anonymous. Federal Register. 43 37361-37363 (1978).

6. Wilson, B.W., Ishikawa, Y., Chow, E. and Cisson, C.M. Neurotox. In Press.

7. Aldridge, W.N. Biochem J. 56, 185-189 (1954)

8. Johnson, M.K. Arch. Toxicol. 114, 711-717 (1969).

9. Abou-Donia, M.B., Othman, M.A., Tantawy, G., Khalil, A.Z. and Shawer, M.F. Experientia. 30, 63-64 (1974).

10. Dudek, B.R. and Richardson, R.J. Biochem. Pharmacol. 31, 1117- 121 (1982).

THE SIGNIFICANCE OF INHIBITION OF NONSPECIFIC ESTERASES IN THE DEVELOPMENT OF ORGANOPHOSPHORUS-INDUCED DELAYED NEUROTOXICITY

Mohamed B. Abou-Donia, Daniel M. Lapadula, Clark D. Carrington and Amin A. Nomeir

Department of Pharmacology
Duke University Medical Center
Durham, North Carolina 27710
USA

While a single dermal dose of 250 to 1,000 mg/kg S,S,S-tri-n- butyl phosphorotrithioate (DEF) produced a delayed neurotoxicity (OPIDN) in chickens, similar to that caused by tri-o-cresyl phosphate (TOCP), oral administration of the same doses resulted only in a late acute effect similar to that produced by the DEF metabolite n-butyl mercaptan. The differential effects of oral and dermal application of single doses of 100-1,000 mg/kg DEF on esterases and liver metabolism enzymes were investigated one day following the administration. O,O-Diethyl O-4-nitrophenyl phosphorothioate (parathion) and TOCP were used as negative and positive controls for OPIDN. Brain acetylcholinesterase was significantly inhibited with topical doses of 500 and 1,000 mg/kg DEF and with orally and dermally applied parathion. Plasma cholinesterase and liver microsomal carboxylesterase activities were significantly reduced from control in all treatment groups. Neurotoxic esterase (NTE) was significantly decreased from control with topical dosing of 200, 500, and 1,000 mg/kg DEF and with TOCP treatments. Oral doses of DEF increased cytochrome P-450 content 73 to 200% while dermal application caused a 200 to 325% increase over control. p-Chloro-n-methylaniline demethylase was also increased by DEF treatment but to a lesser extent than that of aniline hydroxylase or cytochrome P-450 content. TOCP and parathion had no significant effect on liver microsomal enzymes. These results indicate that dermal application of DEF is a more effective inhibitor of esterases and inducer of liver microsomal drug-metabolizing enzymes than oral administration with toxicity directly related to both the dose and route of administration.

Introduction

Organophosphorus compound-induced delayed neurotoxicity (OPIDN) is produced by some organophosphorus compounds with antiesterase activity in humans and some animal species (1, 2). OPIDN is characterized by leg weakness, ataxia, and paralysis after a latent period of 6-14 days. Clinical signs are associated with Wallerian-type degeneration of axons and myelin in the central and peripheral nervous systems (1, 3). This effect was first demonstrated with tri-o-cresyl phosphate (TOCP), later it was produced by a number of organophosphorus compounds (1). Certain animal species (cats, dogs, cows, and chickens) are susceptible to OPIDN, while others (rodents and some primates) are not. The adult chicken has been used to study this effect.

S,S,S-tri-n-butyl phosphorotrithioate, a cotton defoliant, produced cholinergic, late acute, or delayed neurotoxic effects in hens depending on its dose and route of administration (4-8). Orally administered DEF is metabolized to n-butyl mercaptan (nBM) in the gastrointestinal tract (5). The hematotoxic effects of nBM may contribute to the late acute effect induced by orally administered DEF in hens (9).

Since DEF affects specific enzymes in the nervous system and plasma, and since its toxicologic actions, which are dependent on its route of administration, seem to be influenced by drug metabolizing enzymes, this study was carried out to investigate the effects of oral and dermal administration of DEF on these enzymes.

Methods

Chemicals

The following chemicals were obtained from the corresponding suppliers: technical grade DEF (95%), Mobay Chemical Corp. (Kansas City, MO); TOCP (99%), Kodak Co. (Rochester, NY); O,O-diethyl O-4-nitrophenyl phosphorothioate (parathion, 99%), Pflatz and Bauer, Inc, (Stamford, CT); and nBM (98%), Aldrich Chemical Co., (Milwaukee, WI). Biochemicals and electrophoresis supplies were purchased from Sigma Chemical Co. (St. Louis, MO) and Bio-Rad Laboratories (Richmond, CA), respectively.

Source and Care of Hens

Laying leghorn hens, 14-18 months old and weighing approximately 1.8 kg, were purchased from Featherdown Farm (Raleigh, NC). Hens were housed in cages in humidity (40-60%)- and temperature (20-23°C)-controlled rooms with a 12-hr light cycle before and during the study. Animals were allowed to adjust to their environment for at least a week before treatment. They were given feed (Ralston Purina Co., St. Louis, MO) and water *ad libitum*.

Treatment of Hens

Groups of three to five control and treated hens were used in each experiment. Test compounds were given either orally in gelatin capsules or applied dermally with a micropipette over an area of 10 cm^2 on the back of the hen's unprotected neck. The following controls were included: TOCP (positive for OPIDN), parathion (negative control), and empty gelatin capsule (gelatin capsule control). Hens were weighed weekly and examined every other day for neurologic deficits (10). At termination, all hens were killed by decapitation.

Effect of DEF on producing delayed neurotoxicity in hens. Each of the following doses was orally or dermally administered to a group of five hens: 100-1,000 mg/kg DEF; 500 mg/kg TOCP; or 10 mg/kg parathion. Blood samples (2 ml) were collected from the wing vein in heparinized syringes after 4 hr and on days 1, 2, 7, 14, 21, and 28 after treatment. Hens were killed after 28 days.

Effect of DEF on hen liver microsomal enzymes. Groups of five hens were given the following single oral or dermal doses of 100-1,000 mg/kg DEF, 500 mg/kg TOCP, or 5 mg/kg parathion. All hens were killed after 24 hrs.

Effect of microsomal enzyme inducers. Groups of three hens were treated with a daily intraperitoneal dose, for three consecutive days, of 80 mg/kg sodium phenobarbital (PB) in saline or 40 mg/kg 3-methyl cholanthrene (3MC) in corn oil. A single dermal dose of

1,000 mg/kg DEF was given to a group of three hens. All hens were decapitated 24 hr after the last dose.

Histopathological Procedures

Tissues from the nervous system were dissected for histopathological examination from control and treated hens. Cross and longitudinal sections were prepared from the spinal cord, and sciatic, tibial, and peroneal nerves (11). Methyacrylate (2 μM) or paraffin (8 μM) sections were stained with toluidine blue or hematoxylin and eosin (H and E) with luxol fast blue (LFB), Holmes' silver stain, or Glees stain, respectively.

Enzymatic Analysis

Immediately after decapitation of hens, brain, spinal cord, and liver were removed quickly.

Brain and plasma enzymes. Brain acetylcholinesterase (AChE, EC 3.1.1.7) and plasma butyrylcholinesterase (BuChE, EC 3.1.1.8) activities were determined as described previously (11). Neurotoxic esterase (NTE) was measured by the Johnson (12) method.

Liver microsomal enzymes. Washed liver microsomes were prepared (13), frozen with liquid nitrogen and stored at -70°C. The activity of the following enzymes was assayed: aniline hydroxylase (15), *p*-chloro-*N*-methylaniline (PCMA) demethylase (16), and carboxylesterase using 1-naphthyl acetate as a substrate (17). Cytochrome P-450 (14) and protein (18) contents were also determined.

Sodium Dodecyl Sulfate-polyacrylamide Gel Electrophoresis (SDS-PAGE)

Microsomal proteins from livers of hens treated with DEF and microsomal enzyme inducers were analyzed by SDS-PAGE (19). Protein molecular weight was estimated by coelectrophoresis of microsomal fractions with molecular weight markers. Quantification was carried out using LKB Laser Densitometer.

Statistics

Significance of the difference between enzyme activities of control and treated hens was assessed by the Student's two-tailed *t*-test. A *p*-value of 0.05 or less was considered significant.

Results

Acute Cholinergic Effect

Oral administration. The oral LD_{50} for a single dose of DEF within 8 days of administration is 275 mg/kg. A single oral dose of 250 to 1,000 mg/kg DEF produced cholinergic signs in hens that were dose dependent. Hens receiving 750 or 1,000 mg/kg developed pupil constriction, salivation, and diarrhea within a few hours of administration. These hens became paralyzed and died within two days of treatment. Less severe cholinergic signs were seen in hens given 250 and 500 mg/kg DEF. Most of these hens, however, died within eight days of treatment.

Dermal application. Hens treated with a single topical application of 250 to 1,000 mg/kg DEF developed varying degrees of cholinergic signs. Severity of clinical signs was less than that produced by oral administration. Only one dermally-treated hen died as the result of cholinergic effect.

Hens treated with a single oral or dermal dose of 10 mg/kg parathion developed severe cholinergic effects immediately after dosing, but all recovered with time. Neither oral nor dermal administration of 500 mg/kg TOCP produced any cholinergic signs.

Late Acute Effect

Hens given a single oral dose of 250 to 1,000 mg/kg DEF developed signs of late acute effect. These included sluggishness, loss of appetite, loss of balance, and secretion of yellowish fluid from the mouth. Characteristically, the color of the comb changed from bright red to bluish and then became progressively paler until death. These signs overlapped with and were superimposed on cholinergic signs in hens treated with 500-1,000 mg/kg DEF.

Hens given a single oral 500 or 1,000 mg/kg nBM (a DEF metabolite) showed all signs of late acute effect in a dose dependent manner. Specifically, by 6 hrs after administration, hens given 1,000 mg/kg nBM developed all clinical signs seen in hens treated with large oral doses of DEF, and they all died within 12 hrs. Hens given a single oral dose of 500 mg/kg nBM exhibited mild late acute effect signs and recovered within 7 days.

None of the following treatments produced signs of late acute effect: dermal DEF, oral or dermal TOCP or parathion.

Delayed Neurotoxicity

Oral administration. Hens given a single oral dose of 500-1,000 mg/kg DEF died as the result of cholinergic and late acute effects. Hens given 100 and 250 mg/kg developed mild ataxia that progressed to gross ataxia in the latter group. All TOCP-treated hens developed the ataxia with near paralysis stage, and one of these progressed to paralysis.

Dermal application. Topical application of a single oral dose of 250 to 1,000 mg/kg DEF produced clinical signs of delayed neurotoxicity in hens in a dose dependent manner. Those given 1,000 mg/kg DEF progressed to paralysis. A dermal dose of 500 or 750 mg/kg DEF produced ataxia with near paralysis, with one from each group progressing to paralysis. One hen from the 250 mg/kg treatment group developed near paralysis and progressed to paralysis; the remaining hens from this group exhibited the severe ataxia stage. DEF at 100 mg/kg did not produce signs of delayed neurotoxicity. All hens receiving a single dermal dose of 500 mg/kg TOCP developed paralysis. None of the hens given a single topical 10 mg/kg parathion developed delayed neurotoxicity.

Neuropathological Changes

Spinal cord. No spinal cord changes were seen in surviving hens treated with a single oral dose of 100 or 250 mg/kg DEF. On the other hand, dermal application of a single dose of 500-1,000 mg/kg DEF produced histopathologic lesions in the spinal cord that were dose-dependent. Cross and longitudinal sections of spinal cords from hens treated with high doses of DEF showed extensive loss of myelin with swollen and degenerated axons (Fig. 1). No spinal cord changes were seen in hens given dermal doses of 100 or 250 mg/kg DEF or 10 mg/kg parathion.

Peripheral nerves. The only histopathological changes in peripheral nerves in hens given single oral doses of DEF were seen in those from the 100 or 250 mg/kg groups. These changes were seen as axonal swelling (equivocal changes) in hens treated with 250 mg/kg DEF. Only one hen given 100 mg/kg DEF showed minimal focal demyelination in the peripheral nerves. Dermal application of DEF produced unequivocal degeneration of the peripheral nerves. Again, severity and frequency of histopathologic alterations depended on the dose. These changes included dilated axonal sheaths, myelin balls, macrophages containing myelin debris, axonal dilation, and axonal fragmentation (Fig. 2).

Dermal and oral administration of 500 mg/kg TOCP produced axonal degeneration and demyelination of the spinal cord and peripheral nerve. The morphology and distribution of these changes were identical to those from DEF-treated hens, that developed OPIDN. Histopathologic alterations were more severe in dermally than orally-treated hens.

Plasma BuChE

Oral administration. Plasma BuChE was inhibited in hens treated with an oral dose of 100 to 1,000 mg/kg DEF in a dose-dependent fashion, with activity ranging between 53.8 and 3.8% of control four hours after administration, respectively. Maximum inhibition occurred after 24 hours of dosing. Recovery of plasma BuChE activity began 48 hours after treatment. Complete recovery was seen in the enzymatic activity of the hens that survived the treatment (i.e., those given 100 and 250 mg/kg) by seven days after administration. Plasma BuChE from hens given parathion or TOCP completely recovered by day 14 following inhibition initially.

Dermal application. A single dermal dose of DEF decreased plasma BuChE activity by 86 to 13% of control in hens given 100 to 1,000

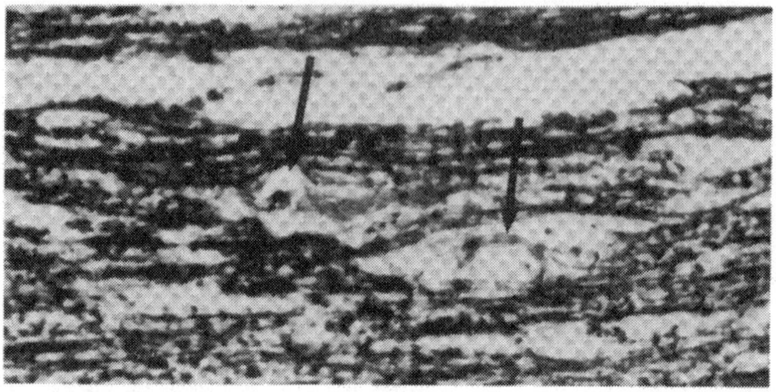

Fig. 1. Thoracic spinal cord from a hen given 1,000 mg/kg dermal dose of DEF. Two of the large swollen axons from the anterior column are seen here in this longitudinal section. Degeneration of axons and myelin is also observed and debris can be identified with macrophages. H and E - LFB, X 400.

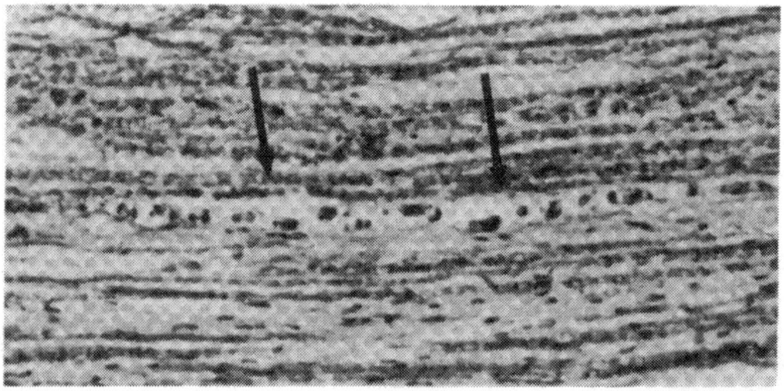

Fig. 2. Peripheral nerve from another hen given a 1,000 mg/kg dermal dose of DEF. Most of the myelinated axons in the figure are normal, while the axon in the center is degenerated and myelin debris can be seen within macrophages. H and E - LFB, X 425.

mg/kg DEF, respectively. Maximum inhibition of enzymatic activity was reached between 2 and 7 days after application. Plasma BuChE activity from hens given 100 mg/kg DEF showed complete recovery by day 21. On the other hand, the enzymatic activity in all other groups given 250 to 1,000 mg/kg was 78 to 15% of control activity.

Plasma BuChE activity in hens given a single dermal dose of TOCP had completely recovered by day 28.

Brain AChE

AChE activity one day after treatment. Brain AChE activity was inhibited to a greater extent when hens were treated dermally rather than orally (Table 1). AChE activity was significantly inhibited in hens given a dermal dose of 500 or 1,000 mg/kg DEF. While TOCP did not significantly inhibit AChE, parathion did.

AChE activity 28 days after treatment. Brain AChE activity of hens that survived 28 days after the oral administration of a single dose of DEF (i.e., 100 and 250 mg/kg) was not significantly different from that of control animals (Table 1). On the other hand, topical administration of 500, 750, or 1,000 mg/kg DEF caused a significant decrease of AChE activity 28 days after administration. Similar results were obtained with a single topical application of 10 mg/kg parathion and 500 mg/kg TOCP.

Brain and spinal cord NTE

NTE activity in the brain and spinal cord of hens treated with a single oral dose of DEF was not significantly different from that of the control (Table 1). By contrast, topical administration of 200, 500, or 1,000 mg/kg DEF caused significant inhibition of brain NTE whereas a 500 or 1,000 mg/kg dermal dose of DEF significantly inhibited spinal cord NTE. Also, while oral and dermal treatment with TOCP inhibited NTE in both brain and spinal cord, neither type of treatment with parathion caused NTE inhibition.

Microsomal Enzymes

Cytochrome P-450. Liver microsomes from untreated hens contained only small amounts of cytochrome P-450: 0.123 ± 0.039 nmole/mg of

TABLE 1

EFFECT OF A SINGLE ORAL OR DERMAL DOSE OF DEF, TOCP, AND PARATHION ON MICROSOMAL ENZYMES AND BRAIN, LIVER, AND PLASMA ESTERASES IN THE HEN[a]

Enzyme	Dose (mg/kg)					
	DEF				TOCP	Parathion
	100	200	500	1,000	500	5
BRAIN						
AChE						
Oral	74 ± 20	83 ± 20	68 ± 10	80 ± 18	68 ± 6	20 ± 3
Dermal	83 ± 12	74 ± 12	56 ± 6*	58 ± 14*	85 ± 12	25 ± 8
NTE						
Oral	109 ± 10	104 ± 7	78 ± 14	65 ± 9	57 ± 1*	112 ± 7
Dermal	54 ± 13	41 ± 4*	19 ± 6*	14 ± 6*	31 ± 8*	129 ± 18
SPINAL CORD						
NTE						
Oral	137 ± 13	100 ± 10	100 ± 7	95 ± 16	17 ± 1*	119 ± 5
Dermal	93± 10	90 ± 8	54 ± 5*	51 ± 7*	48 ± 10*	121 ± 15
LIVER						
Cytochrome P-450						
Oral	173 ± 16*	220 ± 28*	282 ± 24*	300 ± 40*	132 ± 15	109 ± 20
Dermal	302 ± 37*	339 ± 25*	376 ± 20*	443 ± 88*	108 ± 16	112 ± 18
Aniline hydroxylase						
Oral	242 ± 36*	328 ± 56*	340 ± 37*	296 ± 50*	133 ± 17	128 ± 21
Dermal	408 ± 71*	375 ± 36*	407 ± 46*	372 ± 80*	175 ± 21*	155 ± 44
PCMA Demethylase						
Oral	136 ± 9	166 ± 28	176 ± 31*	151 ± 27	151 ± 27	125 ± 29
Dermal	176 ± 31	172 ± 19*	163 ± 10*	157 ± 25	172 ± 33	143 ± 56
Carboxylesterase						
Oral	37 ± 6*	34 ± 4*	33 ± 2*	27 ± 5*	73 ± 8*	58 ± 8*
Dermal	24 ± 5*	23 ± 3*	23 ± 4*	22 ± 3*	56 ± 7*	45 ± 8*

[a] Results are calculated as percentage of control values measured at the same time. Each value represents means ± SEM for at least four hens: AChE, 50.76 ± 6.79 μmole ATCH hydrolyzed/min/mg of protein; brain and spinal cord NTE, 23.77 ± 2.35 and 6.65 ± 0.65 nmole of phenylvalerate hydrolyzed/min/mg of protein, respectively; BuChE, 1.47 ± 0.098 μmoles BUTCH hydrolyzed/min/mg of protein; cytochrome P-450, 0.123 ± 0.039 nmole/mg of protein; aniline hydroxylase, 3.57 ± 0.20 nmole of *p*-aminophenol formed/min/mg of protein; PCMA demethylase, 0.342 ± 0.016 nmole of *p*-chloroaniline formed/min/mg of protein; and carboxylesterase, 1,651.4 ± 92.4 nmole of 1-napthol formed/min/mg of protein.

* Significant difference from control ($p < 0.05$).

protein (Table 1). Cytochrome P-450 production in liver microsomes from DEF treated hens was induced in a dose- and route-dependent manner. Dermal application was more effective than oral administration in inducing cytochrome P-450 content. Single dermal or oral doses of TOCP or parathion did not affect cytochrome P-450 content.

Aniline hydroxylase. Microsomal aniline hydroxylase activity was induced by a single dermal dose of DEF. Although the enzymatic increase was not dose-dependent, it did depend on the route of administration (Table 1). Dermal application of DEF increased aniline hydroxylase activity by 200 to 300% over that of the control animals while oral dosing increased the enzymatic activity 100 to 200%.

PCMA demethylase. The only significant increase of this enzymatic activity was seen with a dermal dose of 200 and 500 mg/kg DEF (Table 1). All other treatments, including those of TOCP and parathion, had no significant effect on the enzymatic activity.

Carboxylesterase. This enzymatic activity in liver microsomes was significantly inhibited by all of DEF, TOCP, and parathion treatments (Table 1). Dermal treatments were more effective than oral treatments, with the greatest decrease occurring with a dermal dose of 1,000 mg/kg DEF.

SDS-PAGE of Liver Microsomal Enzyme Inducers

Protein profiles of liver microsomes from 3MC-, PB-, and DEF-treated hens were distinctly different. Microdensitometry showed a significant increase in protein bands of 49K, 52K, and 53.5K bands in microsomes of hens treated with PB. Microsomes from 3MC-treated hens demonstrated a significant increase in 52K and 55K bands. Microsomes from DEF-treated hens revealed a pattern similar to that of PB-treated animals indicating an induction of cytochrome P-450.

Scans of these microsomes for cytochrome P-450 content revealed a λmax of the Soret peak of the reduced cytochrome P-450 CO complex in PB- and DEF-treated hens to be 451 nm while it was 448 nm in 3MC-treated hens and 451 in untreated hens.

Pharmacokinetics of a single oral and dermal dose of [^{14}C]DEF

The pharmacokinetics of a single oral and dermal 50 mg/kg dose of [^{14}C]DEF have been studied in laying hens. Three hens from each treatment were killed at each time interval: 0.5, 2, 4, 8, and 12 days. Radioactivity disappearance from the plasma followed an exponential curve at rate constants of 0.26 and 0.18 day^{-1}, corresponding to half-lives of 2.7 and 3.8 days for oral and dermal administration, respectively.

Discussion

This report demonstrates that the toxicologic effects of the phosphorothioate compound DEF, the extent and permanence of injury, the progression or improvement of clinical signs, and its biochemical actions depend on the dose and the route of exposure. DEF may produce three toxic effects: (1) acute cholinergic effect, shortly after exposure, as the result of inhibiting AChE; (2) late acute effect, 2-4 days after oral administration of large doses of DEF, resulting from nBM toxicity, which causes hematotoxicity, loss of appetite and weight, weakness, emaciation, paralysis, and death, and is neither related to AChE inhibition nor associated with histopathological changes in nervous tissues; and (3) delayed neurotoxicity, 6-14 days after dermal application, which causes axonal and myelin degeneration accompanied by ataxia, paralysis, and death.

Dermal application of DEF more effectively inhibited AChE than oral administration. AChE inhibition accounts for its acute cholinergic effect. DEF is also a potent inhibitor of both carboxylesterase and BuChE, results which correlate with previous findings (4, 5, 17).

This study demonstrates that neurotoxic dermal doses of DEF significantly inhibited brain NTE. Oral administration of DEF, which failed to produce OPIDN, did not inhibit NTE. It is noteworthy, however, that although NTE inhibition and "ageing" are well correlated with the production of OPIDN, the role of NTE in the mechanisms of delayed neurotoxicity has not been established (1). NTE has not been isolated, its physiologic and biochemical functions are not known (20). Furthermore, NTE is present, inhibited, and aged in young chicks and in rats without subsequent development of OPIDN (20, 21).

The results of this study may explain the role that nonspecific esterases (i.e., BuChE, NTE, and carboxylesterase) play in the pathogenesis of OPIDN. None of these enzymes has a known physiologic function; yet delayed neurotoxic organophosphorus compounds greatly inhibit these enzymes (especially BuChE and NTE) while compounds not capable of causing OPIDN have much lower inhibitory effects. The high affinity of these chemicals for nonspecific esterases may initially contribute to the protection of the exposed animals from the acute effect of these chemicals by reducing their circulating pool. This would allow these animals to survive long enough for freeing of the organophosphorus chemicals, by either a reversible process or in the course of the turnover of these enzymes to take place. Thus, as time passes enough of the neurotoxic organophosphorus chemicals would accumulate at the neurotoxicity target to reach a minimum amount or threshold that causes OPIDN (1).

An important finding in this study is the induction by DEF of chicken liver microsomal cytochrome P-450 content, as well as aniline hydroxylase and PCMA demethylase, the latter two being cytochrome P-450 mediated reactions. Dermal is more effective than oral administration. Neither TOCP nor parathion produced a significant induction of any of these enzymes.

Our results, similar to previous findings, indicate that PB increased the protein band 49K while 3MC increased the higher band 55K (22,23). Since DEF increased the same band as PB, the induction of cytochrome P-450 is indicated. This study confirms previous findings that the content of liver microsomal cytochrome P-450 content in chickens is approximately one-fourth that of the rat (24, 25).

A number of factors may play a role in the differential toxicity of oral versus dermal treatment of animals with DEF. The possibilities include differences in absorption, metabolism, disposition, and elimination of DEF and its metabolites all of which have been seen in other neurotoxic organophosphorus compounds (26). The enhanced effectiveness of dermal exposure - in inhibiting esterases, inducing microsomal enzymes, and conferring OPIDN - may be due to the persistence of DEF or an active metabolite in the hen, in contrast to its' hydrolysis in the gastrointestinal tract upon oral administration. This suggestion is supported by the finding that although DEF is a weak inhibitor of AChE _in vitro_ it is a potent inhibitor of this enzyme _in vivo_. The formation of an active metabolite similar to that demonstrated in TOCP metabolism (26) may account for the increased _in vivo_ inhibition of AChE. Also, pharmacokinetic studies indicate that the biologic t1/2 of radioactivity is longer in plasma of hens given a single dermal dose of [^{14}C]DEF than when the same dose is given orally.

Acknowledgments

The authors thank Mrs. Erna S. Daniel for her secretarial work and Dr. Elmer J. Rauckman for assistance in cytochrome P-450 content determination. The supply of DEF from Mobay Chemical Corp.is acknowledged. This study was supported in part by NIEHS Grant ES02717, NIOSH Grant OH00823, and NIEHS Training Grant T32 ES07031.

References

1. Abou-Donia, M.B.: Ann. Rev. Pharmacol. Toxicol. _21_, 511-548 (1981).

2. Smith, M.I., Elvove, E., Frazier, W.H.: Public Health, Rep. _45_, 2509-2542 (1930).

3. Cavanagh, J.B.: CRC Crit. Rev. Toxicol. _2_, 365-417 (1973).

4. Abou-Donia, M.B., Graham, D.G., Abdo, K.M., Komeil, A.A.: Toxicol. _14_, 229-243 (1979a).

5. Abou-Donia, M.B., Graham, D.G., Timmons, P.R., Reichert, B.L.: Neurotoxicol. _1_, 425-447 (1979b).

6. Baron, R.L., Johnson, H.: Brit. J. Pharmacol. _23_, 295-304 (1964).

7. Casida, J.E., Baron, R.L., Eto, M., Engel, J.L.: Biochem. Pharmacol. 12, 73-83 (1963).

8. Gaines, J.B.: Toxicol. Appl. Pharmacol. 14, 515-534 (1969).

9. Abdo, K.M., Timmons, P.R., Graham, D.G., Abou-Donia, M.B.: Fund. Appl. Toxicol. 3, 69-74 (1983).

10. Abou-Donia, M.B.: Biochem. Pharmacol. 27, 2055-2058 (1978).

11. Abou-Donia, M.B., Pressig, S.H.: Toxicol. Appl. Pharmacol. 35, 269-282 (1976).

12. Johnson, M.K.: Arch. Toxicol. 37, 113-115 (1977).

13. Schenkman, J.B., Ciniti, D.L.: Life Sci. 11, 247-257 (1972).

14. Omura, T., Sato, R.: J. Biol. Chem. 239, 2370-2378 (1964).

15. Mazel, P.: Experiments illustrating drug metabolism in vitro. In Fundamentals of Drug Metabolism and Drug Disposition. pp. 546-582. Williams and Wilkins, Co., Baltimore, MD, 1971.

16. Abou-Donia, M.B., Deickert, J.W.: Toxicol. Appl. Pharmacol. 18, 507-516 (1971).

17. Sultatos, L.G., Costa, L.B., Murphy, S.D.: Toxicol. Appl. Pharmacol. 65, 144-152 (1982).

18. Bradford, M.: Ana. Biochem. 72, 248-254 (1976).

19. Laemmli, U.K.: Nature 277, 680-685 (1970).

20. Johnson, M.K.: Toxicol. Appl. Pharmacol. 61, 480-481 (1981).

21. Johnson, M.K.: Rev. Biochem. Toxicol. 4, 141-202 (1982).

22. Moore, R.W., Welton, A.F., Aust, S.D.: Detection of hemoproteins in SDS-Polyacrylamide Gels. In: Methods of Enzymology Vol. 52, pp. 324-331. Academic Press, New York, 1978.

23. Welton, A.R., Aust, S.D.: Biochem. Biophys. Res. Comm. 56, 898-906 (1974).

24. Lasker, J.M., Graham, D.G., Abou-Donia, M.B.: Biochem. Pharmacol. 31, 1961-1967 (1982).

25. Ehrich, M., Larsen, C.: Comp. Biochem. Physiol. 64C, 383-386 (1983).

26. Abou-Donia, M.B.: Neurotoxicology 4, 113-130 (1983).

THE AGING REACTION OF INHIBITED NEUROPATHY TARGET ESTERASE - FUNDAMENTAL STUDIES AND TOXICOLOGICAL SIGNIFICANCE

Martin K. Johnson
MRC Toxicology Unit, Medical Research Council Laboratories, Woodmansterne Road, Carshalton, Surrey, SM5 4EF, U.K.

Introduction

Organophosphorus (OP) compounds have diverse effects on both the central and peripheral nervous systems. Best known is the inhibition by many OP esters, including insecticides and "nerve gases", of AChE with toxic consequences associated with overstimulation of cholinergic systems. Also AChE inhibitors such as paraoxon may produce a dose-dependent necrosis in rat skeletal muscle: pathological change is initiated at the motor end-plate and, by 24 hr, a generalized breakdown of muscle fibre architecture is evident (1). A critical loss of AChE activity (85%) over a specified period (2 hr) is necessary for this subacute effect to occur (2) and the process is discussed in detail by Dettbarn elsewhere in this volume.

OP-induced delayed neuropathy (OPIDN) is a syndrome distinct from each of the above and is caused by some but not all OP esters. It is characterised by the delay of between one and 3 weeks after intoxication before clinical effects are manifested. It has often, erroneously, been called OP-demyelinating disease. The better terminology of a "dying-back neuropathy" has in its turn been displaced by the title of distal axonopathy implying symmetrical distal axonal degeneration of certain neurons. The resulting paralysis is

Cholinesterases, © Walter de Gruyter & Co., Berlin - New York, 1984

not caused by muscle fibre necrosis but by concurrent degeneration in distal regions of long, large diameter axons in peripheral nerves and spinal cord.

OPIDN has attracted toxicologists for a number of reasons, of which the commercial importance and extent of use of the compounds is but one: numerous potential plasticisers, hydraulic fluids, flame-retardants and pesticides are neuropathic. Further interest exists because the response can be produced by a single dose in man and various larger mammals and in adult hens, yet there is a delay before frank disorder is seen as if a fuse had beeen lit but the dynamite keg were a long way removed. Small rodents do not develop neuropathy in response to single doses of typical neuropathic OP esters such as DFP and hens are the laboratory species of choice.

The subject of OPIDN has been reviewed from different angles a number of times starting with Davies in 1963 (3). The reviews in 1964 and 1973 by Cavanagh (4,5) attended principally to pathology. In 1975 I wrote an extensive review of the biochemical mechanism as then understood and explored the areas illuminated by this understanding (6). That review was coupled with a further article devoted to structure/activity relationships for every OP compound for which neurotoxicity test data were available (7). More is now known in molecular terms about the initiation of OPIDN and biochemical studies on the target protein and toxicological applications of the information gathered thereon have been reviewed recently (8) to show the rationalisation of toxicity testing which has come about as a fruit of understanding. The development of the cellular disorder which follows initiation and precedes clinical expression of neuropathy is still a mystery to be unfolded but understanding the initiation has improved our capacity to suggest rational routes of enquiry.

The target for initiation of OPIDN

1) DFP-Phosphorylation sites. When a typical neuropathic OP ester such as DFP is injected into living hens or incubated with hen brain homogenates *in vitro* many proteins are organophosphorylated. As long ago as 1969 it was shown that a small proportion of the total labelled protein responded to a wide range of OP ester inhibitors in the way required of the target for initiation of OPIDN (9). About 5% of the total [32-P]-DFP-labelling sites were both resistant to paraoxon and sensitive to mipafox *in vitro* and not inhibited *in vivo* by various non-neuropathic OP esters but inhibited when adequate doses of neuropathic esters were administered. The principle of the *in vitro* assay procedure for the Neuropathy Target Protein is shown in Fig. 1. It is

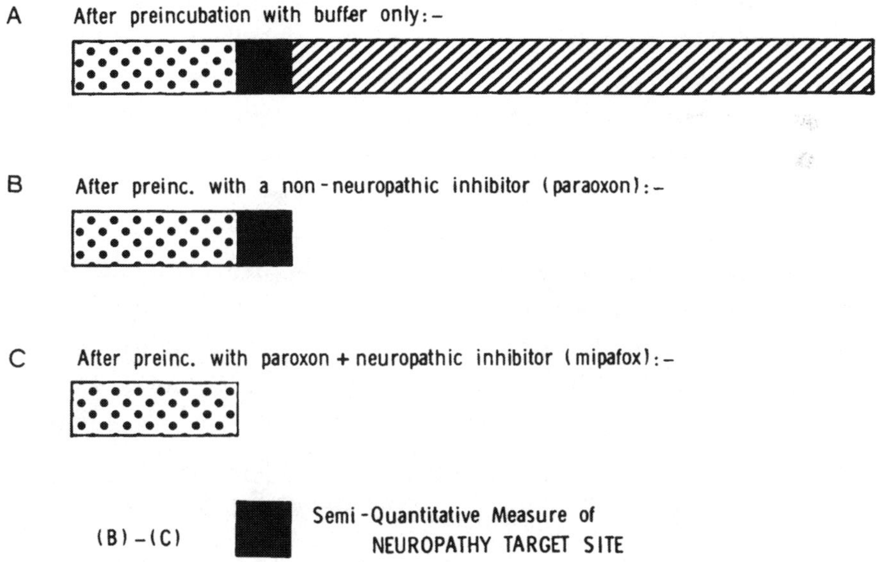

Fig. 1. [32-P]-DFP labelling of sites in hen brain homogenate and identification of OPIDN target site. For details see Refs. 9 and 13.

important to realise that all macromolecular sites open to phosphorylation by DFP were examined in the initial screen (condition (A) of Fig. 1). There is no possibility that the process of "focussing" on the target with selective inhibitors could have overlooked the true target. Crude kinetic analysis suggested that the identified quantity of sites (about 24 µmoles/g brain) was fairly homogeneous but this was not established rigorously.

2) Esteratic activity of the neuropathy target protein. Since it was likely that a protein site phosphorylated by low concentrations of DFP would prove to be the catalytic site of an esterase, screening was undertaken to find potential substrates which should, theoretically, slow the rate of phosphorylation of the target by displacement of DFP from the Michaelis complex. Only phenyl phenylacetate significantly diminished the rate indicating that this ester had preferential affinity for the target protein and suggesting that the target is a phenyl phenylacetate esterase. Active brain enzymes hydrolysing phenyl phenylacetate had previously been identified but they were very sensitive to some non-neurotoxic inhibitors such as paraoxon and TEPP (10) and these enzymes were shown not to be associated with OPIDN (11). However when the total activity against this substrate was examined more carefully using selective preincubations (as was done for the labelling site, Fig. 1) then Fig. 2 shows that a distinct paraoxon-resistant mipafox-sensitive esterase (the unshaded block) was found with responses *in vitro* and *in vivo* to neurotoxic and non-neurotoxic OP esters which correlated well with the responses of the target phosphorylation site (12, 13, 7). The presence of this esterase activity of the target protein can be detected only after selective inhibition of the similar but irrelevant enzymes: it is now commonly called neuropathy target esterase (NTE, formerly neurotoxic esterase). The procedures required to assay the various esterase activities contain precisely

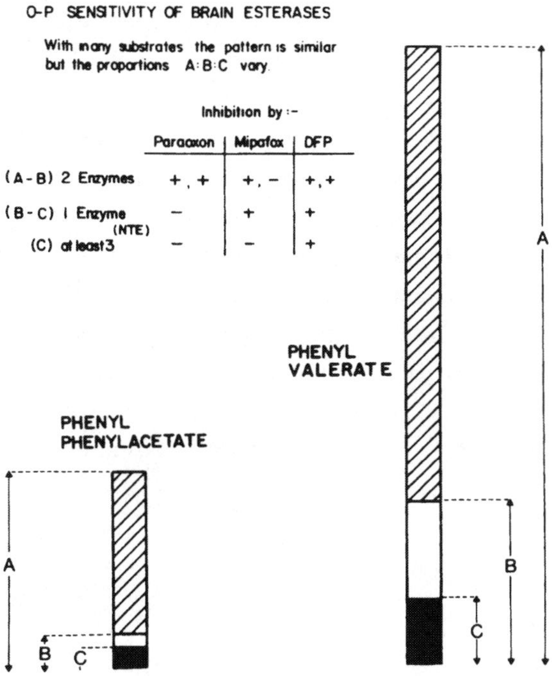

Fig. 2. Differentiation of hen brain esterases by use of selective inhibitors

the same preincubation steps as are indicated for radiochemical assay (compare Figs. 1 and 2). Subsequently it was shown that phenyl valerate is a more convenient substrate for NTE in terms of both sensitivity and specificity although the principle is identical (14). There is an excellent correlation between blocking of the labelling site by a wide variety of compounds both *in vivo* and *in vitro* and inhibition of NTE activity (13).

The exposition above shows that the identification of one particular esterase as the target for initiation of neuropathy has developed from and depended on the unambiguous identification of the target phosphorylation site. If it had been merely a good inspired choice of one out of all possible (known and unknown) esterases then it would be valid to query whether some other esterase (i.e. different protein) might not be the true target since no one knows how many other esterases may occur in brain. Failure to appreciate this logic may account for doubts which have occasionally been expressed about NTE as the target. Confirmation of an entirely different nature concerning the relevance of NTE to OPIDN came from the further mechanistic studies described below.

3) Protection against OPIDN by NTE inhibitors which could not give aged inhibited NTE. It became apparent as early as 1970 that if phenylmethanesulphonyl fluoride (PMSF) was used to acylate the target with concomitant inhibition of NTE then a different but exactly complementary toxicologic response was produced to that caused by DFP: hens dosed with PMSF became resistant to the neuropathic effects of a challenge dose of DFP given in the next few days although the anticholinesterase effects of DFP were unchanged (13). This remarkable effect was significant for 2 reasons:

(1) It confirmed the involvement of the catalytic site of NTE in initiation of OPIDN;
(2) It showed that loss of catalytic activity *per se* was not a sufficient cause of neuropathy.

I then studied certain organophosphates, phosphonates and phosphinates which were close structural analogues and differed only in the possession of 2 or one C-O-P bonds instead of C-P bonds. One example is shown in Fig. 3.

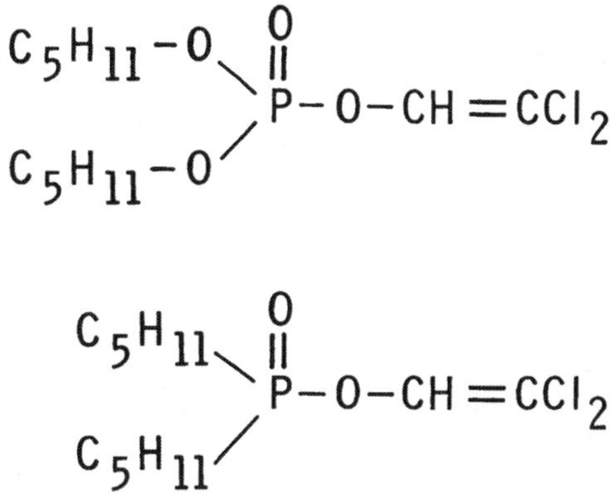

Fig. 3. Analagous organophosphate and phosphinate with complementary toxicological effects. Both are active against NTE (a) _In vitro_ at 10^{-8}M (tested both by binding site and by esterase assays), and (b) _In vivo_ at <5 mg/kg. The upper compound is NEUROPATHIC and the lower is PROTECTIVE. (Data from Refs. 15 and 7).

It was clear that these compounds were equally potent as blockers of the target protein and inhibitors of ester hydrolysis by NTE but the phosphates and phosphonates were neuropathic while the phosphinates were protective (15, 7).

Experiments like the above with a number of protective agents lead to the now generally accepted 2-step initiation process (Fig. 4) which requires absolutely an 'aging' step after the organophosphorylation (or phosphonylation or phosphoramidation) of the catalytic site of NTE. This aging transforms the phosphorylated target to a modified form in which one 'R' group has been cleaved from phosphorus and a negatively charged group remains attached to protein. As

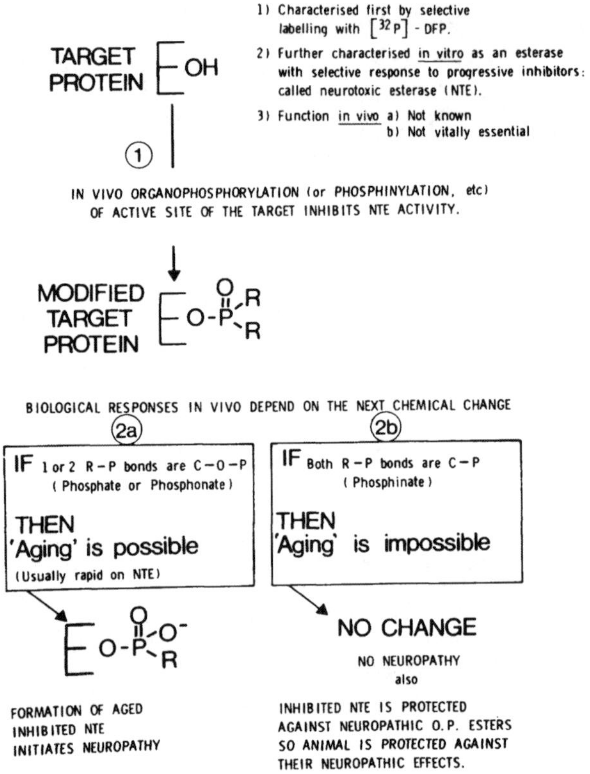

Fig. 4. Alternative chemical modifications (1 and 2a or 2b) of the OPIDN target protein with their complementary responses of NEUROPATHY or PROTECTION (Reproduced from Ref. 8 with permission).

shown in the contrasting boxes (2a) and (2b) of Fig. 4 not all bonds on inhibited NTE can be cleaved so that while aging is possible after inhibition of NTE by some classes of OP esters it is not possible after inhibition by phosphinates (or by sulphonyl fluorides). When aging is not possible the initiation process is aborted but the site remains blocked until fresh enzyme appears by resynthesis or by spontaneous reactivation. Hens in the protected state appear to suffer no ill effect even if the period is extended by repeated doses of a protective agent over 2 weeks (15).

Studies of the aging reaction

1) Demonstration of aging. Although the aging of inhibited NTE was proposed as an absolute necessity for initiation of OPIDN it proved remarkably difficult to demonstrate the reaction. Aging can be studied as, either, a chemical change in the groups attached to the protein or a progressive failure in the response of inhibited enzyme to nucleophilic reactivating agents. It has been shown for AChE treated with DFP that the time course of these 2 reactions is similar (16) and that the chemical change causes the loss of responsiveness to reactivators. Initially we were unable to show either that tritiated material was liberated into solution from [3-H]-DFP-inhibited NTE or to reactivate the inhibited enzyme. However phosphinylated NTE could be reactivated by several nucleophilies including high concentrations of KF at pH 5.2 (17). Our early failures were explained when we found that aging of DFP-inhibited NTE was extremely rapid ($t_{1/2}$ = 3-4 mins at pH 8.0/37°) and also that it was mechanistically different from the better-known aging reaction of AChE (17). Fig. 5 illustrates this difference. For hen brain cholinesterases inhibited by a mixture of [32-P] and [3-H]-labelled DFP the aging process is only half completed in 18 hours during which time bound tritium label is released into solution. For NTE the right-hand side of Fig. 5 shows that although no label is released into solution the nature of the labelled bound material changes with time. Initially the bound group is di-isopropylphosphoryl which can be released

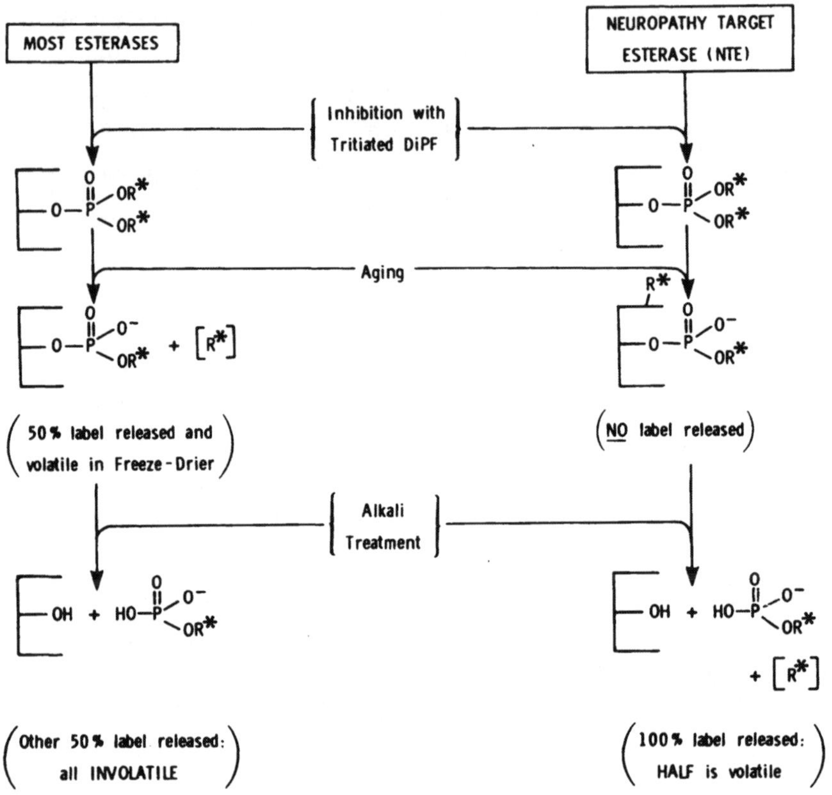

Fig. 5. Contrasting fates of tritiated alkyl group during aging of DFP-inhibited NTE v other esterases.

by alkali as di-isopropyl phosphoric acid (involatile). With a half-life of 3.25 min the bound material is converted to a monoisopropyl phosphoryl group which can be liberated by alkali as involatile acid plus a bound "isopropyl" (? iso-propoxy) group which is also liberated by alkali treatment but in a form which is easily removed by freeze-drying (17).

Further tests showed that NTE inhibited by DFP within 2 min could largely be reactivated if nucleophile was added immediately but that the rapid chemical change of bound groups was accompanied by loss of reactivatibility.

2) How does chemical structure of the bound group relate to aging and is the mechanism similar with all inhibitory OP esters? It is difficult to predict whether aging of NTE inhibited by other OPs will always involve transfer of the cleaved group onto a secondary site. Unless large quantities of purified enzyme become available the direct monitoring of the aging process will require radiolabelled inhibitor. With one other tritiated inhibitor we showed that aging of di-*n*-pentyl phosphoryl NTE also occurred with transfer of half the tritium to another macromolecular site and the reaction half-life was <1 min (18). Since the rate and pH dependance were similar for the chemical change and the loss of reactivatibility, the latter characteristic was used to monitor aging of NTE after inhibition by attachment of a variety of inhibitory groups. Table 1 shows that the process is rapid in many cases so that the mechanism may well be similar. Since aging is 2 orders faster for simple di-*n*-alkyl phosphates than for the highly branched pinacolyl group in soman it is unlikely that the mechanism is S_N1 as was demonstrated for soman-inhibited AChE (19). Unfortunately phosphoramidated esterases (not only NTE) appear to be refractory, even before aging, to the reactivation procedures which we have used. We are therefore unable to show that bond-cleavage with or without group transfer occurs in this case.

Rates of aging with the phosphates were so high that no ranking or relating of structure to activity was possible except to note that the bis-2-chloroethoxy derivative (compound 7) aged more slowly than the ethoxy derivative

Table 1. Approximate half-time for aging of neurotoxic esterase inhibited by various organophosphorus esters (RR^1P-O-esterase)

	Structure		Approx. $t_{1/2}$[a] (min)
	R	R^1	
	Phosphates		
(1)	MeO	Same as R	< 2
(2)	EtO	Same as R	< 5
(3)	PrO	Same as R	< 5
(4)	Pr^iO	Same as R	3-4
(5)	BuO	Same as R	< 2
(6)	$C_5H_{11}O$	Same as R	< 1
(7)	2-ClEtO	Same as R	10
(8)	PhO	Same as R	< 5
(9)	$2\text{-}Pr^iPhO$	Same as R	< 10
(10)	$C_5H_{11}O$	MeO	< 2
(11)	PhO	$2\text{-}HOPhCH_2O$	Very short
	Phosphonates		
(12)	Me	MeO	5
(13)	Me	$(Me)_3C\text{-}CH(Me)O$	600
(14)	Et	EtO	3
(15)	Et	2-ClEtO	300
(16)	Ph	MeO	10
	Phosphinate		
(17)	C_5H_{11}	C_5H_{11}	Aging not detected[b]

[a] Aging rates *in vitro* were determined as the rate of loss of ability to be reactivated by treatment with KF and (for 4 and 6) radiochemically; for (11) the evidence was indirect.

[b] Theoretically no aging is expected.

Data from Ref. 18.

(compound 2). In general, phosphonates aged more slowly than did phosphates, but further comparisons are limited since all the phosphonates were racemic mixtures and it does not necessarily follow that the same optical configuration of groups was achieved in the phosphonylated active site in each case; indeed, it is not certain whether only one isomer was responsible for most of the inhibition produced in any particular case. However, it is worth noting that the chloroethoxy ester (compound 15) aged about 100-fold more slowly than did its unsubstituted analogue (compound 14).

As shown in the accompanying poster at this meeting (20) aging of inhibited NTE is extremely slow after inhibition by any one of the 4 resolved isomers of soman: racemic soman is compound No. 13 in Table 1. The reaction is the more interesting since some spontaneous reactivation of the enzyme occurred after inhibition by the two P(-) isomers but not with P(+). The only other cases of spontaneous reactivation of inhibited NTE which have been described involve carbamylated enzyme (21) or the unusual inhibitor phenylmethanephosphonyl difluoridate (Ref 8 and see below).

3) Is the group transfer intermolecular or intramolecular?
No tritium could be trapped in solution by conducting aging of DiP-NTE in presence of a mixture of glutathione and imidazole (17). Williams separated the [^{3}H]-DFP labelled proteins of brain by gel electrophoresis and also by gel filtration (22, 23). He showed that mipafox-sensitive sites were not quite homogeneous. A minor component is probably not relevant to OPIDN since it is comparatively insensitive to a protective phosphinate. This minor component was of lower MW (about 92K) compared with the phosphinate-sensitive major mipafox-sensitive peak (MW about 155-178K). After aging of NTE almost exactly 50% of tritium attached to the major polypeptide could be liberated in volatile form by treatment with alkali whereas negligible volatile radioactivity was obtained from the minor component or from any

other labelled macromolecule. These 2 observations strongly suggest that the major peak of mipafox-sensitive labelling represents NTE and that the site which receives the group transferred during aging is on the NTE macromolecule.

4) Is NTE unique in aging with group transfer? In an extension of his study mentioned above, Williams labelled proteins of brain, spinal cord, liver, kidney and spleen from hen and, also, human placenta. Using the same technique as above he showed that in a 40 min. aging period (37° and pH 8.0) group transfer occurred only with a mipafox-sensitive component which was present in each tissue and which had a MW of about 178K in SDS (23). Also NTE-like esteratic activity in these tissues was such that the Catalytic Centre Activity for NTE in each tissue was very similar ($1.42-1.85 \times 10^5 min^{-1}$).

5) Can the variable sensitivity of different species to OPIDN be attributed to differences in the aging reaction? Man and the hen are 2 species in which OPIDN can be caused by a single dose. Single doses of OP compounds which are neuropathic in hen are not usually effective in rat and even multiple dosing over a period produces an uncertain response (24). For the rat I have shown that it is easy to inhibit brain NTE totally *in vivo* and to maintain inhibition for 2 weeks (8) with some OP esters. Also aging *in vitro* of DiP-NTE from rat brain occurs at the same rapid rate as for the hen enzyme (8). No studies on aging of inhibited NTE from human brain has been done but the human placenta NTE aged substantially in Williams' 40 min. experiment. There seems no reason to suppose that differences in aging characteristics will account for species sensitivity. It seems likely that initiation occurs in all species but that in some species the development does not occur unless the initiation signal is very prolonged. These species differences may be

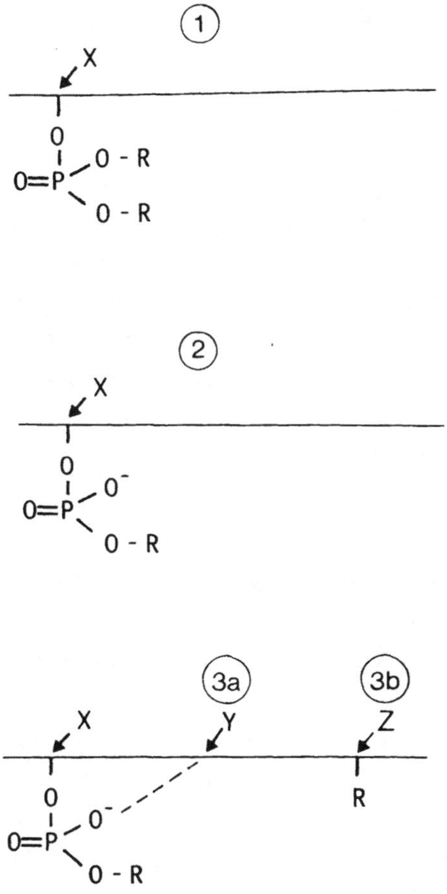

Fig. 6. The proven steps (1 and 2) of initiation of OPIDN with proposed alternative (3a or 3b) consequences. Step (1): organophosphorylation occurs at X causing inhibition of catalytic activity of NTE; (2): cleavage of one R-O-P bond to form a negatively charged group with concomitant aging of inhibited NTE; (3a): negative charge at X disrupts normal (unknown) function of another site, Y, OR (3b): transfer of R to a site, Z, during aging disrupts the normal (unknown) function of Z. (From Ref. 8, with permission).

linked with the size and configuration of nerve axons and their repair capacity: they are discussed further in the article by Richardson which follows in this volume.

6) Toxicological implications: Is the charged residue or the transferred group the focal point for initiation of neuropathy? I proposed that nerve degeneration ultimately occurs because of the formation of the charged group attached to the NTE molecule and that this charge upsets a normal physiological process of the neurone (15, 25). However, the possibility must be considered that, in every case of aging of inhibited NTE, the group lost during aging may be transferred to a secondary site.

Figure 6 shows the alternatives available as Step 3 of Initiation (the beginning of the Development Phase) of OPIDN. During the aging of NTE which had been inhibited by either tritiated DFP or di-*n*-pentyl 2,2-dichlorovinyl phosphate it was found that the label associated with the alkoxy groups which were removed from phosphorus was not liberated into solution but became attached to another macromolecular site (labelled "Z" in Fig. 6) (17, 18). This was in contrast to the liberation of small molecular-weight products into solution during aging of inhibited brain cholinesterases (17). Without a complete range of radio-labelled neurotoxic esters it is impossible to show whether this efficient transfer occurs when every variety of chemical group takes part in the aging reaction. It seems unlikely for, say, phosphoramidates or for phenoxy substituents. However, many unexpected reactions can occur in special environments such as may be provided by an enzyme active centre and if such a transfer does occur when NTE is inhibited by any neurotoxic ester then modification of the receiving site Z could be proposed as the event which precipitates neuropathy with formation of the charged group on the aged enzyme having no direct consequence.

Two approaches have been made to try to choose the correct interpretation (3a or 3b of Fig. 6). The first was to synthesise an inhibitor which could age but which would liberate a group intrinsically unsuited to attachment at Z: fluoride seemed such a group. Several compounds were synthesised and phenylmethanephosphonodifluoridate was found to inhibit NTE at easily tolerable doses *in vivo*. It must be assumed that one fluoride atom was lost during inhibition leaving the other P-F bond as the only bond available for cleavage during aging. However although P-F bonds are not intrinsically very stable very little aging was detected in inhibited NTE of brains removed from hens 2 days after dosing and considerable spontaneous reactivation had occurred (8). It seems possible that unless site Z has some ability to "pull" the relevant group off phosphorus and onto itself then aging of NTE is no longer facile. During the 2-3 days necessary for NTE activity to return to 80% of normal the hens were resistant to challenge doses of DFP just the same as if the target had been covered by a compound which could not age instead of by one which could but didn't (8). These observations confirm the absolute necessity of Step 2 for initiation but fail to show whether an effect at Site Y or Site Z is the key to OPIDN. The second approach has been to attempt to block Site Z directly instead of by transfer from phosphorus attached to X. Several chloromethyl ketones or N-substituted haloacetamides have been synthesised to resemble phenyl phenylcarbamate or phenyl benzylcarbamate which are both acylating inhibitors of NTE. Thus far the ketones inhibit NTE *in vitro* but are too reactive and corrosive to be used *in vivo* while the amides are surprisingly uninhibitory (8). It has also been shown that 4-bromophenylacetylurea, a neuropathic compound with some formal similarity to phenyl phenylcarbamate (26), appears not to modify Site (Z) *in vivo* since predosing with this compound does not alter the ability of rat brain NTE inhibited by DFP to undergo the aging reaction (8).

Although both the above rational approaches have failed to resolve the problem some recent studies in my laboratory (unpublished) have shown that modification of the target site in vivo by attachment of a phosphoromonoamidate in which the $-NH_2$ group is unsubstituted has unusual effects - possibly the negativity of the negatively charged oxygen is moderated in some way and a part-protected state is brought about. Further studies with related model compounds are under way.

7) What happens to aged inhibited NTE during the development stage of OPIDN? After inhibition of NTE by several different compounds (both neuropathic and protective) reappearance of active enzyme occurs with a half-life of 4-5 days (15, 27) so that about 70% normal levels of activity may be present by the time clinical signs of neuropathy are seen. Since aging has occurred for the neuropathic compounds this activity is presumed to be freshly-synthesized. It will require immunochemical methods to trace the persistence, redistribution, transport or disappearance of the aged NTE. However some progress could be made in deciding whether phosphinylated NTE persists in vivo since this could be identified by differential assays before and after treatment of tissue with an appropriate reactivator.

It is intriguing that clinical signs in a hen which developed severe neuropathy after a neuropathic dose of soman isomer were not seen until the 12th day after dosing (J. Willems, private communication): after DFP signs can be seen on the 9th day. It may be that the initiation signal was not actually given until aging was complete which certainly takes 3-4 days with the NTE-inhibitory isomers of soman (20). A possible corollary is that although aging was slow the inhibited NTE was not disposed of during this latent period.

Conclusion

The aging of inhibited NTE appears to be mechanistically unique among mammalian tissue esterases. The molecular basis for this characteristic is worthy to be pursued: the chemical nature of site Z is not yet proven.

The toxicological implications of the aging of NTE are considerable. Already it is possible to devise structures having pesticidal activity with no capability to cause delayed neuropathy and protective mixes are possible. Further study of the influence of chemical structure on both inhibition and aging of NTE may be fruitful in increasing our understanding of enzyme mechanisms and in our control of toxic hazard.

References

1. Wecker, L., Dettbarn, W.D.: Experimental Neurol. 51, 281-291 (1976).
2. Wecker, L., Kiauta, T., Dettbarn, W.D.: J. Pharmacol. Exp. Therap. 206, 97-104 (1978)
3. Davies, D.R.: Neurotoxicity of organophosphorus compounds. Hanbuch der experimentellen Pharmakologie, Erganzungswerk, vol. XV, G.D. Koelle, pp. 860-882, Springer, Berlin-Heidelberg-New York, (1963).
4. Cavanagh, J.B.: Int. Rev. exp. Path. 3, 219-267 (1964).
5. Cavanagh, J.B.: Crit. Rev. Toxicol. 2, 365-417 (1973).
6. Johnson, M.K.: Crit. Rev. Toxicol. 3, 289-316 (1975b).
7. Johnson, M.K.: Arch. Toxicol. 34, 259-288 (1975a).
8. Johnson, M.K.: Rev. Biochem. Toxicol. 4, 141-212 (1982).
9. Johnson, M.K.: Biochem. J. 111, 487-495 (1969a).
10. Poulsen, E., Aldridge, W.N.: Biochem J. 90, 182-189 (1964).
11. Aldridge, W.N., Barnes, J.M.: Biochem. Pharmacol. 15, 541-548 & 549-554 (1966).

12. Johnson, M.K.: Biochem. J. 114, 711-717 (1969b).

13. Johnson, M.K.: Biochem. J. 120, 523-531 (1970).

14. Johnson, M.K.: Biochem. Pharmacol. 24, 797-805 (1975c).

15. Johnson, M.K.: J. Neurochem. 23, 785-789 (1974).

16. Berends, F., Posthumus, C.H., v.d. Sluys, I., Deierkauf, F.A.: Biochim. Biophys. Acta. 34, 576-578 (1959).

17. Clothier, B., Johnson, M.K.: Biochem. J. 177, 549-558 (1979).

18. Clothier, B., Johnson, M.K.: Biochem. J. 185, 739-747 (1980).

19. Michel, H.O., Hackley, B.E., Berkowitz, L., List, G., Hackley, E.B., Gillilan, W., Pankau, M.: Arch. Biochem. Biophys. 121, 29-34 (1967).

20. Johnson, M.K., Read, D.J., Benschop, H.P.: Interaction of the resolved isomers of soman with chicken brain acetylcholinesterase and neuropathy target esterase (NTE). In: Abstracts of Second Int. Meeting on Cholinesterases, Bled, Yugoslavia, p. 145 (1983).

21. Johnson, M.K., Lauwerys, R.: Nature 222, 1066-1067 (1969).

22. Williams, D.G., Johnson, M.K.: Biochem. J. 199, 323-333 (1981).

23. Williams, D.G.: Biochem. J. 209, 817-829 (1983).

24. Majno, G., Karnovsky, M.L.: J. Neurochem. 8, 1-16 (1961).

25. Johnson, M.K.: Fed. Proc. 35, 73-74 (1976a).

26. Johnson, M.K.: Brit. Med. Bull. 25, 231-235 (1969c).

27. Caroldi, S., Lotti, M.: Toxicol. App. Pharmacol. 62, 498-501 (1982).

DIRECT COMPARISON OF THE DISTRIBUTION OF NEUROTOXIC ESTERASE AND ACETYLCHOLINESTERASE IN RAT AND HEN BRAIN

P.J. Hollingsworth, B.R. Dudek, C.B. Smith and R.J. Richardson

Toxicology Research Laboratory, School of Public Health, and Department of Pharmacology, The University of Michigan, Ann Arbor, Michigan 48109 USA

Introduction

Neurotoxic esterase (NTE) is strongly implicated as the target protein in the initiation of organophosphorus-induced delayed neurotoxicity (OPIDN), yet marked differences in susceptibility to OPIDN exist among species possessing neural NTE with seemingly identical phosphorylation characteristics _in vitro_ and _in vivo_. Since nothing is known about the physiological function of NTE or the basis of species differences in susceptibility to OPIDN, and since the highest concentration of NTE in any given species is found in brain, it was of interest to determine the degree of homogeneity of NTE distribution in brain, to compare the NTE distributions of susceptible (hen) and nonsusceptible (rat) species, and to compare these distributions with those of a better understood esterase, AChE.

Methods

Animals used. Male, Sprague-Dawley rats, weighing 175-320 g, and White Leghorn hens (spent hens), weighing 1.5-2.8 kg, were used. Rats and hens were killed by decapitation, and their brains were rapidly removed. Rat brains were dissected as described previously (1). Areas of the rat brain were identified by the use of the atlas of the rat brain by König and Klippel (2). Homologous areas of the hen brain were selected on the basis of physiological function, anatomical interrelationships and the distribution of specific neurotransmitters as identified by chemical and histochemical techniques (3-6). Areas of the hen brain were identified by the use of the atlas of the chicken brain by van Tienhoven and Juhasz (7). Homologous areas of the hen brain and the rat brain are listed in Table 1.

Table 1. Homologous brain areas of rat and hen.

Rat[1]	Hen[2]
Cerebellum	Cerebellum
Brainstem	Brainstem
Hypothalamus	Hypothalamus
Amygdala	Archistriatum
Hippocampus	Hippocampus
Parietal Cortex	Hyperstriatum ventralis
Caudate Nucleus	Paleostriatum augmentatum

1 Areas of the rodent brain as described by König and Klippel (2).
2 Areas of the avian brain as described by van Tienhoven and Juhasz (7).

NTE activity assay. NTE activity was assayed by a

modification of the method described by Johnson (8). Tissues from specific rat or hen brain areas were homogenized in a volume of ice-cold, 50 mM Tris-HCl/2 mM EDTA incubation buffer (pH 8.0 at 25°C) sufficient to give a final concentration of 6 mg of tissue (wet weight) per ml of buffer. Phenyl valerate was used as substrate to give a final calculated concentration of 1.4 mM, although the actual concentration was difficult to estimate since the substrate was present in the form of a detergent micelle. The phenyl valerate dispersion was prepared by adding a solution of Triton X-100 (0.03% in H_2O, 30 vol) to a solution of phenyl valerate (15 mg/ml) in redistilled dimethyl foramide (1 vol). The paraoxon-sensitive activity was measured in the presence of 40 µM paraoxon. IRE activity was then determined in the presence of both paraoxon, 40 µM, and mipafox, 59 µM. NTE activity is the difference between IRE activity and the activity measured in the presence of paraoxon alone.

AChE assay. AChE activity was assayed by a modification of the method described by Ellman *et al*. (9). Tissues were homogenized in a volume of ice-cold , 50 mM Tris-HCl/2 mM EDTA buffer sufficient to give a final concentration of 20 mg of tissue (wet weight) per ml of buffer. AThCh, 75 mM, was used as substrate. Iso-OMPA, 0.1 mM, was used to inhibit BuChE.

Protein determinations. The protein content of all samples was determined by a modification of the method of Lowry *et al*. (10) in which bovine serum albumin was used as the protein standard.

Analysis of results. All values represent means ± the standard error of the mean. For statistical evaluations

Student's t-test was used, and P values are given in parentheses.

Results

<u>Distribution of NTE activity in rat brain.</u> NTE activity is distributed unevenly within the rat brain (Table 2). The highest activity was found in homogenates of the hypothalamus (9.1 ± 0.9 nmol/min/mg protein, n=7) and in homogenates of the brainstem (8.0 ± 0.6 nmoles/min/mg protein, n=7). The lowest activity was found in the homogenates of the hippocampus (5.0 ± 0.5 nmoles/min/mg protein, n=7) and of the cerebellum (5.2 ± 0.7 nmoles/min/mg protein, n=6). NTE activity in the various areas of the rat brain was distributed as follows: hypothalamus > brainstem > amygdala > cortex > caudate nucleus > cerebellum > hippocampus. The caudate nucleus, an area which has the highest AChE activity in the rat brain (see below) had a low NTE activity similar to that found in the cerebellum and hippocampus. NTE activity for whole brain homogenates was 5.6 ± 0.4 nmoles of phenyl valerate hydrolyzed/min/mg protein (n=4).

<u>Distribution of IRE activity in the rat brain.</u> Unlike NTE activity, IRE activity is distributed evenly throughout all areas of the rat brain except for the cerebellum (Table 2). Values ranged from 7.3 ± 0.3 nmoles/min/mg protein (n=7) for homogenates of caudate nucleus to 8.1 ± 0.4 nmoles/min/mg protein (n=7) for the hypothalamus. This represents an 11% difference and is not statistically significant. However, IRE activity was significantly higher in the cerebellum (10.1 ± 0.6 nmoles/min/-mg protein, 25% higher, n=7, $P < .025$) than in the hypothalamus, the next highest area.

Table 2. Distribution of NTE and IRE activity in rat brain

Area	NTE Activity[1]	n	IRE Activity[1]	n
Hypothalamus	9.1 ± 0.9	7	8.1 ± 0.4	7
Brainstem	8.0 ± 0.6	7	7.8 ± 0.7	7
Amygdala	7.0 ± 0.5	6	7.8 ± 0.4	6
Parietal Cortex	5.8 ± 0.6	7	7.6 ± 1.0	7
Whole Brain[2]	5.6 ± 0.4	4	7.3 ± 0.1	4
Caudate Nucleus	5.5 ± 0.3	7	7.3 ± 0.3	7
Cerebellum	5.2 ± 0.7	6	10.1 ± 0.6	7
Hippocampus	5.0 ± 0.5	7	7.7 ± 0.3	7

[1] nanomoles phenylvalerate hydrolyzed/min/mg protein. Each value is the mean ± standard error of n observations.

[2] Whole brain refers to the brain less the cerebellum. NTE activity in the hypothalamus was 82 percent greater than that found in the hippocampus ($P < .005$).

Distribution of NTE activity in hen brain. There is little information available as to the distribution of NTE in the central nervous system of the hen even though this is the species most frequently studied in the evaluation of neurotoxic organophosphorus compounds. As in the rat brain, in the hen brain NTE is distributed unevenly (Table 3). The areas with the highest activity were the the hyperstriatum ventralis (homologous to the rat parietal cortex, 19.6 ± 1.1 nmoles /min/mg protein, n=6) and the paleostriatum augmentatum (homologous to the caudate nucleus, 19.5 ± 1.5 nmoles/min/mg protein, n=5). Lowest NTE activity was found in homogenates made from the brainstem (8.8 ± 0.4 nmoles/ min/mg protein, n=6) and from the hypothalamus (9.7 ± 0.5 nmoles/ min/mg protein, n=6). NTE activity in homogenates of the hyperstriatum ventralis and the paleostriatum augmenta-

Table 3. Distribution of NTE and IRE activity in hen brain.

Area	NTE Activity[1]	n	IRE Activity[1]	n
Hyperstriatum ventralis	19.6 ± 1.1	6	6.9 ± 0.3	6
Paleostriatum augmentatum	19.5 ± 1.5	5	7.0 ± 0.4	5
Archistriatum	15.1 ± 0.6	6	5.9 ± 0.3	6
Hippocampus	15.0 ± 1.3	6	6.5 ± 0.3	6
Cerebellum	13.9 ± 1.3	6	6.5 ± 0.5	6
Hypothalamus	9.7 ± 0.5	6	6.8 ± 0.2	6
Brainstem	8.8 ± 0.4	6	6.9 ± 0.2	6

[1] See Table 2 for details.

tum was more than twice that found in homogenates of the brainstem ($P < .0005$) and the hypothalamus ($P < .0005$). NTE activity in the various areas of the hen brain was distributed as follows: hyperstriatum ventralis = paleostriatum augmentatum > archistriatum > hippocampus > cerebellum > hypothalamus > brainstem.

Distribution of IRE activity in the hen brain. As in the rat brain, IRE activity is distributed fairly evenly throughout all areas of the hen brain (Table 3). Values ranged from 5.9 ± 0.3 nmoles/min/mg protein (n=6) for homogenates of archistriatum to 7.0 ± 0.4 nmoles/min/mg protein (n=5) for homogenates of the paleostriatum augmentatum. This represents a 20% difference ($P < .05$).

Distribution of AChE in rat brain. AChE activity was measured in those areas of the rat brain and spinal cord in which NTE activity was determined. The purpose of these experiments was to ascertain whether the distribution of the enzyme responsible for inactivation of neurogenically released ACh had a pattern of distribution similar to that found for NTE. The variations in the activity of AChE in the rat nervous system were much greater than those observed for NTE. Highest AChE activity was found in homogenates of the anterior caudate nucleus (86.0 ± 3.9 nmoles/min/mg protein, n=5, Table 4). This activity was three-fold greater than that found in the amygdala (29.0 ± 1.3 nmoles/min/mg protein, n=4), the area with the next highest activity. The lowest AChE activity was found in homogenates of the cerebellum (6.0 ± 0.3 nmoles/min/mg protein, n=3) and the parietal-occipital cortex (9.5 ± 0.8 nmoles/min/mg protein, n=5). Acetylcholinesterase activity was fourteen-fold greater in homogenates of the anterior caudate nucleus than in those from the cerebellum. AChE activity in homogenates from the various areas of the rat brain was distributed as follows: caudate nucleus > amygdala > brainstem > hippocampus > hypothalamus > parietal cortex > cerebellum.

Table 4. Distribution of AChE activity in rat brain.

Area	AChE Activity[1]	n
Caudate Nucleus	86.0 ± 3.9	5
Amygdala	29.0 ± 1.3	4
Brainstem	20.5 ± 0.5	5
Hippocampus	13.3 ± 0.3	5
Hypothalamus	13.2 ± 1.2	5
Parietal Cortex	9.5 ± 0.8	5
Cerebellum	6.0 ± 0.3	3

[1] nanomoles acetylthiocholine hydrolyzed/min/mg protein. Each value is the mean ± standard error of n observations.

<u>Distribution of AChE in hen brain.</u> In marked contrast to the rat brain, the highest AChE activity in the hen brain was found in homogenates from the cerebellum (93.0 ± 0.2 nmoles/ min/mg protein, n=3, Table 5) and the lowest activity was found in homogenates from the brainstem (27.9 ± 4.1 nmoles/min/mg protein, n=3), hippocampus (27.2 ± 3.1 nmoles/min/mg protein, n=3) and hypothalamus (27.1 ± 2.9 nmoles/min/mg protein, n=3). As in the rat, homogenates of hen amygdala had rela-

Table 5. Distribution of AChE activity in hen brain

Area	AChE Activity[1]	n
Cerebellum	93.0 ± 0.2	3
Archistriatum	63.7 ± 7.6	3
Paleostriatum augmentatum	41.2 ± 9.1	3
Hyperstriatum ventralis	32.7 ± 3.1	3
Brainstem	27.9 ± 4.1	3
Hippocampus	27.2 ± 3.1	3
Hypothalamus	27.1 ± 2.9	3

[1] nanomoles acetylthiocholine hydrolyzed/min/mg protein. Each value is the mean ± standard error of n observations.

tively high activity (63.7 ± 7.6 nmoles/min/mg protein, n=3). AChE activity in homogenates from the various areas of the hen brain was distributed as follows: cerebellum > archistriatum > paleostriatum augmentatum > hyperstriatum ventralis > brainstem = hippocampus = hypothalamus. AChE activity in the cerebellum was approximately threefold greater than in the hypothalamus, hippocampus and brainstem, and 1.5 times greater than in the archistriatum.

Discussion

Marked differences exist between the distribution of NTE activity in the hen and in the rat nervous system. The absolute amount of activity was about the same in homogenates made from the hypothalamuses of the two species; however, relative to other brain areas, activity in the rat brain was highest in the hypothalamus and in the hen brain was very low in the hypothalamus. NTE activity was higher in every area of the hen brain than in any area of the rat brain with the exception of the brainstem. The following differences existed between activities in homologous areas of the rat and hen brain (when activity in hen brain is expressed as a percentage of the activity in rat brain): cerebellum (hen 235%, $P < .005$); amygdala (hen archistriatum 216%, $P < .0005$); caudate nucleus (hen paleostriatum 355%, $P < .0005$); parietal cortex (hen hyperstriatum ventralis 340%, $P < .0005$); hippocampus (hen 300%, $P < .005$); hypothalamus (hen 107%, N.S.) and brainstem (hen 110%, NS). These differences in the distribution of NTE in the brains of the two species might be related to the differences in the sensitivity of the rat and the hen to OPIDN.

No clear correlation appeared between the distribution of AChE activity and that of NTE in the rat nervous system. The anterior caudate nucleus, the area with the highest AChE activity had one of the lowest NTE activities. The hypothalamus, the area which had the highest NTE activity had an intermediate AChE activity. Homogenates of cerebellum showed low activity for both esterases. With the exception of the cerebellum, AChE activity in the hen nervous system was better correlated with NTE activity than it was in the rat nervous system. Relatively high values for the activity of both esterases were found in the hyperstriatum ventralis, paleostriatum augmentatum and archistriatum. However, even in the hen nervous system the correlation between AChE and NTE activity is not particularly good. These observations indicate that NTE is not merely a variant of AChE which is distributed in the same manner as AChE but which has a different substrate specificity.

Acknowledgements

This study was supported in part by USPHS grants MH-36226 and ES-01611.

References

1. Smith, C.B., Garcia-Sevilla, J.A., Hollingsworth, P.J.: Brain Research 210, 413-418 (1981).
2. König, J.F.R., Klippel, R.A.: The Rat Brain. A Stereotaxic Atlas of the Forebrain and Lower Parts of the Brain Stem, The Williams and Wilkins Company, Baltimore, Maryland 1963.
3. Jurio, A.V., Vogt, M.: J. Physiol. London 189, 489-518 (1967).
4. Ikeda, H., Gotoh, J.: Japan. J. Pharmacol. 21, 763-784 (1971).
5. Dube, L., Parent, A.: J. Comp. Neurol. 196, 695-708 (1981).
6. Northcutt, R.G.: Ann. Rev. Neurosci. 4, 301-350 (1981).
7. van Tienhoven, A., Juhasz, L.P.: J. Comp. Neurol. 118, 185-197 (1962).
8. Johnson, M.K.: Arch. Toxicol. 37, 113-115 (1977).
9. Ellman, G.L., Courtney, K.D., Andres, V., Jr., Featherstone, R.M.: Biochem. Pharmacol. 7, 88-95 (1961).
10. Lowry, O.H., Rosebrough, N.F., Farr, A.G., Randall, R.J.: J. Biol. Chem. 193, 265-275 (1951).

UNIFYING MECHANISMS IN ACHE REGULATION AND ORGANOPHOSPHATE INDUCED NEUROPATHY OF THE CHICKEN

Barry W. Wilson, Yuji Ishikawa[1], Edward Chow, Mark G. McNamee, William R. Randall[2], Gary T. Patterson[3], Richard K. Entrikin and Pamela S. Nieberg.

University of California at Davis, Davis, California, USA, 95616

1. Permanent Address; Department of Anatomy, Chiba University, Chiba, Japan. Present Addresses: 2. Department of Biochemistry, Imperial College, London, England; 3. Oak Ridge Research Institute, Oak Ridge, Tennessee, USA

Introduction

Much recent research on AChE uses it as a "model" molecule, investigating the synthesis, movement, localization, and degradation of its multiple molecular forms (1). In addition, the toxic effects of inhibiting AChE activity with compounds like organophosphate esters (OP's) have led to much research on inhibitors of the enzyme such as DFP, paraoxon, and mipafox that react with the serine residue at the active site, and, after a rearrangement known as "aging", cause its irreversible phosphorylation (2). Less attention has been given to phosphorylations of other esterases with serine-active sites. One such interesting and somewhat controversial esterase is the "neurotoxic esterase, NTE"; its inhibition by some OP's has been proposed by Johnson and his colleagues (3) to initiate an insidious delayed axonal neuropathy (organophosphate induced delayed neuropathy, OPIDN) in sensitive animals like man, the dog and the chicken. (3,4). Our research on OP's has recently expanded from an emphasis on regulation of AChE to include studies of NTE activity and the biochemical bases for OPIDN (5). This chapter highlights what we have recently learned about AChE regulation and NTE, including some speculations on mechanisms that may be common to both areas.

Early appearance of the small globular forms of AChE (4,7, and 11-12S in birds) during development,(1), reports of the absence of large collagen-tailed forms (20S in quail and chicken) in muscle cultures derived from non-innervated embryonic muscle (6), and reports that neurons and neural extracts stimulate the appearance of the collagen-tailed forms in culture (7) support the idea that expression of the small forms is intrinsic to the developing muscle fibers and that innervation "induces" formation of the tailed forms. However, recent research shows that some sera, notably horse serum (the one preferred by many for the culture of muscle cells), inhibit appearance of the 20S form

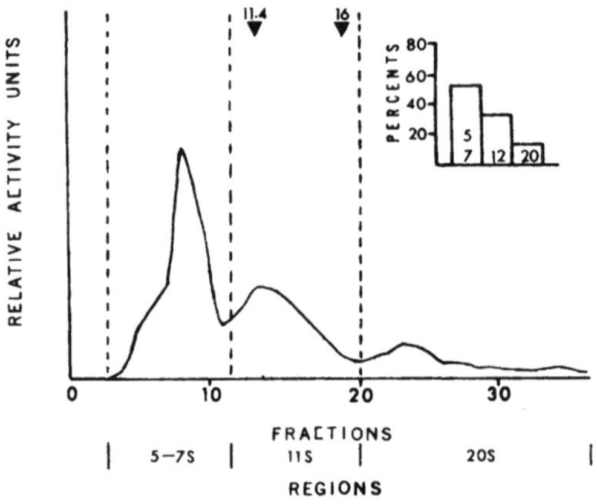

Figure 1. Sucrose sedimentation of AChE from quail muscle cultures grown 14 days in complete medium. Cultured from 9 day quail embryo pectoral muscle in 88% MEM, 2% EE and 10% horse serum. AChE extracted in .05 M Tris-HCl, pH 7.3, 1% Na cholate, 0.5M $MgCl_2$, layered on a 5-20% sucrose gradient in 0.05M Tris-HCl, pH 7.3, 1.0 M NaCl, 0.5% Triton X-100 and 0.2 mM EDTA. Inset; percent of AChE activity in 5-7,11 and 20S regions of the gradient.

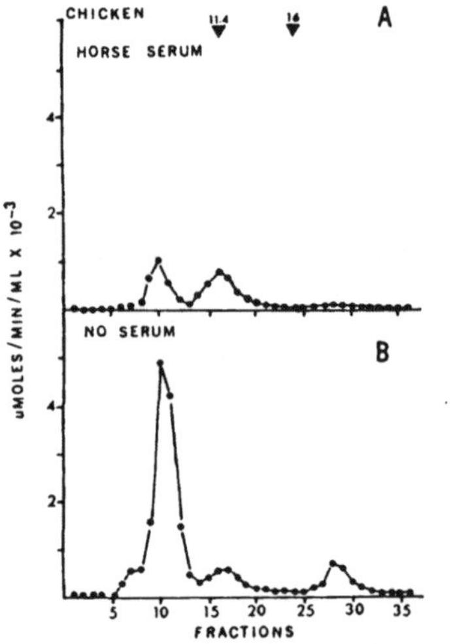

Figure 2. Sucrose sedimentation of AChE from a chicken muscle culture of cells from 11 day chick embryo pectoral muscle. A. 10 day culture in complete medium. B. 10 day culture in serumless medium for 24 hours.

regardless of the age of the donor tissue (8). The effect of serum is made even more apparent by the use of a cholate-based extraction buffer that releases more of the 20S form from muscle cultures than the Triton-based extraction buffers commonly used to solubilize AChE (8,9).

Data on AChE forms are shown here as the extent of hydrolysis of radioactive ACh (10) for each fraction of the gradients (Fig. 1) and (inset, Fig. 1) as the relative activity of each region of the gradients containing separable AChE forms calculated by determining the areas under the curves. Nine 9 day quail embryo cells, unlike those from comparably aged chick embryo cells (8,11), are an excellent source of cells that readily produce the 20S form of AChE in culture even in the presence of horse serum (Fig. 1).

Fig. 2 shows that removal of horse serum for 24 hours from the culture medium of chick embryo muscle from an 11 day embryo causes an increase in

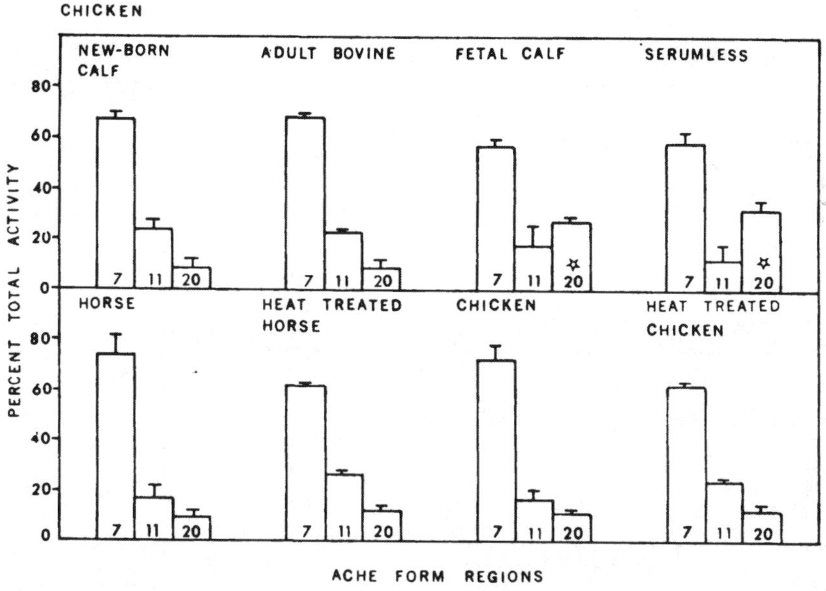

Figure 3. Effect of different sera on AChE forms from cultured chick embryo muscle. Prepared from 11 day embryo pectoral muscle grown 12 days in culture and exposed for 48 hours to media containing different sera. * indicates statistical differences to the level of the 20S form in control (horse serum) cultures.

AChE activity and the appearance of relatively large amounts of the 20S form in the absence of innervation or of special extracts. (The activity of the 20S form also increases in quail cultures under similar conditions.) Dr. Patterson's thesis research (12) showed the inhibitory factor (or factors) responsible was highest in horse serum, lowest in fetal calf serum (Fig. 3) and larger in size than 100K daltons (Fig. 4). (It is interesting that the cultures in which Kato et al.(13) noted the presence of 20S AChE in chick embryo muscle were grown in media containing calf and not horse serum.) Whatever is present in the sera does not affect the AChE forms in spinal cord motor neuron cultures; levels of the smaller globular AChE forms they contain did not increase after removal of serum (data not shown).

Dr. Randall's thesis research examined the AChE patterns of cell cultures derived from muscle primordia at different stages of development. Fig. 5 shows the shift in pattern of AChE from small forms to large forms during development of quail muscle. (Note the presence of considerable 20S activity in 9 day embryo muscle, the age used to prepare the cultures in Fig. 1.) The experiments confirmed in the rat (6) and showed in the

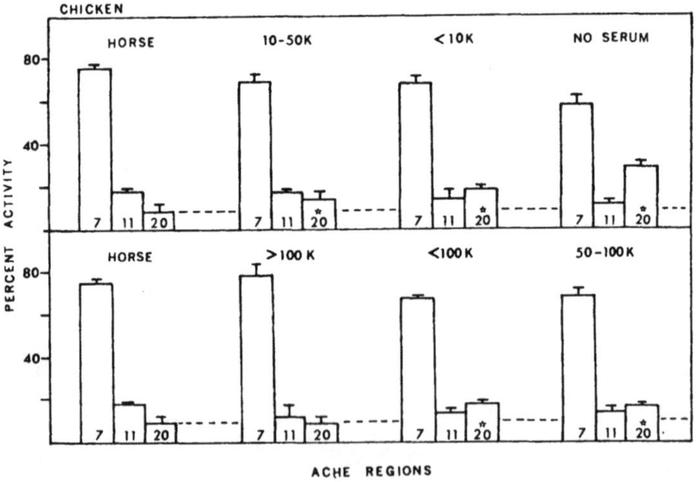

Figure 4. Effect of different horse serum fractions on cultured chick embryo muscle AChE forms. Fractions prepared with Diaflo membranes and added on an equal protein basis compared to unfractionated horse serum. In no case were the fractions more than 15% of the medium. * statistic as in Fig.3.

quail that cultures from early embryos before innervation did not exhibit large collagen tailed forms - so long as the medium contained horse serum (Fig. 6,14). When serum was removed, collagen-tailed forms soon appeared in the same cultures.

It is as if the factors in serum are there to prevent assembly of collagen-tailed AChE in the absence of motor end plates. One might imagine the Schwann cells that invest the forming motor end plates isolate them from tissue fluid during development, permitting collagen-tailed AChE to form freely there and reducing its formation

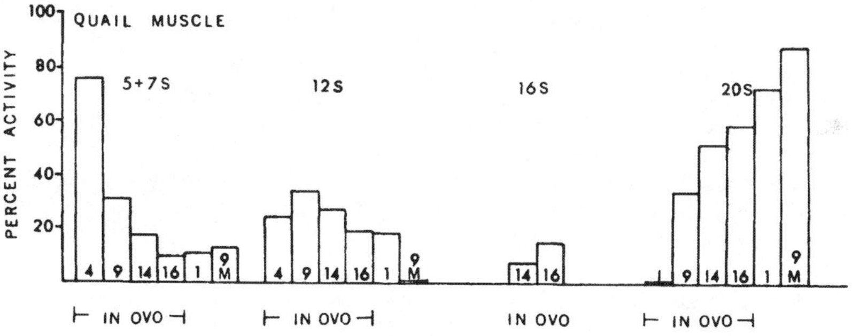

Figure 5. Relative levels of AChE forms in developing quail pectoral muscle. 4,9,14,and 16 day embryo, 1 day and 9 month post-hatch muscle samples.

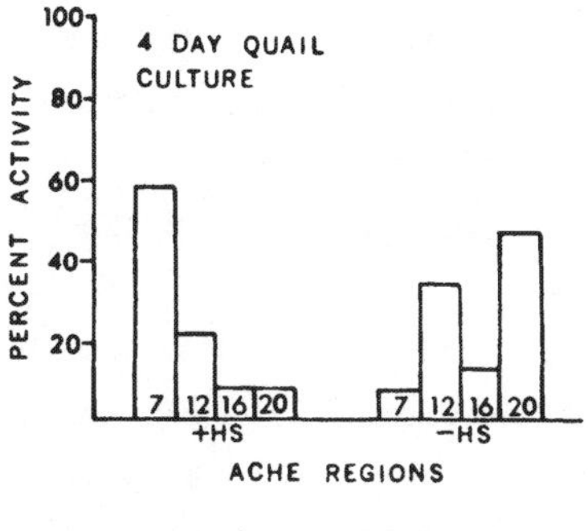

Figure 6. Relative levels of AChE forms in cultured quail muscle from 4 day limb buds. 12 days in culture.

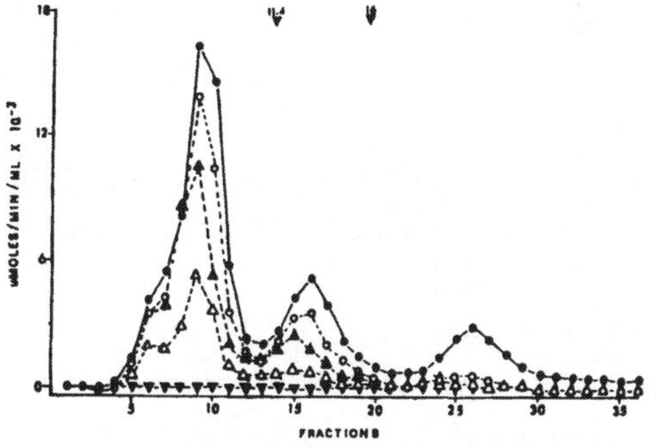

Figure 7. Recovery of cultured quail muscle after DFP. 12 day muscle culture treated for 15 minutes with 10^{-4} DFP. ▼ 0; △ 2; ▲ 4; ○ 8; ● 24 hours after treatment.

elswhere along the fibers. For example, a set of instructions intrinsic to the muscle fibers could control synthesis of the small AChE forms and basement membrane substances and an exogenous one could regulates assembly of one form from another. Regardless, the results warn against accepting evidence that innervation and neural factors are directly involved in the regulation of AChE in culture if the experiments have not been done in serum-free media.

TABLE 1
PROPERTIES OF ACHE RECOVERY FROM OP'S
IN MUSCLE AND NERVE CULTURES

New AChE from synthesis of new protein.
New AChE rapidly synthesized, rapidly degraded.
AChE synthesis greater than controls.
Recovery rate proportional to inhibition.
The smaller the form the more rapid its recovery
New 20S AChE is both inside and outside the cell.

Recovery Of Cells From OP Treatment

Brief treatment of muscle and nerve cultures with OP's inhibits existing AChE, permitting study of the newly synthesized AChE that takes its place (15). Fig. 7 illustrates the process with a quail muscle culture in which AChE was inhibited by a brief treatment with DFP and the recovery of the several molecular forms was followed over time with sucrose gradient density sedimentation. Such data with both cultured chicken and quail muscle, indicate that the small forms recover more rapidly than the large ones (16).

The recovery process shows several interesting features (Table 1); for example, the level reached by the newly formed enzyme is invariably higher than in the untreated cultures and the greater the initial inhibition, the more rapid is the rate of recovery . One interesting possibility is that phosphorylated AChE regulates the rate of AChE resynthesis (5).

Even though nerves may not be necessary for the synthesis and assembly of AChE in embryo muscle, innervation is important to maintain proper AChE levels and molecular forms in a functional muscle fiber. Previous work of ours (17,18) and others (19) has shown that levels of small AChE forms and extrajunctional staining increase greatly and the 20S form disappears in denervated fast twitch muscle of the chicken. We are currently using denervated biceps brachii (BIC) and posterior latissimus dorsi (PLD) muscles of young chicks to study the action of glucocorticoids such as corticosterone-21-acetate (C21A) on AChE regulation <u>in situ</u>.

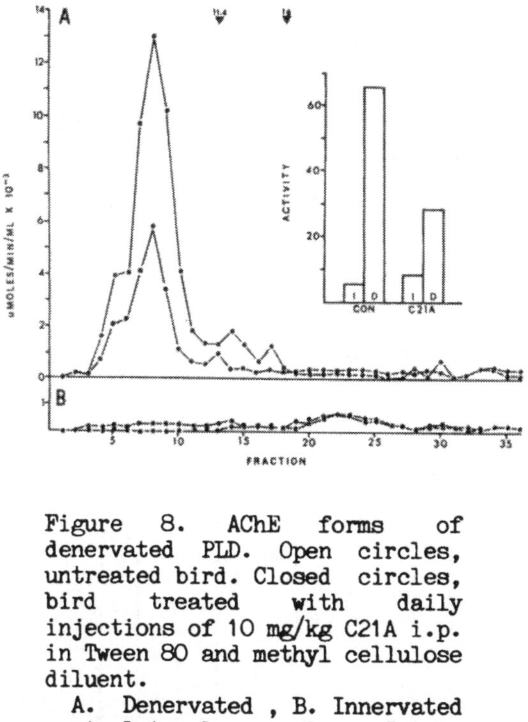

Figure 8. AChE forms of denervated PLD. Open circles, untreated bird. Closed circles, bird treated with daily injections of 10 mg/kg C21A i.p. in Tween 80 and methyl cellulose diluent.

A. Denervated, B. Innervated contralateral muscle. Inset, total AChE activity of the muscles. Note difference in units of activity. 5-6 week old birds denervated 14 days before sampling.

Figure 9. Extrajunctional AChE in denervated PLD. A. Innervated; B. Denervated untreated; C. Denervated C21A. Conditions as in Fig. 8. 10X objective.

Fig. 8 shows the results of an experiment where birds were given C21A the day before and daily after denervation of the right PLD muscle. In this case (and in other experiments on the biceps) C21A treatments prevented some of the increase in levels of the low molecular weight forms, but did not affect loss of 20S AChE activity. The most striking difference was cytochemical; extrajunctional AChE levels, determined by staining cryostat sections for AChE (20), were much reduced in C21A treated denervated muscles compared to denervated muscle from untreated birds (Fig. 9). Whether the action of C21A is directly upon the muscle, or upon regrowth of the severed axons is under study.

One of the reasons for testing the action of corticosteroids on AChE regulation in denervated muscle was an earlier finding that these chemicals reduce the abnormally high total AChE levels and extrajunctional localization of AChE in muscles from chicks with inherited muscular dystrophy along with alleviating other symptoms of the disorder (21,22). Fig. 10 shows the results of an experiment where dystrophic chicks were injected with C21A for five weeks. The decrease in AChE levels of C21A-treated dystrophic muscle was reflected in a decrease in the small, globular molecular forms, bringing the enzyme pattern of the muscles closer to that of normal muscle.

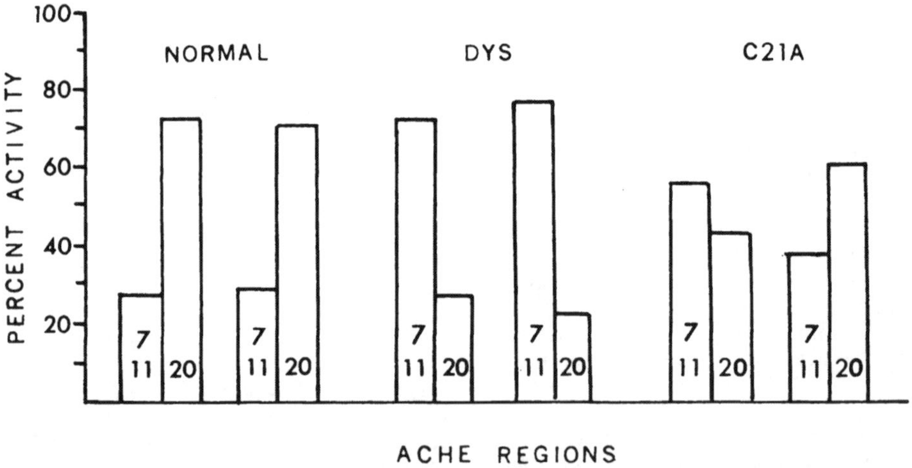

Figure 10. AChE forms of C21A treated dystrophic muscle. Bars represent pairs of 5 week old normal Line 412, control dystrophic Line 413 and dystrophic given daily injections of C21A (10 mg/kg) from hatch.

The way that OP's such as DFP, mipafox, sarin and TOCP cause OPIDN is not known; one theory proposes that the first step in the process is analogous to the way OP's inhibit AChE, hypothesizing that neurotoxic OP's preferentially inhibit a single protein, NTE, and that the

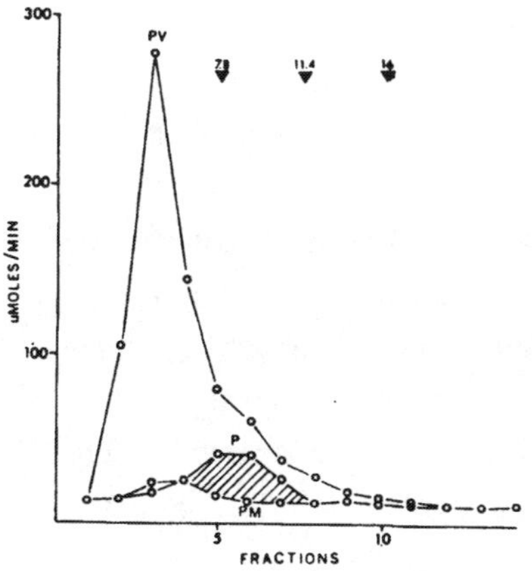

Figure 11. Phenyl valerate hydrolysis of chick embryo brain homgenate. Sample homogenized (1:4 w/v) in 1 mM Tris-HCL, 0.5M NaCl and 0.2% Triton X-100; centrifuged at 100,000 xg and the supernatant run on a 5-20 % sucrose gradient with 1mM Tris-HCl, pH 7.2, 0.5 M NaCl and 0.025 Triton X-100 for 16 hours at 150,000 xg. Colorimetric phenyl valerate hydrolysis determination without inhibitors (PV), with 40 uM paraoxon (P) and 40 uM paraoxon plus 50 uM mipafox (PM). NTE activity in barred region.

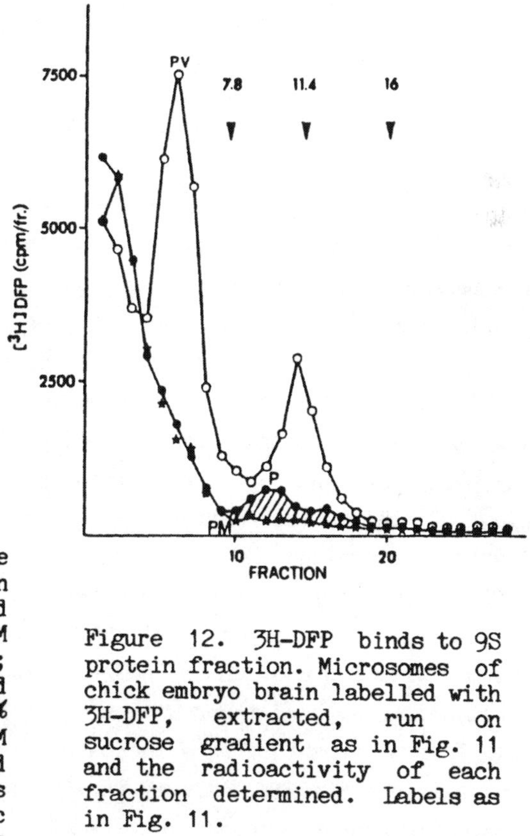

Figure 12. 3H-DFP binds to 9S protein fraction. Microsomes of chick embryo brain labelled with 3H-DFP, extracted, run on sucrose gradient as in Fig. 11 and the radioactivity of each fraction determined. Labels as in Fig. 11.

phosphorylated protein "ages" to form the active neurotoxic molecule (3,23). Much evidence for the existence of NTE has been circumstantial; its natural substrate is unknown; the assay to determine NTE activity consists of measures the extra inhibition brought about by the addition of a neuropathic OP (mipafox) to that caused by a non-neuropathic OP (paraoxon) in the hydrolysis of phenyl valerate. Recently we modified the techniques we use to study AChE forms and obtained evidence for an NTE-like enzyme that migrates in the 9S region after sucrose density gradient centrifugation (5 ,24).

Fig. 11 shows the distribution of phenyl valerate hydrolase activity on a 5-20% sucrose density gradient of chick embryo brain. Most of the activity inhibited by the non-neuropathic OP paraoxon peaked in the 4S region; enzyme activity specifically inhibited by the neuropathic OP mipafox peaked in the 9S region. Similar results were obtained for spinal cord, spleen and adult brain. Recently, we have been conducting more experiments to test whether the 9S mipafox sensitive form corresponds to the hydrolase activity designated as NTE. In one set of experiments Dr. Ishikawa labeled microsomal fractions of chick embryo brain with ^{3}H-DFP (a neuropathic OP) and unlabeled mipafox and/or paraoxon following the technique of Williams and Johnson (25), solubilized and subjected them to ultracentrifugation and SDS-PAGE. Proteins labelled with DFP in the presence of unlabelled paraoxon migrated in the 9S region of the gradients (Fig. 12) as expected of NTE, and, in confirmation of the results of Williams and Johnson (25), a 160K protein was preferentially labeled under these conditions with the labeled neurotoxic OP (data not shown). In another set of experiments Dr. Ishikawa and Mr. Chow examined the decrease in brain NTE activity _in vivo_ that accompanies treatment of an animal with a neuropathic agent. Fig. 13 shows sucrose gradients from homogenates of brains of animals that had been treated with the neuropathic CBDP (the active product of TOCP) and the non-neuropathic paraoxon. Only the brains from the animals treated with the neuropathic OP showed a decrease in the mipafox sensitive activity in the 9S region.

TABLE 2
SIMILARITIES OF 9S ACTIVITY AND NTE

Sensitive to mipafox, DFP; insensitive to paraoxon.
Labeled by ^{3}H-DFP following unlabeled paraoxon.
Labelling accompanied by label of 160K protein.
Activity decreases in brain from CBDP poisoned hens.
Activity unchanged in brain from paraoxon poisoned hens.

The data support the conclusion that an enzymatically active protein (or perhaps proteins) migrating as 9S form(s) behaves as expected of NTE. We are currently working on isolating and purifying the protein(s) as a prelude to studying its function and role in OPIDN.

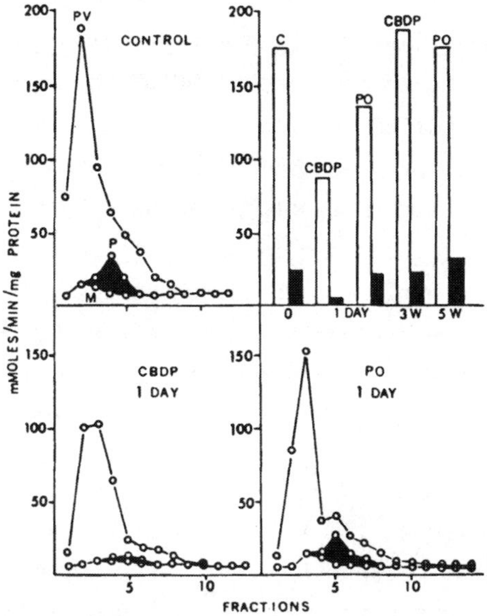

Figure 13. Phenyl valerate hydrolysis of chicken brain after exposure in situ to organophosphates. Adult hens were pretreated with 40 mg/kg atropine and then injected s.c. with 20 mg/kg CBDP or 1.0 mg/kg paraoxon (PO) and sampled at the times indicated. C is uninjected 0 time control. Open bar, 4S paraoxon-sensitive activity peak; dark bar, 9S NTE activity peak.

The experiments discussed here and past findings of others lead to the testable hypothesis that phosphorylation of glucocorticoid-like receptor molecules in nerve and muscle is involved in the regulation of AChE and the production of OPIDN. For example, if molecules like phosphorylated forms of AChE, NTE and similar molecules were mistaken for regulatory substances by the body, then phosphorylated AChE might stimulate synthesis of more AChE, and phosphorylated NTE might enter the motor neuron nucleus and kill the cell.

Binding of dexamethasone to glucocorticoid receptors has been reported to increase in denervated and dystrophic chicken muscle (26,27); glucocorticoid treatments delay some of the electrophysiological changes that accompany denervation (Hall 28). As early as 1960 (29), there have been reports that steroid treatments blocked OPIDN in the chicken. Ehrich and Gross (30) found administration of dietary cortisone reduced symptoms of malathion poisoning and the clinical signs of neuropathy caused by TOTP. Recently, Drakontides et al.(31) presented several reports that triamcinolone reduces the severity of OPIDN in the cat. Of course, other less exciting explanations to the actions of C21A here may obtain. For example, C21A merely may act nonspecifically to reduce the overall protein synthesis of denervated and dystrophic muscles, decreasing their capacity to make new enzymes or proteases to destroy them.

The worth of unifying hypotheses lie in the experiments they generate. Whether or not the ideas presented here are borne out by future experiments, they serve to emphasize that the actions of OP's and other chemical agents can be taking place on the long-term synthetic and genetic machinery of the cells as well as on its short-term metabolism.

Acknowledgements

The authors thank Dr. J. Seiber, Mr. M. Hooper, Mr. M. McChesney and Ms. J. Sonada for their assistance. Supported in part by the NIH, MDA, NIHR and the Northern California Occupational Health Center.

References

1. Massoulie, J. and Bon, S. Ann.Rev. Neurosci. 5, 57-106, (1982)

2. Aldridge, W.N. and Reiner, E. Enzyme inhibtiors as substrates. North-Holland Publishing Company, Amsterdam, 1972.

3. Johnson, M.K. Crit. Rev. Toxicol. 3, 289-316 (1975).

4. Abou-Donia, M.B. Ann. Rev. Pharmacol. Toxicol. 21, 511-548 (1981).

5. Wilson, B.W., Ishikawa, Y., Chow, E. and Cisson, C.M. Neurotox. In Press.

6. Rieger, F., Koenig, J. and Vigny, M. Dev. Biol. 76, 358-365 (1980).

7. Markelonis, G.J., Kemerer, V.F. and Oh, T.H. J. Biol. Chem. 255, 8967-8970 (1980).

8. Bulger, J.E., Randall, W.R., Nieberg, P.S., Patterson, G.T., McNamee, M.G. and Wilson, B.W. Dev. Neurosci. 5, 474-483 (1982).

9. Barat, A., Escudero, E., Gomez-Barriocanal, J. and Ramirez, G. Neurosci. Lett.10, 205-210 (1980.

10. Johnson, C.D. and Russell, R.L. Analyt. Biochem. 64, 229-238 (1975).

11. Emmerling, M.R., Johnson, C.D., and Lipton, B.H. Neurosci. Abs. 5, 478 (1979).

12. Patterson, G.T., Hayman E.G. and Wilson, B.W. In Vitro 19, 272 (1983).

13. Kato, A.C., Vrachliotis, A., Fulpius, B. and Dunant, Y. Dev. Biol. 76, 222-228 (1980).

14. Randall, W.R. and Wilson, B.W. In Vitro 18, 324 (1982).

15. Wilson, B.W., Nieberg, P.S., Walker, C.R., Linkhart, T.A. and Fry, D.M. Dev. Biol. 33, 285-289 (1973).

16. Wilson, B.W. and Nieberg, P.S. Biochem. Pharm. 32 911-918 (1983).

17. Wilson, B.W., Kaplan, M.A., Merhoff, W.C., and Mori, S.S. J. Exp. Zool. 174, 39-64 (1970).

18. Sketelj J., McNamee, M.G. and Wilson, B. W. Exp. Neurol. 60:624-629, (1978).

19. Sillman, I., diGiamberardino, L., Lyles, J., Couraud, J.Y. and Barnard, E.A. Nature 280:160-162 (1979).

20. Karnovsky, M.J. and Roots, L. Histochem. Cytochem. 12, 219-221 (1964)

21. Entrikin, R.K, Patterson, G.T. and Wilson, B.W. Muscle and Nerve. In Press.

22. Entrikin, R.K., Patterson, G.T. and Wilson, B.W. Muscle and Nerve. 5 ,321-327 (1982).

23. Clothier, B. and Johnson, M.K. Biochem. J. 177, 549-558 (1979).

24. Ishikawa,Y., Chow, E., McNamee, M.G., McChesney,M. and Wilson, B.W. Toxicol. Lett. 17, 315-320 (1983).

25. Williams, D.G. and Johnson, M.K. Biochem. J. 199, 323-333 (1981).

26. DuBois, D.C and Almon, R.R. Muscle and Nerve. 4, 370-373 (1981)

27. DuBois DC and Almon RR. Exp. Neurol. 75, 555-565 (1982).

28. Hall, E.D., Baker, T., Riker, W.F. Jr. Ann. Neurol. 1, 263-269 (1977).

29. Glees, P. Ger. Med. Monthly 6, 245-247 (1961).

30. Ehrich, M and Gross, W.B. Neurobehav. Tox. and Teratol. 4, 789-792 (1982).

31. Drakontides, A.B., Baker, T. and Riker, W.F. Jr. NeuroTox. 3, 165-178 (1982).

VII AUTHOR INDEX

IX TITLES OF POSTERS PRESENTED AT THE SECOND INTERNATIONAL MEETING ON CHOLINESTERASES (Bled, Yugoslavia, September, 17th to 21st, 1983)

Session 1: Chemistry and catalytic activity of cholinesterases

1. Reversible inactivation of serum cholinesterase by isocyanates through involvement of an active-site thiol

W.E. Brown, A.H. Green, T.E. Cedel and M.H. Karol

Dept. of Biological Sciences, Carnegie-Mellon Univ., Pittsburgh, PA, 15213 and Dept. of Industrial Environmental Health Sciences, Univ. of Pittsburgh, Pittsburgh, PA 15261 (USA)

2. Effect of cholinesterase inhibitors and substrates on cholinesterase induced luminiscence of luminol

E. Kunec-Vajić[1] and M. Boloban-Sinčić[2]

(1) Zavod za farmakologiju, Medicinski fakultet and (2) SOUR "Pliva", 41000 Zagreb (Yugoslavia)

3. A microfluorometric assay for cholinesterases, suitable for multiple kinetic determinations of picomoles of released thiocholine

R. Parvari[1], I. Pecht[2] and H. Soreq[1]

Departments of (1) Neurobiology and of (2) Chemical Immunology, The Weizmann Institute of Science, Rehovot 76100 (Israel)

4. Rabbit serum (cholin)esterases hydrolysing acetylthiocholine and butyrylthiocholine

V. Simeon

Institute for Medical Research and Occupational Health, 41000 Zagreb (Yugoslavia)

5. Time course of inhibition of cholinesterase by D-tubocurarine

J. Stojan, M. Zorko and M.R. Pavlič

Institute of Biochemistry, Medical Faculty, 61105 Ljubljana (Yugoslavia)

6. Spin labeled esters of fluorophosphonic acid in the study of the microgeography of acetylcholinesterase

A. Štalc[1], M. Šentjurc[2] and S. Pečar[3]

(1) Institute of Pathophysiology, Medical Faculty, (2) Dept. of Physics, "Jožef Stefan" Institute, (3) Dept. of Pharmacy, FNT; Edvard Kardelj University, 61000 Ljubljana (Yugoslavia)

7. Reaction of <u>T. californica</u> acetylcholinesterase with fluorescent thiol-selective reagents

G. Tomlinson, B. Mutus and D.V. Duncan

Department of Chemistry, University of Winnipeg, Winnipeg, Manitoba, R3B 2E9 (Canada)

Session 2: Multiple molecular forms of acetylcholinesterase: Structure, regulation and molecular forms

8. Antigenic and structural differences in the catalytic subunits of the molecular forms of acetylcholinesterase

B.P. Doctor[1] and P. Taylor[2]

(1) Division of Biochemistry, Walter Reed Army Institute of Research, Washington, DC, 20307 and (2) Department of Medicine, University of California, San Diego, La Jolla, CA, 92093 (USA)

9. Solubilization of acetylcholinesterase from Torpedo electric organ by a phosphatidylinositol-specific phospholipase C

A. Futerman[1], M.G. Low[2] and I. Silman[1]

(1) Dept. of Neurobiology, The Weizmann Institute of Science, Rehovot 76100 (Israel) and (2) Oklahoma Medical Research Foundation, Oklahoma City, OK, 73104 (USA)

10. Isolation and characterization of different forms of AChE from <u>Torpedo californica</u>

F. Spillecke and E. Neumann

Max-Planck-Institut f. Biochemie, 8033 Martinsried bei Muenchen (FRG)

11. Acetylcholinesterase molecular forms in <u>Torpedo marmorata</u>: Tissue specificity and hydrophobic character

J.P. Toutant and S. Bon

Laboratoire de Neurobiologie - Ecole Normale Supérieure, 46, rue d'Ulm, 75005 Paris (France)

12. Characterization of the catalytic subunits of acetylcholinesterase from the electric organ of Torpedo marmorata

V. Witzemann

Abt. Neurochemie, Max-Planck-Institut f. biophysikalische Chemie, 3400 Goettingen (FRG)

13. Comparative studies on acetylcholinesterase from Torpedo marmorata

S. Stieger and U. Brodbeck

Medizinisch-chemisches Institut, University of Bern, CH-3000 Bern (Switzerland)

14. The salt soluble forms of acetylcholinesterase in human nucleus caudatus

K. Gennari and U. Brodbeck

Medizinisch-chemisches Institut, University of Bern, CH-3000 Bern (Switzerland)

15. An immunological study of mammalian acetylcholinesterase using anti-rat serum

J. Grassi[1], D. Marsh[2], M. Vigny[2] and J. Massoulié[2]

(1) Laboratoire d'Études Radioimmunologiques, Départment de Biologie, Centre d'Etudes Nucléaires de Saclay, 91191 Gif sur Yvette, Cedex (France) and (2) Laboratoire de Neurobiologie, Ecole Normale Superiéure, 45, rue d'Ulm, 75005 Paris (France)

16. Hydrodynamic properties and detergent interactions of the molecular forms of mouse acetylcholinesterase. Sedimentation coefficients, partial specific volumes, molecular weights and frictional ratios

L.H. Tran, P. Dreyfus, A. Friboulet and F. Rieger

Groupe de Biologie et Pathologie Neuromusculaires, INSERM U. 153, 17, rue du Fer-à-Moulin 75005 Paris (France)

17. AChE in the different fibre types of mammalian muscle. I. Relationships of AChE molecular forms to the fibre types

J. Lai, J. Pizzey and E.A. Barnard

Department of Biochemistry, Imperial College of Science, London SW7 (UK)

18. AChE in the different fibre types of mammalian muscle. II. Effects of denervation

J. Lai, J. Pizzey, D. Green and E.A. Barnard

Department of Biochemistry, Imperial College of Science, London SW7 (UK)

19. Molecular forms of the cholinesterases inside and outside endplates in slow-tonic chicken muscle fibres

J. Jedrzejczyk, I. Silman and E.A. Barnard

Department of Biochemistry, Imperial College of Science, London SW7 (UK)

20. Molecular forms of acetylcholinesterase (AChE) inside and outside endplates in mammalian muscle fibres

J. Jedrzejczyk, J. Pizzey and E.A. Barnard

Department of Biochemistry, Imperial College of Science, London SW7 (UK)

21. Asymmetric molecular forms of AChE in muscles of different mammals

J. Sketelj, M. Pavlin, M. Peršič, M. Rus and M. Brzin

Institute of Pathophysiology, 61105 Ljubljana (Yugoslavia)

22. Acetylcholinesterase and acetylcholine receptor modulation in rat sternocleidomastoid muscle after denervation at birth

B. Blondet, F. Rieger and J. Gautron

Groupe de Biologie et Pathologie Neuromusculaire, INSERM U. 153, 17, rue du Fer-à-Moulin, Paris (France)

23. Latency and amplitude of the changes in the major molecular forms of acetylcholinesterase after denervation of the adult mouse sternocleidomastoid muscle in the motor endplate (MEP)-rich and -free regions

D. Goudou, B. Blondet and F. Rieger

Groupe de Biologie et Pathologie Neuromusculaires, INSERM U. 153, 17, rue du Fer-à-Moulin, 75005 Paris (France)

24. Relationship of collagen-tailed acetylcholinesterase with basal lamina components: Absence of binding with laminin, fibronectin and collagens type IV and V and lack of reactivity with different anti-collagen antisera

J. Grassi[1], J. Massoulié[2] and R. Timpl[3]

(1) Laboratoire d'Etudes Radioimmunologiques, Départment de Biologie, Centre d'Etudes Nucléaires de Saclay, 91191 Gif sur Yvette (France) (2) Laboratoire de Neurobiologie, Ecole Normale Supérieure, 45, rue d'Ulm, 75005 Paris (France) (3) Max Planck, Institut f. Biochemie, Martinsried bei Muenchen (FRG)

25. Intracellular and extracellular molecular forms of acetylcholinesterase in primary cultures of chick embryo myotubes

F. Vallette and J. Massoulié

Laboratoire de Neurobiologié, Ecole Normale Superiéure, 46, rue d'Ulm, 75005 Paris (France)

26. Biochemical evidences for two types of myoblasts during chick embryogenesis

J.P. Toutant[1] and M. Toutant[2]

(1) Laboratoire de Neurobiologie, Ecole Normale Supérieure, 46, rue d'Ulm, 75005 Paris (France) and (2) E.R. 107 CNRS, 17, rue du Fer-à-Moulin, 75005 Paris (France)

27. Acetylcholinesterase assembly during development of quail muscle in culture

W.R. Randall and B.W. Wilson

University of California Davis, Davis, CA (USA)

28. Evolution of acetylcholinesterase molecular forms in the electric lobes and in the electric organs during development of *Torpedo*

S. Bon

Laboratoire de Neurobiologie, Ecole Normale Supérieure, 46, rue d'Ulm, 75005 Paris (France)

29. Brain acetylcholinesterase (AChE) in its molecular forms in *Acomys cahirinus* during early post-natal life

H. Michalek, S. Fortuna, A. Pintor and G.M. Bisso

Laboratorio di Farmacologia, Istituto Superiore di Sanità, 00161 Roma (Italy)

30. Acetylcholinesterase molecular forms in rat brain subcellular fractions (including axonal membranes)

L. Settimi[1], N. Mucci[1] and H. Savolainen[2]

(1) Istituto Superiore di Sanità, Roma (Italy) and (2) Institute of Occupational Health, Helsinki (Finland)

31. Activity and molecular forms of cholinesterases in the liver and plasma of the rat

J. Sketelj, M. Snoj, L. Šekoranja and M. Brzin

Institute of Pathophysiology, 61105 Ljubljana (Yugoslavia)

Session 3: Sub-cellular localization, transport and secretion of cholinesterases

32. Acetylcholinesterase and cholinacetyltransferase activities in different microscopical areas of chick embryo spinal cord.

E. Bronzetti[1], G. De Renzis[2], L. Felici[1] and L. Fumagalli[3]

(1) Dept. Scienze Neurologiche, Università "La Sapienza", Roma, (2) Istituto Anatomia Umana Normale, Università Cattolica, Roma, (3) Dept. Biologia Cellulare, Università di Camerino (MC) (Italy)

33. Ultrastructural demonstration of acetylcholinesterase activity in the corpus geniculatum laterale, pars dorsalis, of the rat

H.J. Lüth[1] and M. Brzin[2]

(1) Paul-Flechsig-Institute of Brain Research, Karl-Marx-University, Leipzig (GDR) and (2) Institute of Pathophysiology, 61105 Ljubljana (Yugoslavia)

34. ACh-system in the longitudinal and circular muscle layer of guinea-pig vas deferens

Ž. Majcen

Institute of Pathophysiology, 61105 Ljubljana (Yugoslavia)

35. Differential axonal transport of acetylcholinesterase forms in the nerves of fast and slow-twitch muscles

F. Bacou[1] and J.Y. Couraud[2]

(1) Station de Physiologie Animale, I.N.R.A., 34000 Montpellier and (2) Départment de Biologie, C.E.N. Saclay, 91191 Gif-sur-Yvette (France)

36. Membrane-bound acetylcholinesterase on the external side of nerve-terminals plasma membrane

C. Bon and Z.Y. Li

Unité des Venis, Institut Pasteur, 28, rue du Dr. Roux, 75013 Paris (France)

37. Regulation of secretion of acetylcholinesterase from neuronal cell cultures

C.A. Lucas and G.W. Kreutzberg

Max Planck Institute for Psychiatry, Department of Neuromorphology, D 8000 Munich 40 (FRG)

38. Turning behaviour following microinjection of acetylcholinesterase and dopamine antagonists into one substantia nigra

J. Weston and S.A. Greenfield

University Laboratory of Physiology, Parks Road, Oxford OX1 3PT (UK)

39. Ultrastructural localization of acetylcholinesterase at the neuro-muscular junction. Immunocytochemical and biochemical study using monoclonal antibodies

P. Mailly[1], M. Vigny[2] and H.L. Koenig[1]

(1) Lab. Cytologie, Université P. et M. Curie, Paris VI, (2) Lab. Neurobiologie, E.N.S., Paris (France)

40. Synaptic antigens defined by monoclonal antibodies

S.E. Moore, O. Hurko, S. Brown and F.S. Walsh

Institute of Neurology, Queen Square, London WC1N 3BG (UK)

41. Acetylcholinesterase focalized at neuromuscular contacts: Neuronal or muscular origin ?

S. De la Porte[1], D. Marsh[3], J. Grassi[4], F. Vallette[3], M. Vigny[3] and J. Koenig[1,2]

(1) INSERM U. 153, 17, rue du Fer-à-Moulin, 75005 Paris (2) Université P. et M. Curie, Paris (3) Lab. de Neurobiologie, E.N.S., Paris, (4) Dept. Biologie, LERI, CEN Saclay, (France)

42. Acetylcholinesterase localization in fast and slow muscles of normal and dystrophic mice

H. Stephens and V. Gisiger

Dépt. d'Anatomie, Université de Montréal, Montréal H3C 3J7 (Canada)

Session 4: Biological functions of acetylcholinesterase and butyrylcholinesterase, and changes in disease states

43. AChE in stimulated fast-twitch avian muscle

J.C. Jarvis, J. Lai and P.J. Barnard

Department of Biochemistry, Imperial College of Science, London SW7 (UK)

44. The molecular forms of cholinesterases in human muscle from dystrophic and hypotonic patients

G. Poiana[1], S. Biagioni[2], F. Leone[1], A. Longstaff[1] and G. Scarsella[1]

(1) Dipartimento di Biologia Cellulare e dello Sviluppo, Università "La Sapienza", Roma, (2) Istituto di Istologia ed Analisi di Laboratorio, Università di Urbino (Italy)

45. Muscle acetylcholinesterase activity and molecular forms from normal and dystrophic mice

G. Poiana[1], S. Biagioni[2], M. Giorgi[1], F. Leone[1], G. Scarsella[1] and M.I. Senni[3]

(1) Dipartimento di Biologia Cellulare e dello Sviluppo and (2) Istituto di Istologia ed Embriologia Generale, Università "La Sapienza", Roma, (3) Istituto di Istologia ed Analisi di Laboratorio, Università di Urbino (Italy)

46. Denervation of sternocleidomastoid muscle in trembler dysmyelinating mutant as compared to control mouse

N. A. Do Thi[1], H.L. Koenig[1] and M. Vigny[2]

(1) Lab. de Cytologie, Université P. et M. Curie, Paris (2) Lab. de Neurobiologie, ENS, Paris (France)

47. Molecular forms of AChE, glucocorticoids and denervation of chicken muscles

B.W. Wilson, P.S. Nieberg, R.K. Entrikin and Y. Ishikawa

Avian Sciences, University of California, Davis, CA, 95616 (USA)

48. Does the nerve cell produce and release only one transmitter ?

R. Pavlin and D. Sket

Institute of Pathophysiology, 61105 Ljubljana (Yugoslavia)

49. Short-term effects of electroconvulsive shock treatment upon acetylcholinesterase levels of several brain areas in the rat.

M. Appleyard, A.R. Green and A.D. Smith

Departments of Pharmacology and Clinical Pharmacology, University of Oxford, Oxford (UK)

50. Acetyl- and butyryl-cholinesterase in Alzheimer-type dementia: Selective loss of the G4 form of acetylcholinesterase

J.R. Atack, E.K. Perry and J.R. Bonham

Department of Pathology, Newcastle General Hospital, Newcastle upon Tyne NE4 6BE (UK)

51. Change in the distribution of acetylcholinesterase molecular forms in the peripheral nerves of rabbits with experimental allergic neuritis

Z. Rakonczay[1], G.K. Molnár[2] and P. Kasa[1]

(1) Central Research Laboratory, Medical University, H-6720 Szeged (Hungary) and (2) Department of Neurology, University Turku, SF-20520 Turku (Finland)

52. Rectal mucosal acetylcholinesterase in Hirschprung's disease

G. Dale, J. Bonham and J. Wagget

Dept. Biochemistry, Newcastle General Hospital, Newcastle upon Tyne NE4 6BE (UK)

53. Regulation by beta-endorphin and derivatives of the activity and distribution of acetylcholinesterase molecular forms in cultured rat myotubes

L.W. Haynes and M.E. Smith

Dept. of Physiology, The Medical School, University of Birmingham, Vincent Drive, Birmingham B15 2TJ (UK)

54. Active transport by acetylcholinesterase

K. Kaufmann

Max-Planck-Institut f. biophysikalische Chemie, D-3400 Goettingen (FRG)

55. The effect of purified acetylcholinesterase added to the bathing fluid on end-plate potentials

D. Šuput and M. Brzin

Institute of Pathophysiology, 61105 Ljubljana (Yugoslavia)

56. Study of non-specific cholinesterase synthesis in rat

J. Iván and K. Vass

Department of Pharmacodynamics, University Medical School, 6720 Szeged (Hungary)

57. Differences between AChE and non-specific ChE (nsChE) in rat superior cervical ganglion (SCG) and plasma

B. Klinar, Lj. Kamarić and M. Brzin

Institute of Pathophysiology, 61105 Ljubljana (Yugoslavia)

58. Interactions of neuroactive drugs and multivalent cations with purified human serum cholinesterase (ChE)

J.K. Marquis

Department of Pharmacology and Experimental Therapeutics, Boston University School of Medicine, Boston, MA, 02118 (USA)

59. Activity and molecular forms of human serum cholinesterase and prolonged succinylcholine action

G. Scarsella[1], S. Biagioni[4], G. Toschi[1], C. Santolamazza[2], A. Novelletto[2], G. Cermele[3] and G. Modiano[2]

(1) Dipartimento della Biologia Cellulare e dello Sviluppo, (2) Istituto di Genetica, (3) VI Clinica Chirurgica, Università "La Sapienza", Roma and (4) Istituto di Istologia ed Analisi di Laboratorio, Università di Urbino (Italy)

60. Modulation of sperm propulsion: Role of cholinesterase

L. Nelson

Department of Physiology, Medical College of Ohio, Toledo, OH, 43699 (USA)

Session 5: Anticholinesterases: Toxicology and structure-function relationship of inhibitors and antidotes

61. Inhibition kinetics for some irreversible inhibitors in the reaction with acetylcholinesterase from electric eel

A. Forsberg and G. Puu

Division of Experimental Medicine, National Defence Research Institute, Department 4, S-901 82 Umea (Sweden)

62. Peripheral site(s) of action of an organophosphorous compound, a methylphosphorothiolate derivate, on skeletal muscle acetylcholinesterase. Evidence for irreversible and reversible reactions on the extracted and immobilized enzyme

A. Friboulet, D. Goudou and F. Rieger

Groupe de Biologie et de Pathologie Neuromusculaires, 17, rue du Fer-à-Moulin, 75005 Paris (France)

63. Interaction of organophosphates with "extra-catalytic" sites on bovine brain acetylcholinesterase (AChE)

J.K. Marquis

Department of Pharmacology and Experimental Therapeutics, Boston University School of Medicine, Boston, MA, 02118 (USA)

64. Ranitidine is a rapidly reversible inhibitor of acetylcholinesterase

P. Mantovani, A. Galli and G. Pepeu

Department of Pharmacology, University of Florence, Viale G.B. Morgagni 65, Florence (Italy)

65. Bambuterol, a terbutaline carbamate prodrug, as substrate and inhibitor for cholinesterase in human blood

A. Tunek

AB Draco, Box 1707, S-22101 Lund (Sweden)

66. Properties of cholinesterase inhibitors of some fractions isolated from impurities of industrial solvents causing neuropathies

E. Vilanova and J.L. Vicedo

Department of Physiology and Biochemistry, Faculty of Medicine, University of Alicante, Alicante (Spain)

67. Reactivators of phosphorylated and phosphonylated cholinesterases. Dicarbamoyl bis-pyridinium mono-oximes

I. Bregovec[1], M. Maksimović [2], V. Deljac[1] and Z. Binenfeld[1]

(1) Laboratory of Organic Chemistry and Biochemistry, Faculty of Natural Sciences and Mathematics, University of Zagreb, Strossmayerov trg 14, 41000 Zagreb (Yugoslavia), (2) Military Technical Institute, Medical Department, Katanićeva 15, 11000 Belgrade (Yugoslavia)

68. Protection of acetylcholinesterase by eseroline against inactivation by DFP and carbamates in vitro and in vivo

A. Galli, M. Nocchi, R. Bartolini, P. Aiello-Malmberg, G. Renzi (+) and A. Bartolini

Department of Pharmacology and (+) Department of Pharmaceutical Sciences, University of Florence, Florence (Italy)

69. The detoxication capacity of rat liver at soman concentrations, present in the tissue after application of sublethal doses

Z. Grubić, J. Sketelj and M. Brzin

Institute of Pathophysiology, 61105 Ljubljana (Yugoslavia)

70. Detoxification of organophosphorus compounds

S.H. Sterri and F. Fonnum

Norwegian Defence Research Establishment, Division for Environmental Toxicology, N-2007, Kjeller (Norway)

71. One teh reactivation of soman-inhibited cholinesterase

G. Bucht and G. Puu

Division of Experimental Medicine, National Defence Research Institute, Department 4, S-901 82 Umea (Sweden)

72. The effect of HI-6 on soman- induced muscle lesions

A. Dekleva[1], D. Sket[2], J. Sketelj[2] and M. Brzin[2]

(1) Institute of Anatomy and (2) Institute of Pathophysiology, 61105 Ljubljana (Yugoslavia)

73. Interaction of the resolved isomers of soman with chicken brain acetylcholinesterase and neuropathy target esterase (NTE)

M.K. Johnson[1], D.J. Read[1] and H.P. Benschop[2]

(1) Medical Research Council, Carshalton, Sy. (UK), (2) T.N.O. Rijsvijk (The Netherlands)

74. Stereospecific reactivation by some Hagedorn-oximes of acetylcholinesterase from various species including man, inhibited by soman

L.P.A. de Jong and G.Z. Wolring

Prins Maurits Laboratory TNO, Rijsvijk (The Netherlands)

75. AChE reactivation potency of mono- and bis-pyridinium oximes: Peripheral versus central effectiveness in the rat

D. Pantelić and M. Maksimović

Military Technical Institute, 11000 Belgrade (Yugoslavia)

76. Stability of oxime HI-6 in acidic solution

I. Pilipović[1] and I. Vukušić[2]

(1) Pharmaceutical, Chemical and Supplies Industry, W.O. "TSNP", Jukićeva 35, 71000 Sarajevo (Yugoslavia), (2) Institute for the Control of Drugs, Moše Pijade 160, 41000 Zagreb (Yugoslavia)

77. On the in vitro interaction of sarin and soman with PAM-2, HI-6 and HGG-12

D. Rakin[1], B. Toković[2] and B. Bošković[1]

(1) Military Technical Institute, Katanićeva 15, 11000 Belgrade and (2) Military Medical Academy, 11000 Belgrade (Yugoslavia)

78. HI-6 against inhibition of AChE in the rat brain

D. Sket and M. Brzin

Institute of Pathophysiology, 61105 Ljubljana (Yugoslavia)

79. Some aspects of AChE reactivation by HI-6 after soman poisoining in the rat

D. Sket, J. Sketelj, B. Klinar and M. Brzin

Institute of Pathophysiology, 61105 Ljubljana (Yugoslavia)

80. The presynaptic modulatory effect of the oxime HI-6 at the neuromuscular junction

B. Stamenović and V. Brajović

Military Medical Academy, 11000 Beograd, Crnotravska bb (Yugoslavia)

81. Inhibition of acetylcholinesterase by some bispyridinium compounds

M. Škrinjarić-Špoljar

Institute for Medical Research and Occupational Health, 41000 Zagreb (Yugoslavia)

82. IR study of interaction of oximes HI-6, PAM-2C1 and HGG-12 with soman, in vitro, in the presence and absence of cholinesterases

B. Toković, S. Ćušić, P. Radošević and J. Kojić

Zavod za preventivnu medicinu, VMA, 11000 Beograd (Yugoslavia)

83. A comparative study of the ageing of DFP-inhibited serine hydrolases

A.C.M. van der Drift

Medical Biological Laboratory TNO, P.O. Box 45, 2280 AA Rijsvijk (The Nétherlands)

84. Electrophoretic studies of the aged soman-inhibited butyrylcholinesterase

P. Masson, B. Marnot, J.-Y. Lombard and P. Morélis

Centre de Recherches du Service de Santé des Armées, Division de Chimie et Pharmacologie, 108 Bouleväard Pinel, 69275 Lyon (France)

85. Effects of soman on Renshaw cell responses to antidromic ventral root stimulation

R. Anastasijević, B. Stamenović, M. Stanojević and J. Vučo

Institute for Medical Research, Bul. JNA 10, 11000 Belgrade and Military Medical Academy, Crnotravska bb, 11000 Belgrade (Yugoslavia)

86. Muscarinic and nicotinic cholinergic mechanisms involved in seizures induced by cholinesterase inhibitors (ChEI)

A. Simonić, H. Krutak-Król and E.F. Domino

Department of Pharmacology, University of Michigan, Ann Arbor, MI, 48109 (USA)

Session 6: Anticholinesterases and neurotoxic esterase : Mechanism of delayed neurotoxicity

87. Sucrose density gradient sedimentation of Mifapox sensitive and Paraoxon esterases

Y. Ishikawa, E. Chow, M.G. McNamee and B.W. Wilson

Avian Sciences, University of California, Davis, CA, 95616 (USA)

88. Neurotoxic esterase: Comparision between human lymphocyte and platelet activity

M. Maroni[1] and M.L. Bleecker[2]

(1) Institute of Occupational Medicine, University of Milan, via S. Barnaba 8, 20122 Milan (Italy) and (2) Johns Hopkins Medical Institutes, Department of Neurology and Environmental Health Sciences, Division of Occupational Medicine, Baltimore, Maryland, 21205 (USA)

89. Neurotoxic esterase in extranervous tissues of man

A. Moretto[1], A. Fassina[2] and M. Lotti[1]

(1) Istituto di Medicina del Lavoro and (2) Istituto di Anatomia Patologica dell Università di Padova (Italy)

90. The unique mode of aging of DiFP-neurotoxic esterase

D.G. Williams and M.K. Johnson

Medical Research Council Toxicology Unit, Carshalton, Surrey, SM5 4EF (UK)

Kolibri 360 GmbH
Ferdinand-Jühlke-Straße 7
99095 Erfurt, Deutschland
produktsicherheit@kolibri360.de